ETHICS IN COUNSELING & THERAPY

*This book is dedicated to my lifelong best friend and spouse Carmen;
my wonderfully practical daughter Clarissa; my two grandchildren Ian and
Soraya, who provide pleasure and inspiration with their innocence; and my sensitive,
thoughtful, and scholarly daughter Serena who is a colleague in the profession.*

—RH

To Amy, Sara, and Nick.

—ST

ETHICS IN COUNSELING &THERAPY

developing an ethical identity

Rick A. Houser
Stephen Thoma

The University of Alabama

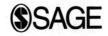

Los Angeles | London | New Delhi
Singapore | Washington DC

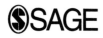

Los Angeles | London | New Delhi
Singapore | Washington DC

FOR INFORMATION:

SAGE Publications, Inc.
2455 Teller Road
Thousand Oaks, California 91320
E-mail: order@sagepub.com

SAGE Publications Ltd.
1 Oliver's Yard
55 City Road
London EC1Y 1SP
United Kingdom

SAGE Publications India Pvt. Ltd.
B 1/I 1 Mohan Cooperative Industrial Area
Mathura Road, New Delhi 110 044
India

SAGE Publications Asia-Pacific Pte. Ltd.
3 Church Street
#10-04 Samsung Hub
Singapore 049483

Acquisitions Editor: Kassie Graves
Associate Editor: Eve Oettinger
Editorial Assistant: Courtney Munz
Production Editor: Catherine M. Chilton
Copy Editor: Barbara Corrigan
Typesetter: C&M Digitals (P) Ltd.
Proofreader: Jennifer Gritt
Indexer: Ellen Slavitz
Cover Designer: Anupama Krishnan
Marketing Manager: Katie Winter
Permissions Editor: Adele Hutchinson

Printed in the United States of America

Library of Congress Cataloging-in-Publication Data

Houser, Rick A.
Ethics in counseling and therapy : developing an ethical identity / Rick A. Houser, Stephen Thoma.

p. cm.
Includes bibliographical references and index.

ISBN 978-1-4129-8137-8 (cloth)

1. Counseling—Moral and ethical aspects. I. Thoma, Stephen. II. Title.

BF636.67.H68 2013
174′.91583—dc23   2011043526

This book is printed on acid-free paper.

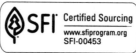

SFI label applies to text stock

12 13 14 15 16 10 9 8 7 6 5 4 3 2 1

CONTENTS

FOREWORD

Most writers in the counseling profession are likely to acknowledge that it is
an honor to be asked to write a foreword for a new book on counseling ethics. I must admit that it is a particular honor when the request is to write a foreword for a book of such importance as this one, authored by Drs. Rick Houser and
Steve Thoma, titled *Ethics in Counseling and Therapy: Developing an Ethical
Identity.* Before describing why this book represents a significant resource for
counselor educators, practitioners, and graduate students, it is useful to first briefly
comment on the sort of ethical issues and related topics that have been discussed
or have failed to be addressed in previous books and articles.

As professional counselors, we are expected to provide helping services that
reflect our commitment for effectiveness, cultural competence, and ethical practices. These three factors represent the cornerstones of the work counselors are
expected to do in the field.

The importance of the latter point is reflected in the noticeable increase in the
number of books and articles that have been published in the counseling profession during the past several years that focus on professional ethics. These publications typically focus on two main areas of relevance for counseling ethics.

One of these major areas involves describing the specific ethical standards
that have been developed and endorsed by numerous professional counseling
associations. This includes the publication of ethical standards and revisions of
existing codes of ethics by the American Counseling Association, American
Association for Marriage and Family Therapy, American School Counseling
Association, Commission on Rehabilitation Counseling Certification, and
Counselors for Social Justice, to name a few. A second major area of attention
in previous publications on counseling ethics involves a description of steps that
counselors are encouraged to take when making ethical decisions in their professional practices.

Although both of the above-stated areas are important in understanding our ethical responsibilities as professional counselors and in making ethical decisions in our work, there are two missing links that have not been thoroughly addressed in past publications. These missing links include the lack of attention to (a) the process and content of counselors' ethical identity development and (b) a comprehensive analysis of cultural considerations as they relate to ethical decision making.

These missing links have resulted in counselor educators', practitioners', and graduate students' focusing more narrowly on ethical issues than what is arguably needed when working in a complex, rapidly changing, and increasingly diverse 21st-century society. The publication of *Ethics in Counseling and Therapy: Developing an Ethical Identity* effectively addresses these issues in ways that can create a sea change in how many persons in the counseling profession have previously thought about their professional ethical responsibilities and actions.

The authors break new ground by exploring the notion of ethical identity development in the first section of the book. Their efforts to illuminate the relevance and importance of counselors' development in this area is clearly reflected in the effective way the authors synthesize many concepts associated with counselors' moral and cognitive development as they relate to their own ethical identity development. While these concepts are new in discussions about ethical decision making, the authors go further by exploring how counselors' emotions, intuitions, and social compassion affect their ethical perspectives.

Counselor educators, practitioners, and graduate students will predictably feel themselves becoming more empowered, personally and professionally, by learning about the ways that these factors affect their own and other persons' ethical decision-making abilities and preferences. As a result of being more empowered when learning about these issues in the first section of this new book, counselors will be better positioned to act more intentionally and with a greater level of cognitive complexity when faced with ethical dilemmas in their work.

Another major aspect of this book that distinguishes it from others is the attention it directs to multicultural issues as they relate to ethical decision making. Given the transformative changes that the multicultural counseling movement has effected and continues to effect in the mental health profession, it is both surprising and disappointing to note the dearth of information included in previous publications that focuses on the relevance of culturally diverse perspectives as they relate to ethics in counseling. The authors address the dearth of information in these areas by writing the first book I am aware of that provides substantial information that will greatly extend readers' understanding of culturally diverse perspectives of ethics and ethical decision making.

The authors summarize how they address the two missing links described above early in this new book. They do so by clearly stating that much of the book describes "a hermeneutic model of ethical decision making" that includes "a culturally sensitive framework." This latter framework is built on a broad range of culturally diverse ethical principles, values, and perspectives to foster the reader's own ethical identity development. More specifically, the culturally sensitive model the authors describe in this book includes succinct presentations of Western, Eastern, Middle Eastern, Native American, Latino/Hispanic, and African American ethical perspectives.

Although *Ethics in Counseling and Therapy* breaks new ground in addressing the missing links described above, the authors do not shy away from exploring traditional issues related to counseling ethics. As a result, this book incorporates discussions of several foundational issues as they relate to ethical challenges many counselors commonly face in their work. This includes presenting numerous ethical dilemmas that require one to reflect on the ways he or she might address boundary issues, questions about a counselor's competence, confidentially issues, and ethical dilemmas associated with clients' right to autonomy. What makes the presentation of these ethical dilemmas different from more traditional approaches to such ethical concepts and responsibilities is that the authors frame their exploration of these principles within the scope of ethical identity development theory and culturally competent ethical practices.

After reading this book, I was excited by its potential to assist counselor educators, practitioners, and graduate students realize more complex levels of ethical identity development as well as complement their ongoing journey to becoming culturally competent mental health professionals. I am confident that you will experience advancements in your own professional, personal, and ethical development as a result of reading this book. For all of these reasons I want to honestly say that if I were in a position to read only one book about counseling ethics this year, *Ethics in Counseling and Therapy: Developing an Ethical Identity* is the one I would choose and recommend to others.

Michael D'Andrea
Seton Hall University
and
National Institute for Multicultural Competence

PREFACE

Interest in and study of ethics has grown significantly during the past two decades in the counseling field. As you will see in reading this text, we emphasize a cultural perspective that is not limited to a Western orientation. The book *Culturally Relevant Ethical Decision-Making in Counseling* (Houser, Wilczenski, & Ham, 2006) first introduced a broader perspective in applying ethical theories in counseling beyond a Western view. In this book we expand the perspective introduced by Houser et al. (2006) and present in much more detail how moral psychology helps in understanding ethical decision making. In particular we discuss how developing a professional ethical identity is a critical step in becoming an ethical counselor. Developing a professional ethical identity provides a much stronger foundation for making sound decisions than a somewhat haphazard approach that is situation specific. We encourage you to think about your own personal development and ethical development and pursue it over the course of your professional career. A hermeneutic model of ethical decision making is introduced, and a culturally sensitive model of incorporating a range of theories is offered. We present information on Western, Eastern, Middle Eastern, Native American, Latino/Hispanic, and African American theories, which provide you with a broad understanding of the various perspectives that clients may bring to counseling.

ACKNOWLEDGMENTS

We want to acknowledge a number of individuals who made significant contributions to the development and preparation of this book. First, Kassie Graves, acquisitions editor–human services for Sage Publications, has been, as usual, extremely helpful and supportive. Her suggestions and feedback were excellent and we feel significantly improved the book. Allen Wilcoxon, University of Alabama, also provided helpful feedback, and we appreciate his willingness to share his knowledge and expertise. We want to thank the reviewers who provided helpful feedback and also improved the quality: Suzanne Mayer, Neumann College–Aston; Madelyn Isaacs, Florida Gulf Coast University–Ft. Myers; and Kathleen Woods, Chadron State College. We want to thank Dr. Michael D'Andrea for a thoughtful, detailed Foreword. Many who write a book's Foreword give a cursory review, but Dr. D'Andrea shares comments that provide a good introduction to the book. Finally, we want to thank the copy editor, Barbara Corrigan, for her detailed and excellent editing. She diligently worked through the manuscript with a careful eye, and she made excellent suggestions for improving the readability of the text.

ABOUT THE AUTHORS

Rick Houser is the department head in educational studies in psychology, research methodology, and counseling at the University of Alabama. He has been a professor, department chair, and associate dean in the College of Education at the University of Massachusetts. Rick Houser has taught graduate-level ethics courses for more than 15 years. He received his doctorate from the University of Pittsburgh in rehabilitation counseling with a minor in research methodology. He conducts research in ethical decision making, stress and coping, and the use of virtual reality in counseling.

Steve Thoma is a professor and the coordinator of the Educational Psychology Program at the University of Alabama. He received his doctorate from the University of Minnesota in 1986 with an emphasis in personality and social development and a focus on moral psychology. He conducts research on the measurement of moral judgment.

SECTION I

INTRODUCTION AND FOUNDATION OF ETHICAL REASONING AND DECISION MAKING

Chapter 1

INTRODUCTION

The introduction of ethical reasoning and decision making in the professional practice of counseling has grown dramatically during the past 15 years (Bradley & Hendricks, 2008; Bryceland & Stam, 2005; Corey, Corey, & Callanan, 2007; Detert, Trevino, & Sweitzer, 2008; Houser, Wilczenski, & Ham, 2006; Welfel, 2006). In addition, there are several textbooks that address ethics in counseling (Corey et al., 2007; Cottone & Tarvydas, 2006; Welfel, 2006). These ethics texts typically focus on ethical issues and give little attention to ethical theories and decision making. The American Counseling Association (1996) provided a brief guide for practitioners on ethical decision making. The guide includes a discussion of ethical principles such as beneficence, justice, and fidelity and proposes a model of identifying the problem, applying codes, and identifying courses of action. It is presented as a linear decision-making model: Step 1 being identify the problem, Step 2 being apply codes of ethics, and so forth. One step is considering the nature and dimensions of the problem, and this may involve consulting the professional literature. The problem for the counselor is that he or she may be confronted with a dilemma that requires a rather immediate response, and multiple factors may require a more simultaneous review of relevant issues and the dimensions of the ethical issue. Also, an ethical dilemma may be seen from a different perspective once additional information is gathered, and the initial conclusion that it was an ethical issue may be removed.

Others have noted the limitations of teaching and making ethical decisions based only on limited and narrowly focused guidelines such as professional codes of ethics and laws (Cottone, 2001; Cottone & Claus, 2000; Lunt, 1999). Freeman (2000) stated that "ethical standards are self-imposed regulations that provide rough guidelines for professional behavior and attempt to specify the nature of the ethical responsibilities of the members, at least minimally" (p. 19). Others have suggested that stringent application of professional codes and structuring of the counseling relationship through professional codes can have a negative impact on the counseling relationship (Bryceland & Stam, 2005). Knapp, Gottlieb, Berman, and Handelsman (2007) stated, "Psychologists may need to choose between following the law and protecting the welfare of their patients, or an ethical value" (p. 58). It is clear that simply using professional codes and/or laws to guide practice is limiting and does not provide a solid foundation to make ethical decisions that are founded on sound ethical reasoning. Frame, Flanagan, Gold, and Harris (1997) wrote that not only is making ethical decisions "complex, but it is also a potential mine field" (p. 107). Counselors on a daily basis make decisions about clients that involve ethical decisions and potentially can harm the client and/or others (family members). An important underlying question is, How does one provide a framework and/or a model for training or developing an ethical identity and behaving in an ethical way, for example, making reasoned, sound ethical decisions.

Before answering the above question about a framework for making sound ethical decisions, it is important to start with a definition of ethics and morals. *Ethics* and *morality* are common terms in both our everyday lives and our professional lives. The definitions of *ethics* and *morals* may not be as readily distinguishable. *Ethics* has been defined as "a generic term for several ways of examining the moral life" (Beauchamp & Childress, 1989, p. 9). *Merriam-Webster's Collegiate Dictionary* (2005) defines *ethics* as "the discipline dealing with what is good and bad and with moral duty and obligation. A set of moral principles." Corey et al. (2007) stated, "Ethics pertain to the beliefs we hold about what constitutes right conduct. Ethics are moral principles adopted by an individual or group to provide rules for right conduct" (p. 12). Professional associations typically establish the ethical standards for a profession. Rest (1983) defined morality as "standards or guidelines that govern human cooperation—in particular, how rights, duties, and benefits are to be allocated" (p. 558). Corey et al. (2007) wrote that morality is "concerned with perspectives of right and proper conduct and involves an evaluation of actions on the basis of some broader cultural context or religious standard" (p. 12). Houser et al. (2006) noted that

> a difference between these two concepts concerns to some degree the objective versus subjective interpretation of right behavior, in the case here professionally acceptable or desirable behavior. Ethics, theoretically, is generated from a more general standard set of guidelines outlined and set forth by professional organizations, whereas morality is more narrow and based on cultural and possibly religious beliefs. (p. 1)

Professional organizations have used broad ethical theories to develop codes that have been based to a significant extent on cultural and religious beliefs (morality).

Storch and Kenny (2007) recalled the development of early medical ethics and the influence of religion on medical ethics. Medical ethics have influenced psychology and counseling ethics. Based on the premise that morality has influenced the development of ethics, we want to suggest that ethics includes morality. Consequently, ethics are founded in part on cultural and religious beliefs, as well as broader perspectives that are sanctioned by professional organizations, including professional ethical codes. We will discuss ethics as the primary focus of this text, but simultaneously we will use research and writings about the influences of morals on professional ethics.

The definitions offered above of ethics and morals are founded in Western perspectives. Eastern and Native American perspectives of ethics include consideration of the effects of and one's responsibility to nature. We believe it is necessary to expand the definition of ethics and morals to include being responsive to nature, which includes caring about all living things and our impact on life in general. Also, such a definition expands the view to consider how one's behavior may affect the community and the environment in which one lives. Later discussion will focus on the development of professional ethical identity, which theoretically should include a broad perspective and consideration of one's effect on nature and responsibility to the world in which one lives.

ETHICAL DEVELOPMENT AND ETHICAL IDENTITY

The intent of this book is to combine theoretical and practical understanding of ethical reasoning, counselor ethical development, and counselor professional ethical identity development. A key foundation of this book is the perspective that good counselor ethical practice is found not in teaching ethical decision making alone but in combination with the counselor's ethical development. A model focusing on counselor ethical development is grounded in the perspective that ethical practice is not a sole event such as a cognitive event utilizing reasoning alone but is developmental and stems from a dynamic interaction between the counselor's values/experiences and professional training/professional socialization. This perspective views counselor ethical development as dynamic and continuous, never stopping. Professions have recently noted the importance of developing a moral/ethical identity (Bebeau, 2008; Hamilton, 2008; Sheppard, Macatangay, Colby, & Sullivan, 2008). Bebeau (2008), for example, in describing the important role of educating professionals, stated the following: "Broad and deep understanding of the public purposes and core values of one's profession is essential to students and colleagues alike" (p. 367). Counseling has not developed a clear understanding of professional ethical/moral identity of counselors (Hendricks, 2008). Counseling is clearly recognized as a profession (Ponton & Duba, 2009), but a clear understanding of what constitutes a moral/ethical professional identity is not clearly defined. Other professions such as law, dentistry, and medicine (Bebeau, 2008; Sheppard et al., 2008) have begun to introduce the development of professional ethical identity into the education and training of students.

The presentation of both ethical reasoning and counselor ethical development will be accomplished by providing a foundation for understanding ethical reasoning and development. The focus on counselor ethical development will include discussion of professional identity and moral identity (Hardy & Carlo, 2005; Reynolds & Ceranic, 2007). Recently, moral identity has been discussed as a major factor in motivation and behaving ethically (Hardy & Carlo, 2005; Hart, 2005). A counselor's acquisition of a strong moral identity as an ethical professional potentially plays a critical role in actions the counselor practices. There will be a careful review and understanding of the major issues confronting professional counselors including such ethical dilemmas as counselor competence, client confidentiality, informed consent, client autonomy, multicultural competence, the use of technology in counseling, supervision, professional demeanor, dual relationships, and professional codes and legal issues. The next section covers philosophical ethical theories that can be used in ethical decision making. Cases will be used throughout the text to illustrate theoretical perspectives and practical issues such as dual relationships. There are reflection questions at the end of each chapter that are important to address and that should foster your own ethical development.

MULTIDIMENSIONAL MODEL

The models of ethical decision making that have been proposed in most professional ethics texts have been linearly focused, and they have employed a problem-solving orientation. Also, the developers of these models have suggested that ethical decision making is an abstract, nonemotional analysis. The model we are proposing incorporates four important elements, three elements addressing ethical development and one focusing on ethical reasoning. The first three focus on counselor ethical development, and the fourth addresses ethical reasoning. The three that focus on ethical development are the role of social identity development (professional identity/moral identity), ethical sensitivity, and motivations to act ethically in taking ethical actions. The fourth element is ethical reasoning, which is primarily cognitive and includes a nonlinear approach, hermeneutics. All four of these elements provide a dynamic and interactional model of ethical reasoning and counselor ethical development.

the branch of knowledge that deals with interpretation, esp. of the Bible or other literary, wisdom & philosophical texts.

Rest (1984) proposed an early ethical decision-making model. He suggested a four-component model for identifying moral or ethical behavior that can help in understanding the relevant components identified in the decision-making model proposed here, for example, hermeneutics and social comparison. The four components include moral sensitivity, moral judgment, moral motivation, and moral character. Moral sensitivity refers to an awareness of a situation involving an ethical or moral dilemma. If one does not know there is a problem, he or she will ignore cues suggesting there is or can be a problem. In part the moral sensitivity component concerns an awareness of how one's actions can affect other people. A second component is moral judgment (Rest, 1984). This component involves moral reasoning or understanding of options and choices that are to be made. The third component is moral motivation, and this involves the prioritizing of values or beliefs, what is most important versus least important (Rest, 1984). The last component of Rest's model contributing to moral behavior is moral character. Moral character concerns a person's having virtues or characteristics that contribute to moral behavior. An example of moral character is standing up for one's values against others, ethical identity. The components proposed by Rest can be helpful in understanding and explaining the four elements of the proposed ethical/moral reasoning and decision-making model presented in this text (see Table 1.1).

Table 1.1 Rest's Four-Component Model

Component	Description
Ethical sensitivity	Concerns awareness of contextual clues and ability to comprehend alternative courses of action
Ethical judgment	Involves the assessment of actions and choice of the most ethical option
Ethical motivation	Concerns the centrality of ethical values and perceptions, how important it is to act ethically
Ethical action	Involves an awareness of the steps to carry out the ethical actions necessary to behave ethically, may involve having the perseverance to follow through on an ethical action

Source: Adapted from Crowell, Narvaez, and Gomberg (2004).

The first element that provides a basis and foundation for ethical development is professional identity or moral identity (Hendricks, 2008). Hendricks (2008) proposed that ethics is part of the identity of the counselor; in other words, ethics is something that is part of the counselor and is who he or she is. Hart (2005) noted the importance of including identity and moral identity to understanding and explaining ethical and moral behavior. Professional identity also fits with Rest's (1984) components of moral character. Socialization of the counselor into the profession includes socialization in ethics and an identity that incorporates a certain perspective. The perspective includes an understanding of emphasizing the welfare of the client and not focusing just on one's own welfare. The professional counselor is socialized into the profession and acquires the values necessary for practice. Hendricks suggested that the development of a professional identity as a counselor is influenced by ethics and ethical codes. The development of a professional identity is typically accomplished during academic training for the profession, and a focus on ethical decision making and ethics should pervade this socialization. Chapter 2, "Professional Identity and Ethics," will include a discussion of moral identity and professional identity. Differences between professional identity/moral identity and personal identity will be presented for clarification.

Chapter 3 is a discussion of ethical sensitivity and ethical motivation. The second element of a foundation for ethical development is ethical sensitivity and ethics (Haidt, 2001; Rest, 1984). Rest (1984) identified moral sensitivity as a component of moral behavior, and emotions/intuitions fit within his perspective. Rest and Narvaez (1994) believed that an awareness of one's impact on another influences an awareness in regard to ethical sensitivity. Another perspective on moral sensitivity is found in the social intuitionist model (Haidt, 2001). Much of the current theory originates from social psychology, and counseling has essentially ignored an important element of understanding how emotions affect ethics and ethical decision making. Haidt (2001) and others (Keltner & Haidt, 2003; Saltzstein & Kasachkoff, 2004; Schnall, Haidt, Clore, & Jordon, 2008) have suggested that morals are not based on reasoned thought but are more likely associated with intuition and emotion (or a gut reaction). According to the social intuitionist view, morals develop from inherent and/or inherited (evolutionary) processes (Haidt, 2001). Haidt described the primary theme of the social intuitionist model and stated, "Moral judgment is caused by quick moral intuitions and is followed (when needed) by slow, ex post facto moral reasoning" (p. 817). Essentially, moral decision making in the social intuitionist view is a gut reaction to an event or situation, more like an aesthetic judgment (Schnall et al., 2008). Reasoning enters into moral or ethical decision making only after the initial reaction and conclusion about the quality of response (moral or ethical response). This view is particularly important for counselors because if there is any truth to the hypothesis that morals or ethics is based on intuition or emotions, then counselors need to be aware of their own reactions. Second, any awareness can be followed by a reasoned decision-making approach.

The third element of the model presented here, ethical motivation, involves identification of the centrality and importance of ethics and the use of social comparison to determine ethical behavior. Moral motivation, according to Rest (1984), involves the influence and importance—the centrality—of values and beliefs. For example, a counselor may emphasize promoting autonomy as a central value. Another perspective accounting for ethical motivation is that one can be influenced to behave ethically as a consequence of comparison with others based on one's view that he or she is an ethical person. Comparison with others may either confirm or refute a professional ethical identity. Frequently, conclusions about the efficacy of an ethical decision are based on what a "reasonable person or counselor" would do in such a situation or ethical dilemma, a social comparison. Also, many have suggested that consulting with peers is a good practice in making ethical decisions (Houser et al., 2006). Novicevic, Harvey, Budkley, and Fung (2008) described the process of social comparison as it can relate to ethical decision making: "Social comparison can occur as a result of individuals' need to evaluate their positions or opinions and behavior relative to others" (p. 1064). A third influence on motivation to act ethically is the role of social responsibility and empathy. Staub (2005) proposed that the motivation to assist others originates from the process of empathy. Humans are motivated to seek approval from others for helping, avoid punishment if they do not help, expect a benefit or reciprocal benefit from helping, have a desire to reduce others' discomfort, and hold values that promote the welfare of others. There is a benefit to developing empathy skills to use in being motivated to act ethically.

The fourth element is ethical/moral reasoning (Rest, 1984), presented in Chapter 4. Ethical and moral reasoning can be traced back to Socrates, who concluded that "an unexamined life is not worth living" (Church, 1956, p. 56). More recent views on moral reasoning can be found in a variety of moral and ethical theories (C. Harris, 1997; Houser et al., 2006; Rest, Narvaez, Bebeau, & Thoma, 1999a; Shanahan & Wang, 2006) and in Lawrence Kohlberg's work on the development of moral stages (Rest et al., 1999a). Rest et al. (1999a) proposed that moral judgment and reasoning are key components of behavior and choices of action. Reflection is based in part on one's schema and stage of development. C. Harris (1997) outlined primarily Western perspectives of moral reasoning focusing on theories such as utilitarian theory, virtue ethics, respect for persons, and natural law. Shanahan and Wang (2006) and Houser et al. (2006) have expanded the view of ethical reasoning to include Eastern and Middle Eastern perspectives and theories. These broader perspectives give ethical reasoning a culturally sensitive model. In this text we will use a hermeneutic model that is nonlinear and presents ethical reasoning as interaction between relevant elements of a horizon or elements that interact to help in understanding and making an ethical decision. Betan (1997) first suggested the use of a hermeneutic model of ethical decision making. For example, elements of the horizon in counseling and ethics may include a counselor's personal values, a supervisor's values, the client's values, professional codes, and so forth (Houser et al., 2006). Consequently the horizon provides the counselor with a picture of the elements of the ethical dilemma and facilitates the ethical decision. A key component of the hermeneutic model we propose involves variation that combines the hermeneutic model with social comparison (moral motivation) and cognitions and reasoning (moral judgment). The hermeneutic model involves the use of interpreting and decision making combined with a heavy emphasis on social comparison or consultation with others, sharing cognitions about the decision (a counselor's sharing with a supervisor or colleague his or her thoughts/cognitions in making the decision), the use of metacognition, and reflecting on the decision-making process as it is implemented. Another perspective that needs to be included in the discussion of clinical judgment in ethical decision making is a focus on intuition (Kahneman & Klein, 2009; Schnall et al., 2008). Kahneman and Klein (2009) noted that the natural decision-making approach involves an understanding of the cues and environment in which an intuitive decision is made. The hermeneutic model is consistent with this view, and there is an attempt to identify and be aware of those relevant cues in making decisions and clinical judgments.

TEXT FORMAT

A summary of the text format may be helpful. The first section of the text includes an introduction to and a discussion of the foundations of ethical reasoning and ethical development; there are four chapters. Chapter 2 involves an introduction to theories and how they apply to professional identity specifically as well as ethics. The third chapter is an introduction to ethical sensitivity. Theoretical views of various contributors to sensitivity will be presented, such as how emotions and intuitions relate to ethics and moral sensitivity. The third chapter also includes a review of motivations to act ethically and will include discussion of relevant theories, cognitive dissonance, and social responsibility and empathy. Chapter 4 is an introduction to cognitions and reasoning or moral judgment. Theory and research on cognitive moral reasoning are presented. This chapter also includes an integration of the previous chapter's theories as they relate to the integrated model of ethical decision making and reasoning through a hermeneutic approach.

The next section focuses on ethical issues in counseling. State licensure boards, professional associations, and professional journals have reported the most frequent ethical issues, and this section is an attempt to introduce and address these issues. There is a chapter on each of these frequently occurring ethical dilemmas. One ethical dilemma (see Chapter 5) facing counselors is the decision to promote autonomy (Houser et al., 2006). This concerns freedom to choose one's own course of action. A question for the counselor is the person's competency to make such decisions. Another issue or ethical dilemma involving autonomy that is a common concern for counselors is confidentiality. Confidentiality may need to be breeched when issues of safely are a concern, but the decision to break confidentiality is not always clear. Informing clients of the limitations of confidentiality is important. A second issue (see Chapter 6) is a concern about dual relationships and boundaries (Houser et al., 2006). Such dual relationships may include bartering, self-disclosure, professional demeanor, and sexual relationships. Another dilemma is counselor competence (see Chapter 7) and may involve the counselor's engaging in activities for which he or she is not trained. An important question here is what constitutes an adequate level of training to be competent. A similar ethical dilemma about general counselor competence is multicultural competence (see Chapter 8). There are specific and unique issues related to multicultural competence that are different than general counselor competence. Consequently, there is a discussion and presentation addressing multicultural competence. The next ethical dilemma is the use of technology. Technology may be used in several ways in counseling, such as Internet counseling (see Chapter 9). This is a new dilemma, and many of the issues involving the use of technology are still being identified, for example, the use of cloud drives. There are unique ethical issues for both the counselor and his or her supervisor involving supervision and ethics, and these are addressed in Chapter 10. There may be issues of dual relationships, sexual relationships, and so forth that arise surrounding supervision, and ethical issues may develop. The next issue addressed in this section is the use of professional (research) knowledge (see Chapter 11). The dilemma here concerns the extent to which counselors should use and apply findings from the professional counseling literature. One expects his or her physician to be up to date in the most recent medical procedures, and a similar view is required for counselors. The last issue or ethical dilemma is the use of professional codes of ethics and adherence to the law (see Chapter 12). The interpretation and understanding of professional codes of ethics and the law are essential to the practice of counseling. For example, there are both state and federal laws that may apply to counseling, and we provide a review of how such laws and court cases apply in counseling.

The next section introduces ethical theories. We make an effort to distinguish between ethical theories that are centered on reasoning and those centered on intuition. Reasoned ethical theories are found in Western theories such as virtue ethics, natural law, and utilitarian ethics. The Western theories (see Chapter 13) presented include virtue ethics, natural law ethics, utilitarian ethics, respect for persons ethics, feminine and feminist ethics, and Native American ethics. More intuitive approaches may be found in Eastern theories such as Confucian ethics and Taoist ethics. We discuss the following Eastern theories (see Chapter 14): Confucian ethics, Taoist ethics, Hindu ethics, and Buddhist ethics. In addition, there are chapters focusing on Middle Eastern ethical theories (see Chapter 15): Jewish ethics and Islamic ethics. The last chapter, Chapter 16, involves discussion of Southern Hemisphere ethical theories such as pan-African ethics and Hispanic/ Latino ethics.

We want to restate the purpose of this text, which is to provide information that is relevant to understanding counseling and ethics/morals. A second major purpose is to facilitate the development of a professional counseling ethical/moral identity. However, the process of developing a professional ethical/moral identity is ongoing and should be a continuous process throughout one's professional career. The challenge a professional counselor has is to engage and foster his or her own professional ethical identity development and to do so in a dynamic and continuous way. Most important, we are encouraging the development of ethical reasoning, not just a cookie-cutter approach to applying professional codes and laws to ethical dilemmas. Ethical dilemmas are complex and require thoughtful and reflected reasoning. Each client and circumstance requires thoughtful consideration. We hope you enjoy the challenge of discovering and promoting your own ethical development.

Additional Recommended Readings

Burke, A., Harper, H., & Kruger, G. (2007). Moving beyond statutory ethical codes: Practitioner ethics as a contextual, character-based enterprise. *South African Journal of Psychology, 37*(1), 107–120.

Crowell, C. R., Narvaez, D., & Gomberg, A. (n.d.). *Moral psychology and information ethics: Psychological distance and the components of moral action in a digital world.* Retrieved from http://www.nd.edu/~ccrowell/Moral%20Psychology%20and%20IE .pdf

Chapter 2

PROFESSIONAL IDENTITY AND ETHICS

ETHICAL DEVELOPMENT—MORAL CHARACTER

CHAPTER OBJECTIVES

- Understand the theoretical and practical factors contributing to developing a professional ethical identity
- Acquire an understanding of how to develop a professional ethical identity
- Identify one's own personal level of ethical development and how it relates to making ethical decisions

---

Case

Mary is a second-semester intern; she is completing a master's program in rehabilitation counseling. Mary is 24 years old, and she is Native American. She is the youngest of four children, and she grew up in the Midwest outside an American Indian reservation. Her parents practiced traditional Native American values, respecting nature and the universe. Mary's parents encouraged her to be respectful of traditions, but they also encouraged her to question traditions and laws since they noted that in the past laws have been used to injure and impair opportunities for Native Americans. Mary took the Defining Issues Test (DIT) and learned that her moral stage of development is Stage 2 of postconventional and is founded on universal principles. She respects laws and codes of ethics but believes there are universal laws and principles beyond conventional societal perspectives. Mary has a faculty advisor who she believes is an ideal ethical role model.

Her faculty advisor is clear about boundaries between herself and students. She is respectful of students, but she does not hold any dual relationships. Also, Mary has shared personal information with the advisor, and she is confident that the advisor is maintaining confidentiality. The faculty advisor does not impose her own personal values on students and encourages students to grow and develop within their own abilities and skills. At the same time the faculty advisor has communicated high expectations for student performance in practicums and internships. Students who do not demonstrate necessarily skills must repeat courses or assignments.

During their master's training, the program's students are encouraged to become active in professional counseling organizations. Mary did so, and she was elected the vice president of the student counseling association at her university, which may be interpreted as including individual identity and group identity. She felt that serving in this role furthered her commitment to developing a professional ethical identity; she did not want to embarrass herself or her program through any ethical violation. These feelings provided Mary with a moral/ethical motivation. Mary has taken a graduate-level course in professional ethics, and she has determined that she is likely to emphasize two principles—beneficence and fidelity—over other ethical principles such as autonomy. The emphasis on beneficence fits well with her own personal values, which are based in part on Native American perspectives and responsibility to the community and others. Mary values truth and keeping one's word; fidelity again is a key component of her personal values. Through reflection, Mary also discovered that she may experience countertransference from working with clients who are overly needy. She finds that she pushes away people who show such personality characteristics, for example, someone diagnosed with borderline personality disorder. She recognizes that she needs to be extra sensitive when working with such types of clients and maybe even consider referring them to other counselors.

INTRODUCTION

A key foundation of good counseling ethical practice is found in teaching ethical decision making in combination with the counselor's ethical development/identity. The model we are proposing here is based on the perspective that ethical practice is not a sole event such as a cognitive event utilizing reasoning alone but is developmental and stems from a dynamic interaction between the counselor's values/experiences and professional training socialization. An example of socialization is the feedback students receive during practicums and internships, which typically is focused on self-reflection and evaluation of counseling efforts and strategies. This perspective provides a view of counselor ethical development as dynamic and continuous. Professions have recently noted the importance of developing a moral/ethical identity (Bebeau, 2008; Hamilton, 2008; Sheppard, Macatangay, Colby, & Sullivan, 2008). The development of a professional ethical identity fits within Rest's (1984) four-component model, development of moral character. An understanding of ethical identity may be understood in part by a review of social identity theory.

INTRODUCTION TO SOCIAL IDENTITY THEORIES

There are several models of social identity (Capozza & Brown, 2000; Taijfel, 2010). A basic premise of social identity theory is that individuals seek out positive identities—in the case here, a positive ethical identity (Taijfel, 2010). Another important premise of the development of social identity was described by Sinnott (2009), who stated, "The formation of the self and identify is an ongoing process across the lifespan" (p. 129). Social identity can involve a fairly closed and strict access to a specific identity, or it can be acquired freely. The U.S. Congress is a unique and special group to which to belong. There are a considerable number of steps one has to complete before claiming the identity of a member of Congress. The same may be true in part for acquiring the identity of a Harvard law school graduate. However, acquisition of the identity of an Alabama Crimson Tide football fan is not so rigorous; one can simply buy a sticker, a T-shirt, or a flag to display, and others notice the identity. There is little one has to do to acquire such as identity. Certainly, there can be degrees to which one holds the identity of an Alabama football fan, such as wearing Alabama clothing and decorating one's home with Crimson Tide logos. A professional therapist's acquisition of a social identity is somewhere between the processes of the Harvard law school graduate and the Alabama football fan. A professional therapist must go through considerable training and pass licensure exams before claiming entrance into the profession and professional identity as a therapist. However, this still does not provide the therapist with a professional ethical identity, a component of overall professional identity. It is hoped that a professional ethical identity began to emerge along the way, but there are fewer obvious and overt signs of one's professional ethical identity. An important question that we need to address is, How does a professional ethical identity develop, and how can it be observed or demonstrated? This question will be discussed in a subsequent section of this chapter.

Blasi (1983) provided a model of ethical identity that consists of three elements: judgment of responsibility, centrality of moral identity, and self-consistency. He proposed that first one needs to judge that a situation is within one's responsibility: Can I be responsible for a homicide that takes place in Seattle if I live in Boston? I may have empathy for the family, but for moral action to occur, I must believe

I have a responsibility for the outcome. Second, how important or how central is moral/ethical behavior to my sense of self or identity? When I see a counseling issue, such as a counselor's talking in the lunch room about a client and breaking confidentiality, does this concern me? Do I see this as a problem quite readily, or do I enter into the conversation without seeing the issue? Last, is my ethical/moral behavior dependent on the context or situation? How consistent am I in thinking and acting morally/ethically? Blasi believed that moral identity was based in part on a desire or a motivation to maintain self-consistency in moral behavior.

Worchel, Iussini, Coutant, and Ivaldi (2000) suggested there are four types of identity that may affect a person's behavior. These include personal identity (personal characteristics), group membership, intragroup identity, and group identity. Erik Erickson (1968) has made significant contributions to the identification and understanding of personal self-identity (see Table 2.1). Erickson proposed a stage model of identity development, psychosocial stages of development, that focuses on resolution of conflicts in different stages. These include the conflicts of trust versus mistrust, autonomy versus shame and doubt, initiative versus guilt, industry versus inferiority, identity versus role confusion, intimacy versus isolation, generativity versus stagnation, and ego integrity versus despair (see Table 2.1). The resolution of these stages at various points in one's life contributes to the development and formation of the person's identity. Worchel et al. (2000) further suggested that personal identity is composed of specific person characteristics that may include age, gender, culture, and physical appearance. However, simply having a set of personal characteristics does not necessarily result in an exact identity. Social interaction and responses from others around the individual influence how the identity develops (Worchel et al., 2000). An example is how society treats and views gender. Most cultures have long-held views of specific gender roles (Eagly, 2009). Eagly proposed that prosocial behavior is influenced by gender and specific gender roles. I may have unresolved issues of intimacy versus isolation, and this can affect how I interact with others and my identity as a counselor. I may see my clients as friends or people who provide opportunities for social interaction that I may not have in my personal life.

The second type of identity, according to Worcel et al. (2000), is intragroup identity, which refers to the role the person holds within a group. For example, counselors are aware of certain types of group roles in group therapy: scapegoat, monopolist, help seeker (Gladding, 2007; Yalom & Leszcz, 2005). The role or identity within a group may be positive or negative (Capozza & Brown, 2000). Also, the role in a particular group may be unique to that group and not be transferred to other groups. So a person may play the role of scapegoat in a work group, but in a religious group, he or she may have the role of leader. What does this

Table 2.1 Erikson's Psychosocial Stages of Development and Identity Development

Stage	Issue/Concern	Elements of Stage
Infancy	Basic trust versus mistrust	The infant develops a sense of trust (basic trust) for those who are caretakers or does not develop such a trust (mistrust).
Early childhood/toddlerhood	Autonomy versus shame/doubt	The child learns that he or she has control over the environment or feels he or she does not have control over the environment (free will or not).
Preschool age	Initiative versus self-doubt	The child begins initiating activities and gains self-confidence in self-initiated activities, or the child does not feel he or she can initiate activities through his or her own actions and develops self-doubt.
School age	Competence versus inferiority	The child begins to assess his or her competence (physical, intellectual, and social skills), most often in the context of school-related activities.
Adolescence	Identity versus role confusion	This is the most relevant for counselor identity, which includes occupational identity along with gender identity, sexual identity, social identity, and so forth. The alternative is not developing a clear set of identities, and for counselors this may mean confusion about occupational/counselor identity.
Young adulthood	Intimacy versus isolation	This involves the development of an intimate relationship with another; the alternative is a feeling of isolation if closeness cannot be developed.
Adulthood	Generativity versus stagnation	The element of this stage is the integration of one's identity and intimacy and promotion of the welfare of others, passing along or generating opportunities or caring for others. Certainly counselors have an opportunity to promote generativity. Alternatively it is possible for the individual to stagnate and not promote the welfare of others, the community, and so forth. A counselor may become burnt out and not contribute to his or her client welfare.
Old age	Ego integrity versus despair	This stage is characterized by a reflection on the contributions one has made. There is a feeling that one has made the best of his or her life. Despair may happen if the individual does not feel he or she has fulfilled expectations or made the best of his or her life.

mean for the counselor's professional ethical identity? A counselor may take on the role of promoting ethical behavior in a school or an agency. In essence the person may be the voice of ethical behavior within an organization of counselors or professionals. This role is his or her intragroup identity. At a larger professional level, a counselor may serve on the American Counseling Association Ethics Committee (Ethics and Professional Standards Office) and be involved in the development of revisions to professional ethics or evaluate ethical misconduct. More often the professional counselor may have an opportunity to express his or her professional ethical identity in the school or community organization in which he or she works, but a clear professional ethical identity is important at either a micro (local school or community organization) or macro (national) level of participation.

A third possible type of identity is group membership (Worchel et al., 2000), which refers to an identity of belonging to a group. For example, he belongs to social fraternity [name of fraternity], and these students are [generalization about fraternity members]. Association with and membership in a group allows for a categorization of the person by self and others. It allows for differentiation from others. Most people are members of a number of groups, and each membership may hold different values and beliefs within a community. Those members who attend or have attended a particular university and have stickers on their cars identify each other through the symbol displayed. Certainly they pay particular attention to those who are identified with that particular university. There are hundreds of other such examples, such as belonging to a social group such as the Lions or Masons and displaying a sticker or ring to denote membership. A counselor may be a member of the American Counseling Association, the state entity of the American Counseling Association, or the American Rehabilitation Counseling Association. Another possible professional membership is belonging to a group of those licensed in a state as professional counselors. One can search for members of this group through state registries. Typically state associations of the American Counseling Association are more active and may include more social interaction and frequency of interaction than other types of group membership such as licensure groups.

A fourth type of identity is group identity, and this refers to the identity of a particular group relative to other groups (Worchel et al., 2000). Social dominance and social comparison theories enter into an understanding of this type of identity. Brewer and Gardner (1996) interpreted group identity from an evolutionary model and suggest that collective identities may be understood as "bands (small interacting communities), and tribes (macro-bands characterized by shared identity and communication without continual face-to-face interaction)" (p. 84). One may interpret this type of group identity for therapists as differences between social workers, counselors, psychologists, or psychiatrists. What are the identities and social comparisons that may be made? Certainly there have been significant disagreements over the years between these groups about who can practice what. In addition, state licensure laws have been influenced by one professional group's blocking the recognition of another. These actually are good examples of collective identities and maybe even tribes that band together to maintain status and even financial well-being.

THE CONCEPT OF ETHICAL/MORAL IDENTITY

The development of a professional ethical identity is in some ways associated with a perception that counseling is a valuable and ethical profession. An important question is, What is a positive professional ethical identity? Can one just identify a well-respected practitioner in the counseling field and seek to emulate the individual? The problem with this view is that as is true with developing a particular counseling theory to guide practice, one needs to discover his or her own personal theory. The same is true for developing a professional ethical identity.

Schlenker (2008) provided an interesting definition that can be applied to professional ethical identity. He stated,

> An ethical ideology is an integrated system of beliefs, values, standards, and self-images that define the individual's orientation toward matters of right and wrong. It provides moral schemas and scripts for assessing events and behaving in them, and a moral identity that describes one's ethical character. (p. 1079)

The inclusion of moral schemas and scripts provides a concrete way to understand the development of a professional ethical identity.

A discussion and understanding of how schemas and scripts develop may be helpful to understand how one thinks ethically/morally (Taijfel, 1982; Taijfel & Turner, 1979). Fiske and Taylor (1991) stated that a schema is "a cognitive structure that represents knowledge about a concept or type of stimulus" (p. 98). Aquino, Freeman, Reed, Lim, and Felps (2009) proposed that moral identity functions based on a set of identity schemas within the social-cognitive view. Essentially we develop identity schemas, mental structures of roles and situations that associated with our understanding of the world in various aspects of our lives. Blair-Loy (2001) described a schema as "a socially constructed, cognitive map in people's head" (p. 689). Moral identity schemas are components of our professional identities. Aquino et al. (2009) stated, "Moral identity, which we conceptualize as the cognitive schema a person holds about his or her moral character, is a powerful source of moral motivation because people generally desire to maintain self-consistency" (p. 124). Associated with schemas are scripts that may be triggered when one is confronted with or alerted to act within the specific identity, for example, moral identity. Scripts are memory structures that become activated when one enters a specific situation and a schema is triggered (Kollar, Fischer, & Hesse, 2006). Scripts are generally developed around specific schemas or views of roles and situations. So when one enters a situation such as being in the role of counselor, the counselor schema is activated. Subsequently, specific scripts are developed and are associated with this counselor schema. The important question is, which ethical/moral identity do you want to have? What are the potential scripts that need to be developed? Finally, Aquino and Reed (2002) proposed that specific values, attitudes, and behaviors are associated with an emphasis on the importance of the individual's moral identity. In other words, the higher the value a person places on his or her moral identity, the clearer are the values, attitudes, and behaviors that compose that identity.

Recently moral identity has been discussed as a major factor in motivation and ethical behavior (Hardy & Carlo, 2005; Hart, 2005). Also, Rest's (1984) four-component model of morality identifies moral motivation as a significant contributor to moral behavior. Moral motivation concerns one's prioritizing moral choices over other types of issues (e.g., career success; Bebeau & Thoma, 1999). Development of a moral/ethical identity may be tied intimately to moral motivation and how one prioritizes the practice of counseling. A therapist's acquisition of a strong moral identity as an ethical professional potentially plays a critical role in the actions he or she takes in practice. For example, Schlenker (2008) related ethical ideology to moral identity and ethical character; Schlenker stated, "An ethical ideology is an integrated system of beliefs, values, standards, and self-images that define the individual's schemas and scripts for assessing events and behaving in them" (p. 1079). A key perspective in this view is the development of individual or counselor schemas and scripts related to ethical decisions. What are the schemas and scripts that are helpful in thinking and acting/behaving as a professional ethical therapist? One script or schema might be the attitude and thought of unconditional positive regard. Automatically the counselor sees the client as a worthy and valued individual. The counselor perceives the client as having the potential to change and respects the client's choices over his or her own life. These are cognitions and schemas the counselor holds.

Forehand, Deshpande, and Reed (2002) further explained a social self-schema and proposed that "an individual's social self-schema (i.e., the sum total of his or her social identities) is a unique knowledge structure in memory" (p. 1086). Scripts, then, are specific cognitions that are associated with schemas or roles that one has. Kollar et al. (2006) further clarified what scripts are: "Cognitive psychology typically views scripts as highly specific memory structures that remain relatively fixed in situations in which the script is activated" (p. 161). For example, as a therapist one may hold a schema about greeting a client in a professional manner. The counselor may specifically recall a script that says, "Good morning, Ms. Jones. How are you this morning?" This is a different script and associated schema than one the therapist would have with a friend. A greeting script with a friend may more likely be, "Hey, Dave. What's happening?" Consequently, there are schemas associated with the various roles one has, particularly within the professional role of therapist. An example of an ethical identity schema may evolve around confidentiality. The moment a counselor walks into a session, he or she develops and holds an attitude that what takes place in the session is confidential (there are circumstances in which this may not be true, for example, involving disclosures of violence or abuse). Once the session is completed, the counselor does not run out and begin sharing the contents of the session with others. At the end of the day if the counselor goes home and a significant other asks him or her how the day went, the specific contents of the session are held confidential because the script for the counselor is one of sharing information only from outside the counseling session. The automatic script and schema that are held may involve monitoring disclosures that would violate confidentiality even to a significant other. Consequently, the comment (script) to the significant other might be, "It was a good day, and I had . . . for lunch."

COGNITIVE DEVELOPMENT AND ETHICAL/MORAL IDENTITY

Another consideration in understanding moral/ethical identity is one's cognitive development and moral development (Kohlberg, 1984a). There have been various approaches to explaining moral/ethical behavior and the motivation to act morally/ethically (Aquino & Reed, 2002; Colby, 2002; Hardy & Carlo, 2005). These various sources include moral reasoning (Kohlberg, 1969; Piaget, 1932), moral emotion (Haidt, 2001), and moral identity (Aquino & Reed, 2002; Aquino et al., 2009). Kohlberg's (1969) views were based in part on Piaget's (1932) model of cognitive development. Consequently Kohlberg (1969) proposed that moral development can best be understood from the perspective of stages of moral development, which are associated with a somewhat stable approach to thinking and viewing a problem. In describing stages of moral development, Kohlberg (1969) concluded, "A given stage response on a task does not represent simply a specific response determined by knowledge and familiarity with that task or tasks similar to it"; rather it represents an underlying thought organization (p. 6). One challenge that a person entering the counseling field must take up in his or her personal ethical identity is moving from a student to a professional who is now solely responsible for his or her actions. Previously, when this person was a student, primary responsibility typically rested on the field supervisor or the university supervisor. The developmental level of the practicing professional potentially affects ethical decisions and may be central to how one's ethical scripts are interpreted. Kohlberg (1984a) identified three levels of moral development and six stages within these levels, two stages in each level (see Table 2.2). The preconventional level consists of two stages: one focused on obedience and punishment as an orientation and a second focused on self-interest. The second level, conventional, consists of two stages: (a) interpersonal conformity and (b) adherence to authority and laws. The third level, postconventional, includes one stage with a focus on social contracts and a second stage focused on universal ethical principles. Kohlberg concluded not that one stage was better than another but simply that a higher level of moral development led to advanced moral decisions. Consequently, a counselor who is primarily in the sixth stage, principled ethics (universal principles), will make more sophisticated and well-thought-out decisions. Based on this view, one is in a specific stage of development, and through experience one can move to a more advanced stage (Kohlberg & Hersh, 1977).

Table 2.2   Kohlberg's Stages of Moral Development

Level	Stage	Characteristics
Preconventional	Punishment and obedience orientation	The person is influenced by the consequences of his or her behavior.
Preconventional	Hedonistic orientation	The individual is aware of other's needs and sees opportunities to meet his or her own needs through satisfying others. A worldview of quid pro quo.
Conventional morality	Interpersonal relationships/authority	The individual acts to please others, particularly authority figures such as teachers, bosses, and so forth.
Conventional morality	Social or group needs	The individual acts to conform to societal or group norms.
Postconventional morality	A social contract	The individual acts in accordance with moral rules founded on societal laws. Social order is protected through adherence to laws.
Postconventional morality	Universal ethical principles or individual principles	The individual acts, morally, based on individual principles that are founded on concepts such as respect for human dignity and social justice. There are universal principles that influence moral/ethical actions.

Source: Kohlberg (1984b).

Kohlberg (1969) assumed that the development of moral principles or moral reasoning motivated one to act morally/ethically. Moral reasoning and moral emotion have been found to be only moderately associated with moral action (Eisenberg & Miller, 1987). Like Rest (1983), Hardy and Carlo (2005) concluded that moral reasoning alone cannot account for one's moral/ethical actions or behaviors. Another factor hypothesized and found to contribute to moral/ethical behavior is moral identity, as we have been discussing (Aquino et al., 2009; Colby, 2002; Hardy & Carlo, 2005). Aquino and Reed (2002) noted that moral identity may be a function of what one emphasizes as important; they stated that "one person may see being compassionate as central to his or her moral identity, another may emphasize being fair and just" (p. 1424). We can use the virtue ethics model of the five principles of ethics (Beauchamp & Childress, 2008)—autonomy, fidelity, justice, beneficence, and nonmaleficence—to illustrate how one may associate a hierarchy in one's moral identity. Which one(s) does one emphasize in practice? You may see protecting the welfare of the client as first and foremost over autonomy of the client. This may be a value and a part of your ethical identity.

There have been consistent findings that through experience and education, one can advance through these moral stages of development (Enright, Lapsley, Harris, & Shauver, 1983; Schlaefli, Rest, & Thoma, 1985). A question for beginning counselors is, What is my level of moral development? How will the level of moral development affect my identity and moral decision making? For example, a counselor who is in Level 1, Stage 2 (self-interest orientation) may view seeing a client with a limited number of counseling sessions based on available insurance as a question of whether providing services to the client is worth doing. The self-interest view that is held may result in the conclusion that the counselor should not see the client because it is not worth the effort. However, a counselor in Level 3, Stage 6 may see the issue based on a principle of fidelity or keeping a promise to the client to see him or her through the issues that brought the client to counseling. The actual outcome and decision may be the same, but the reasoning and self-identity are different. For example, the professional identity of the person in Stage 2, Level 1 may lead the counselor to see himself or herself as promoting counseling services almost in the fashion of selling the service. On the other hand, the therapist in Stage 6, Level 3 may hold onto a professional identity that maintains an integrity of honesty, responsibility, and strong respect for others. Important questions include the following: Are there stages of professional identity formation for counselors? What are the tasks for the counselor in these different stages of professional ethical identity development? Rest, Narvaez, Bebeau, and Thoma (1999a) developed a measure to assess moral development based on Kohlberg's theory: the DIT. There have been more than 30 years of research using the DIT, and it is one of the most commonly used instruments to assess moral development (Thoma, 2006).

We strongly encourage you to take the DIT and receive feedback on your level of moral development. You can access the DIT at the following link: http://www.ethicaldevelopment.ua.edu/. You will receive information about your moral/ethical development level and an interpretation of the results. This information may be helpful to you as you develop your own professional ethical identity. We refer to results on the DIT in reflections in later chapters.

ADDITIONAL FACTORS AFFECTING DEVELOPMENT OF AN ETHICAL IDENTITY

In addition to the therapist's stage of moral development, there are a number of ways of understanding and defining what constitutes an ethical therapist. One factor may be the philosophical theoretical perspective that the therapist holds. A theoretical perspective may include how one emphasizes the philosophical system that is applied or emphasized in the interpretation, understanding, and application of ethics. The philosophical perspective likely even influences how one becomes aware of an ethical issue and how one defines an ethical issue. For example, we will discuss various ethical theory systems later in the text, and one common Western approach is virtue ethics. A perspective in virtue ethics is one proposed by Beauchamp and Childress (2008) that divides ethical decision making into five principles: autonomy, beneficence, nonmaleficence, fidelity, and justice. A therapist may value autonomy over beneficence, which in actual practice may mean that a client's autonomous decision making outweighs interference and helping him or her. Specifically, a client may want to choose not taking medication that is helpful (but whose absence is not life threatening), and the counselor may value that autonomy more than does another counselor who sees the benefits of the medication and helping the client through beneficence; consequently the second counselor may strongly encourage the client to take the medication and intervene in ways to ensure that happens. There are a number of other theories of ethics that are associated with specific perspectives that will be covered in later chapters such as Eastern views including Buddhism, Taoism, Hinduism, and Confucianism. In addition, there are Middle Eastern ethical perspectives such as Judaism and Islam. Native American ethical perspectives will be discussed too. The counselor may choose to value and use any of these perspectives in making ethical decisions. How he or she chooses what to emphasize may be critical in the practice of counseling and the ethical identity that he or she holds.

Another relevant factor that potentially affects a counselor's ethical identity is his or her definition of boundaries. Boundaries may involve a number of issues that the counselor should consider such as the amount and level of counselor self-disclosure in the counseling session and the amount and type of physical contact between counselor and client. A. Wilcoxon (personal communication, 2010) proposed a way of thinking about boundaries in regard to "thickness." A thick boundary may be seen as one that is fairly well established based on role and context. A thin boundary is one that is more permeable and not as well defined. Kottler (1986) concluded in reference to therapist self-disclosure that "there are few therapeutic activities that are so abused under the guise of being helpful. Excessive self-disclosure may be done to relieve the therapist's own discomfort with the inherent inequality in the relationship" (p. 61). There have been mixed results with counselor self-disclosure (Barrett & Berman, 2001; Hendrick, 1990; Thomas, Veach, & LeRoy, 2006). Certainly self-disclosure by the counselor varies depending on the theoretical orientation (Barrett & Berman, 2001). Also, some have suggested that counselor self-disclosure, particularly disclosure of vulnerabilities, can have a negative impact on the counseling relationship (Curtis, 1982). Furthermore, Barrett and Berman (2001) noted that too much self-disclosure by a counselor can take away from client self-disclosure and client time to work on issues. A key to understanding boundaries, ethics, and ethical identity in counseling is the type of self-disclosure. Fisher (2004) discussed therapists' self-disclosing sexual feelings toward the client. He noted that some therapists do consider such self-disclosures appropriate and helpful in therapy. However, Fisher further pointed out that such disclosures bring into question boundary issues. Discussing a counselor's personal sexual attraction with a client may be interpreted as crossing a thick boundary and one that the counselor needs to carefully consider (A. Wilcoxon, personal communication, 2010). Denney, Aten, and Gingrich (2008) discussed the use of spiritual self-disclosure by the therapist. They systematically discussed the pros and cons of self-disclosure in therapy in general. Furthermore, they suggested that the therapist should, most important, consider whether the client would experience positive effects as a result of the therapist's spiritual self-disclosure. Not much research into spiritual self-disclosure has been done to date. Similar to other types of self-disclosures, spiritual self-disclosure is a boundary issue, and a careful and thoughtful consideration of such a disclosure is important before proceeding. Certainly, if a therapist uses the therapy session as a pulpit, this creates a potential violation in boundaries. The question for the counselor in regard to ethical/moral identity is, What are my boundaries around self-disclosure? In part this question is answered based on what the context is (type of facility, e.g., substance abuse center, mental health center, hospital). Facilities such as substance abuse counseling centers consider self-disclosure by the counselor about previous drug or alcohol use important aspects of treatment, whereas counselors in outpatient mental health centers likely do not disclose much personal information to clients. As was mentioned above, the topic of discussion is relevant, and whether the counselor discloses information such as religious views or personal failures is an important consideration of the counselor's ethical/moral boundaries.

There are other types of boundaries that potentially affect the ethical behavior of counselors such as dual relationships. A review of reports of therapist misconduct to state licensure boards discovered that violation of dual relationships was the most frequent complaint (Neukrug, Milliken, & Walden, 2001). There are several types of dual relationships that potentially cause counselors ethical problems. One is the use of touch or physical contact, even sexual contact between therapist and client. The use of physical touch such as a pat on the shoulder after a difficult session may be seen as an example of a thin boundary, one where the clarity of the boundary is less well established (A. Wilcoxon, personal communication, 2010). Other dual relationships may involve providing therapy to friends, relatives, or neighbors. Perkins, Hudson, Gray, and Stewart (1998) noted that such boundary violations for therapists may more often occur in small rural areas where social networks are more connected and less anonymous than they might be in larger urban centers. A final type of dual relationship is the use of bartering, which can result in the therapist's taking advantage of a client and making an exchange that is more beneficial to the therapist, who has more power over the client.

Another factor that potentially affects counselors' ethical identity is personal needs. Corey, Corey, and Callanan (2007) noted that a therapist's personal needs possibly affect ethical behavior, and they categorized those needs as countertransference. Corey et al. (2007) suggested there are several counselor actions based on countertransference that can create problems: overprotection, discouraging clients from expressing strong feelings, rejecting a client for being overly needy, seeking client feedback, overidentification with a client, strong emotional feelings (sexual or romantic) toward a client, and development of social or friendship relationships. Overprotection of a client may mean viewing clients as helpless (maybe you had a sibling or a parent who you felt needed protection, and the client reminds you of this person). I recall a student who reported attending a professional counseling program where someone was given a bandage for overinvolvement in caring for a client, a way to symbolize such overprotection. Discouraging clients from expressing strong feelings is a second potential therapist countertransference reaction (you may have had an earlier experience with someone who was overly expressive, and therefore you avoid such displays). A third potential personal need may be expressed through countertransference, according to Corey et al. (2007), which may involve rejecting a client who is needy. Earlier in your life you may have experienced another person who was overly needy, and this may cause a strong reaction in you. A fourth type of countertransference may be a therapist's seeking constant feedback for therapy progress. This may result from early criticism or a desire to please others. The last type of countertransference, according to Corey et al. (2007), may be overidentification with a client (you see experiences and struggles in a client's life similar to those you have had). Therapists are humans, and clients may attempt to seduce them (similar to lifestyles outside of therapy). Because of personal preferences based on previous experiences, therapists may be more attracted sexually to certain types of clients (Corey et al., 2007). The last countertransference that may occur is the development of a social relationship or friendship with a client. The counselor may see the client as similar to friends he or she has had in the past and want to develop similar kinds of relationships.

What may tie these elements together is the ethical ideology the person holds (Schlenker, 2008). Schlenker (2008) noted that personal commitment to moral principles is an important dimension in developing an ethical identity or ideology. Personal commitment is proposed to be most important, and Schlenker concluded that

> personal commitment to a principled ideology determines the strength of the relationship between moral beliefs and behavior. Commitment links the self-system to the ethical principles, producing an accompanying sense of obligation to perform consistently with those principles, an increased sense of responsibility for relevant actions, and a reluctance to condone and rationalize ethical transgressions. (p. 1080)

Key in this perspective is the view that consistency and commitment lead to action or behavior that is ethical. For a counselor developing an ethical ideology and identity, this is based on a strong commitment to behave a certain way. Whether it means establishing clear professional boundaries or avoiding dual relationships, the counselor seeks to establish a commitment to these principles. As you can see from the discussion, the development of a professional ethical identity is complex and entails consideration of, understanding of, and commitment to a professional ethical identity, not one that may change from situation to situation because it is convenient or expedient.

Case Analysis and Reflection

Reread the case at the beginning of the chapter. Do you think that Mary can act ethically given her emphasis on beneficence and fidelity? She appears to value beneficence or helping others over promoting client autonomy. Should Mary have been elected to an officer role in the student professional organization? Do you think she can relate to students who function at lower levels of moral development and provide good role modeling?

Questions for Further Reflection

1. What are important values you hold, and why are they important?

2. What would an ideal counselor/therapist have as an ethical identity (if you were asked to describe an ethical counselor)? What would friends and colleagues say in describing your ethical identity?

3. Identify examples of scripts and schemas you have, if possible related to counseling and ethics.

4. What professional ethical/moral identity do you currently have? What would you like to have?

5. What can you do to develop an ethical/moral identity that is consistent with your desired/ideal ethical/moral identity?

6. Which stage of moral development would you guess you currently hold? Explain.

7. What are examples of personal identity, group membership, intragroup identity, and group identity for you? How do these relate to ethical identity?

8. Take the DIT2 and obtain your results (http://www.ethicaldevelopment .ua.edu/). Are the results consistent with what you would expect, or are they different? Explain.

9. What is your training program doing to foster the development of a professional ethical/moral identity?

10. What long-term strategy will you use to continue developing your professional ethical/moral identity?

Additional Recommended Readings

Barrett, M., & Berman, J. (2001). Is psychotherapy more effective when therapists disclose information about themselves? *Journal of Consulting and Clinical Psychology, 69*(4), 397–603.

Bebeau, M., & Thoma, S. (1999). "Intermediate" concepts and the connection to moral education. *Educational Psychology Review, 11,* 343–368.

Capozza, D., & Brown, R. (Eds.). (2000). *Social identity processes.* Thousand Oaks, CA: Sage.

Curtis, J. (1982). Principles and techniques of non-disclosure by the therapist during psychotherapy. *Psychological Reports, 51,* 907–914.

Fisher, C. (2004). Ethical issues in therapy: Therapist self-disclosure of sexual feelings. *Ethics & Behavior, 14*(2), 105–121.

Fiske, S., & Taylor, S. (1991). *Social cognition* (2nd ed.). New York, NY: McGraw-Hill.

Forehand, M., Deshpande, R., & Reed, A., II. (2002). Identity salience and the influence of differential activation of the social self-schema on advertising response. *Journal of Applied Psychology, 87,* 1086–1099.

Kohlberg, L. (1984a). *Essays on moral development: Vol. 2. The psychology of moral development.* San Francisco, CA: Harper & Row.

Kohlberg, L. (1984b). *The psychology of moral development: The nature and validity of moral stages.* San Francisco, CA: Harper & Row.

Kollar, I., Fischer, F., & Hesse, F. (2006). Collaboration scripts: A conceptual analysis. *Educational Psychology Review, 18,* 159–185.

Schlaefli, A., Rest, J., & Thoma, S. (1985). Does moral education improve moral judgment: A meta-analysis of intervention studies using the DIT. *Review of Educational Research, 55,* 319–352.

Thoma, S. (2006). Research using the Defining Issues Test. In M. Killen & J. Smetana (Eds.), *Handbook of moral psychology* (pp. 67–91). Mahwah, NJ: Lawrence Erlbaum.

Worchel, S., Iussini, J., Coutant, D., & Ivaldi, M. (2000). A multimodal model of identity: Relating individual and group identities to intergroup behavior. In D. Capozza & R. Brown (Eds.), *Social identity processes* (pp. 15–32). Thousand Oaks, CA: Sage.

Chapter 3

AWARENESS OF AND SENSITIVITY TO ETHICAL ISSUES

DEVELOPMENT OF ETHICAL SENSITIVITY AND MOTIVATION TO ACT ETHICALLY

CHAPTER OBJECTIVES

- Acquire an understanding of how cognitions and emotions contribute to developing ethical sensitivity
- Develop an understanding of how emotions and intuitions provide a source of awareness of ethical issues
- Develop an understanding of the importance of monitoring emotions and intuitions (gut reactions) to ethical situations and an awareness of how such emotions may also hinder understanding of ethical dilemmas/issues
- Acquire an understanding of the factors that influence motivations to act ethically
- Identify the values, beliefs, and professional values that are central to your professional ethical identity and which serve to promote motivation to act ethically
- Develop an understanding of how social comparison theory applies to motivation to act ethically
- Understand how empathy acts as a motivation to behave ethically

---

Case

Joe is a clinical mental health counseling intern in his second semester of internship. He has had a good relationship with his supervisor, and he is feeling more and more confident of his abilities to provide counseling. He took an ethics course as part of his graduate program. Joe has strong beliefs about behaving ethically, and he discusses ethical concerns with his supervisor on a regular basis. He meets with his supervisor to discuss cases and the clock hours he has accrued. Joe notes that he is not getting enough client-contact clock hours, and this concerns him because he wants to graduate this semester. His supervisor assures him that even if he does not get enough hours, he will sign off on the necessary hours so Joe can graduate. Joe has a strong gut reaction to this offer. He appreciates his supervisor's offering to sign off on his hours, but Joe questions whether this is an ethical choice and action. Joe does not want to start his career getting involved in unethical behavior. He is not sure what to do. Is he being overly sensitive, or is this really an ethical issue?

INTRODUCTION TO ETHICAL SENSITIVITY

Welfel (2009) offered a ten-step model of ethical decision making, with the first step's being the development of ethical sensitivity. An important question is, What is moral or ethical sensitivity? Weaver (2007) noted the broad group of professionals, such as those in nursing, medicine, dentistry, and business, who have focused on ethical sensitivity. Weaver cited a problem in the identification and definition of ethical sensitivity around the lack of consistency and agreement on what constitutes the concept of ethical sensitivity. A review of the definitions offered may be helpful in understanding ethical sensitivity. Welfel and Kitchener (1992) noted that the first step in ethical action, "interpreting the situation as a moral one, involves the recognition that one's actions affect the welfare of another" (p. 179). Weaver, Morse, and Mitcham (2008) defined ethical sensitivity as "that which enables professionals to recognize, interpret and respond appropriately to concerns of those receiving professional services" (p. 607). Rest (1984) discussed ethical sensitivity in the following way:

> a person realizes that she/he could do something which would affect the interests, welfare, or expectations of other people. (Realizing that one's actions might be violating some moral norm or principle is one of the ways that a person might realize his/her actions affects the interests, welfare, or expectations of others.) p. 21

Commonalities in these definitions involve the recognition and ability to perceive an impact on another or others. Essentially this involves the practitioner's being able to recognize and make a determination as to the relevancy and significance of cues involving a potential ethical situation and an effect on another person or persons. Ethical issues potentially arise in each counseling session, and counselors can devote considerable time to addressing issues; each counseling session, one hopes, has the potential to affect the client. What does the counselor pursue as possible ethical issues, and what is left? Key is the counselor's ability to perceive or recognize a relevant ethical issue without another's assistance. What are the processes of making such recognitions or perceptions?

Researchers in the professions (e.g., Bebeau, 1994) have focused on the sensitivity component because data indicate that there is a wide range in the ability to see a moral dimension within professional situations. Some professionals and students seem attuned to the moral dimension, whereas others seem very limited in their moral vision, focusing instead on professional practice such as using appropriate techniques and procedures. Researchers have noted that moral sensitivity is somewhat a function of empathic ability (Bebeau, 2002). The benefit of advanced empathy skills for ethical sensitivity centers on the individual's/counselor's being aware of how those involved in a possible dilemma are affected by various actions. Furthermore, evidence from the health professions suggests that in the absence of direct instruction, socialization into a professional field does not guarantee increased moral sensitivity (Bebeau, 2008). It appears that one must have direct involvement in approaching professional experiences from a moral perspective before increased sensitivity occurs.

How we should characterize the processes that support moral or ethical sensitivity is currently a controversial topic and is associated with the major debates within moral psychology. Traditionally, the processes involved with moral sensitivity were defined primarily as cognitive and were focused on how an individual consciously attends to the moral features of a situation (Rest, 1983). This view suggested that with social development, perspective taking in particular, the individual learns to identify cues that highlight issues of harm and areas in which cooperation can be promoted. As was mentioned above, asking oneself questions that can serve as clues can be helpful because ethical sensitivity is associated with advanced empathy. An example of a question in considering an ethical dilemma is, Who will be affected by a particular course of action, and how will he or she be affected? Moral heuristics such as this allow one to become a mature moral agent with the capacity to identify moral issues within daily life and professional exchanges. Although gut feelings are acknowledged and incorporated into the models, for the most part these emotions are not considered a primary focus for traditional models of moral sensitivity, particularly within professional populations. Indeed, for many in this tradition, the sense is that professionals ought to be wary of gut feelings and consciously set them aside in dealing with clients.

COGNITIVE DEVELOPMENTAL PERSPECTIVES

In the traditional cognitive developmental view, sometimes affect and emotions are triggered by situations before one has a good grasp of the events and motives of the involved individual. These strong emotions are viewed as morally neutral because the effect on one's action may or may not further a moral outcome. One may be galvanized into action by one's emotional reaction to a person in need and save a life. Conversely, one may be disgusted by the appearance of a patient and provide fewer services and fail to attend to his or her needs. In both cases strong emotions are triggered perhaps before the person is able to understand why he or she is feeling them, but these strong emotions are in themselves insufficient to define the resulting action as having a moral basis.

Hoffman's work on the development of empathy provides another view of how emotions influence moral sensitivity (e.g., Hoffman, 1981). In Hoffman's view, empathy has its roots in emotional reactions to others. However, Hoffman made clear that across development, an understanding of one's emotions and what they imply for an understanding of social situations marks adult empathy. That is, from emotional roots, Hoffman saw the complex forms of empathy in adults are the result of cognitive processes, particularly the understanding of social phenomena, interacting with emotions.

A number of researchers have developed research programs building off of Rest's description of moral sensitivity; see Chapter 1 for a review of the description of Rest's (1984) four-component model. The primary goal of this work is to assess moral sensitivity in professional populations (Bebeau, 2008). Toward this end, these researchers have developed a methodology that focuses on the student's ability to recognize the moral dimension in a real-life situation nested within the professional field. For instance, in counseling, Volker (1984) developed training audiotapes of counselors interacting with their patients. In each case, embedded within the exchange was a moral issue. Participants in the study were asked to reflect on the exchange, extract the major issues defining the clinical situation, and then interpret them. In addition to collecting technical information, a scoring procedure was developed to assess whether the participant recognized the moral dimension and to what degree. Higher scores were given to those participants who were able not only to recognize the moral situation but also to articulate the moral aspects of the exchange. As expected, Volker found that counseling students varied in their ability to detect moral aspects within professional settings. Furthermore, high scorers on the moral sensitivity measure were independently rated as more effective counselors.

Within dentistry, Bebeau developed a measure (Bebeau, 2008; Bebeau, Rest, & Yamoor, 1985) in which a dental student assumes the role of a dentist in a real-time exchange with a patient. Unlike Volker's (1984) approach in which the participant passively evaluates the recorded clinical session, Bebeau's measure requires students to listen and respond to an actor playing the role of a patient. Consistent with the Volker measure, Bebeau's procedure assesses students on their ability to acknowledge the moral dimension in the situation and whether the student's solution incorporates moral aspects. Over many years of collecting data on moral sensitivity in dental students, Bebeau has found significant variation in students and an absence of growth in the ability to attend to moral content without direct instruction in professional ethics. Furthermore, Bebeau has found that professionals facing remediation for code violations are frequently deficient in moral sensitivity (Bebeau, 2009).

Rest's (1984) description of moral sensitivity has led to a number of research programs and measurement systems. Findings from these studies support the basic features of moral sensitivity as a variable within professional populations and not tied simply to one's socialization into the field. For example, F. Chang (1994) noted that preservice teachers functioned at a conventional level of moral reasoning compared to those in other disciplines; see Kohlberg's (1984b) categories of moral reasoning. Ethical sensitivity is influenced by personal characteristics beyond training and education. However, researchers have developed a methodology to promote ethical professional practice and increase moral sensitivity (Bebeau, 1994). Furthermore, this work has been tied directly to instruction and has highlighted the need to build in a comprehensive ethics education program in professional schools (Bebeau, 1994). Bebeau (1994) discussed a curriculum to increase ethical professional practice, and this included efforts to increase moral or ethical sensitivity. The curriculum, designed to increase ethical sensitivity, included case discussion and role-play among professionals concerning potential ethical issues and what makes them ethical issues.

EMOTIONS AND INTUITIONS

The cognitive development view of moral or ethical development generally and moral sensitivity specifically has recently come under question by researchers who come from outside of developmental psychology and education (Haidt, 2001). These researchers identify evolutionary psychology, cultural psychology, and neuropsychology as their primary affiliations. Building from experimental work and brain-imaging studies, members of this group highlight the role of intuitions and associated emotions. Moral sensitivity is thus primed by "evaluative feeling(s) (like-dislike, good-bad) without the conscious awareness of having gone through steps of search, weighing evidence, or inferring a conclusion" (Haidt & Borkland, 2007, p. 187). For these researchers, emotions play a much more foundational role in our moral orientation and sensitivity. Haidt (2001) in particular has championed the idea that emotions and intuitions are actually the driving force in much of an individual's moral life. In this view, cognitive and conscious processes provide secondary post hoc interpretations of moral actions used in the service of providing a rationale to the individual and others. That is, in Haidt's view, cognitive processes provide the language by which we interpret our behaviors but are not the processes used to construct moral actions. The model that has developed around these ideas is identified as the social intuitionist model. Other models cover similar points. For instance, Hauser (2006) saw moral intuitions as evidence for a moral grammar that provides humans with a rudimentary system that primes human cooperation. Similarly, Greene and Baron (2001) proposed a two-aspect model in which intuitive and deliberative moral processes both contribute to moral functioning. Together, these researchers suggest that moral sensitivity is not simply a cognitive or developmental process but a process that resides more within the emotional system. The question has become the degree to which emotion influences moral phenomena and moral sensitivity in particular. To some (e.g., Haidt and the social intuitionist model), emotion is preeminent. To others, emotion has a role, but it is unclear how central it is to moral functioning—is it an equal partner or a focusing set of processes that lead one to recognize and focus on moral aspects of the situation (Hauser, 2006)? A counselor may have strong feelings about particular issues such as abortion. This may be represented as a gut reaction by the counselor. A counselor working in a public agency may need to be aware of how he or she identifies such an ethical issue. As a group these researchers suggested that Kohlberg's (1984b) model is incomplete as it does not truly incorporate the powerful role of noncognitive intuitions and associated emotions.

The basis of this theoretical system comes from a variety of sources but starts with an analysis of human evolutionary origins. These findings suggest that sensitivity to moral phenomena occurs in other primates and very young children. There is evidence that empathy has been promoted during our evolutionary history; other studies have found that emotions are associated with moral responses to situations (Rozen, Haidt, & McCauley, 1993). When one reasons about a moral issue, it is rarely emotionally neutral. Similarly, perceived moral violations are associated with strong emotions such as shame, disgust, or anger (Rozen et al., 1993). Finally, studies of how the brain processes moral content indicate support for the claim that moral judgments are associated with emotional processing

(Greene & Baron, 2001). Taken together, the evidence is increasingly strong that emotions are implicated in processing moral information and constructing one's action. Furthermore, these researchers are undoubtedly correct that complete models of moral functioning must incorporate the ways in which emotions function. However, the evidence is not strong that emotions trump cognitive understanding of moral phenomena, as has been suggested by some of the social intuitionist model's leading supporters (e.g., Haidt, 2001). As Huebner, Lee, and Hauser (2010) made clear, the field is currently only beginning to tease apart the relative contribution of reasoning and emotion in the service of moral judgments and action. Much of current basic research is directed at this question.

LIMITS OF INTUITION AND EMOTIONAL MODELS ON MORAL/PROFESSIONAL EDUCATION

In addition to the current ambiguity of the findings on the role of emotion on moral functioning, the current models driven by the focus on emotions provide little guidance to educators and professionals about how best one should construct programs to influence moral functioning. Nor do these researchers provide information about how moral functioning develops over time. Developmental information on naturally occurring growth is important to help identify experiences that might guide educational interventions. Instead, researchers such as Haidt (2010) suggested that to influence moral functioning, we should focus on the context in which professionals and students interact and provide situations that occasion prosocial concerns (Haidt, 2010). Like the social psychologists before Kohlberg and the cognitive revolution, Haidt's view is that the situation drives action, and thus he at best minimized the individual's role in the construction of behavior. Compared to the older social psychological models, all that has changed is the mechanism causing growth. That is, now the focus is on emotional triggers as the operative mechanism leading to action rather than the older focus on exposure to social norms through the socialization process. To Haidt (2001), focusing on moral thinking and the individual's role in reasoning about moral issues is a mistake because it is not causal in the construction of moral action. This perspective provides problems for applied researchers and clinicians because if researchers such as Haidt are right, our behavior is irrational, and our choices are nonconscious. Thus, professional ethics courses and moral education are ultimately not very helpful beyond giving students a language with which to interpret their actions. This view has been criticized by others—particularly developmental psychologists (e.g., Turiel & Killen, 2010)—as the "people are stupid" school of psychology because it fails to recognize the contribution of an individual's thinking and decision making to functioning both in any given situation and across time. These researchers, influenced by research on child development, note the strong cognitive underpinnings of growth. Although these researchers acknowledge biological processes such as those that promote social development, what is most striking in this work is the child's reasoning about his or her world and how development is characterized by the integration of emotions and thought in the service of becoming socially competent.

Although the social intuitionist model and other emotion-based models have limitations for professional ethics education and professional practice, there is an important message in this work for counselors and therapists. Particularly important is the clear focus these models place on our tendency to react and quickly judge others. If Green, Hauser, and Haidt are correct, our moral judgments include very automatic and deeply felt emotions that can color our reactions to our clients. Part of our ethics training, therefore, should focus on how we can recognize the ways in which we react and then develop cognitive strategies to help better evaluate our impressions and construct more reasoned responses. As we will see later, Rest's (1984) model anticipates this conflict between moral and nonmoral consideration in moral motivation. Moral motivation, according to Rest, involves the influence of values and beliefs, and these can originate from comparison with others' views. This view of what motivates moral action is not incompatible with the intuitionist perspective on moral functioning that moral development is associated with sentiments but supported and shaped later through social interactions. The influence of social comparison will be introduced in more detail below.

MOTIVATION TO ACT ETHICALLY

There are several perspectives on the sources of ethical motivation (Eisenberg, Cumberland, Guthri, Murphy, & Shepard, 2005; Kagan, 2005; Staub, 2005). These views include centrality of ethical beliefs and congruency, comparison with others and professional standards, and empathy and social responsibility. Kagan (2005) identified one source of moral motivation: "to produce evidence indicating that one's behaviors, thoughts, and feelings are in accord with a representation that the agent regards as good" (p. 1). As discussed, we have proposed in previous chapters the development of professional ethical identity as a goal in training counselors. Evaluating behaviors, thoughts, and feelings consistent with what a professional counselor or therapist considers ethical fits with Kagan's definition. Staub's (2005) view of ethical motivation is similar to Kagan's, and Staub stated, "I see motivation as moral when to some substantial degree its focus is to fulfill or live up to a moral belief, value or principle" (p. 35).

CENTRALITY OF VALUES AND BELIEFS

One's motivation to act in a way that is consistent with one's ethical understanding is central to understanding the conditions under which ethical action occurs. An assumption is that when confronted with an ethical situation, the individual may be asked to address multiple options for ethical action. For instance, a counselor may find ethical considerations in any given situation conflicting with financial concerns, personal relationships, or other belief systems. One theory that explains how ethical motivation may function can be found in cognitive dissonance theory (Festinger, 1957). Festinger (1957) first introduced cognitive dissonance theory, which states that when there is a difference between cognitions and behavior, there is dissonance and discomfort. Consequently when dissonance is present, the individual is uncomfortable and seeks to reduce the discomfort by achieving congruity. Kurtines and Gewirtz (1987) described how self-attribution, similar to social identity, plays a role in ethical behavior. They gave an example of attributional processes and stated,

> The individual attributional processes that occur subsequent to helping may: (1) develop a more altruistic self-image that, because of internal consistency pressures, will enhance the likelihood of future prosocial responding; and (2) view the subjective utility . . . of assisting in future situations differently than previously because of increased negative consequences for one's self-esteem if one acts in a manner inconsistent with one's self-image. (p. 35)

Essentially, Kurtines and Gewirtz proposed that acts of ethical behavior increase future likelihood of such behavior because they increasingly establish the self and ethical identity.

There has been considerable research supporting cognitive dissonance theory (Draycott & Dabbs, 1998). Researchers have found that cognitive dissonance serves as motivation (Elliot & Devine, 1994; Keller & Block, 1999). Essentially, ethical motivation may be interpreted as seeking to maintain cognitive consistency and avoid cognitive dissonance through actions and professional ethical identity. Cognitive dissonance has been related to ethical motivation (McCabe, 1993; Vinski & Tryon, 2009). McCabe (1993) found that students who cheated attempted to reduce cognitive dissonance through rationalizations such as denial, deflecting blame, condemning the accuser, and so forth. Cognitive dissonance theory applies to ethical motivation based on the view that one's professional ethical identity requires maintenance through consistency of self-perceptions and actions, ethical beliefs, and ethical behaviors. Development of a strong professional ethical identity may actually facilitate a motivation to be ethical and to avoid cognitive dissonance—not a bad thing.

Rest (1984) provided another perspective on how one interprets concretely the gathering and understanding of evidence consistent with one's professional ethical identity, that is, maintaining cognitive consistency. According to Rest, moral motivation involves the influence of values and beliefs. Key in the influence of values and beliefs is the centrality they hold in the person's professional ethical identity (Morton, Worthley, Testerman, & Mahoney, 2006; Rest, 1984). Rest and Narvaez (1994) noted that moral motivation concerns "the importance given to moral values in competition with other values" (p. 214). Morton et al. (2006) also defined moral motivation as "prioritizing moral values above other values and taking responsibility for moral outcomes" (p. 389). In addition to placing values and beliefs in a hierarchical order within a professional context, one takes responsibility for the ethical outcome. Consequently the person may evaluate the relevance of these values and beliefs and how they fit with his or her professional identity. Also, there may be an evaluation of his or her responsibility for the outcome of an ethical decision or behavior. A worst-case scenario is behaving in a way that results in one's professional association's or state licensing board's charging misconduct or unethical practice. Kagan (2005) did suggest that the importance or relevance of a particular ethical issue is influenced by the context and era. What is important in a particular context and during a particular era may change over several years and become more or less important. For example, display of overt sexual activity in a public arena, for example, in the media, specifically movies, is more frequently presented today than it was 100 years ago in the United States. Such display even varies today from culture to culture and country to country.

There may be several relevant influences on how one comes to hold certain values or beliefs. One influence is the developmental stage the person holds at a particular time period (review Chapter 2 for a summary of stages of development, or read Kohlberg, 1969). Developmental models note the links between a developing understanding of ethical consideration and the perceived importance and interpretation of various values and beliefs. For example, proponents of the developmental perspective note that individuals prioritize personal considerations as the foundation for ethical behavior. They have a different set of considerations for various beliefs to inform judgment versus individuals who prioritize social norms and conventions, which in turn differ from those who emphasize postconventional considerations (e.g., Rest, Narvaez, Bebeau, & Thoma, 1999b). Thus, developmental models highlight the role of how various belief systems are understood rather than where they originate. For example, all helping professions make mention and teach the notion of informed consent as a foundational principle in professional ethics. However, how this notion is understood is not uniform across students, practitioners, and disciplines (Rest & Narvaez, 1994). Some may view informed consent as a rule one must follow to be in the good graces of and be approved by other professionals. Others may see this concept as an agreed-on consideration that defines client–counselor/therapist relationships, depending to some degree on their states of moral development. Still others employ a perspective that informed consent requirements provide a central check and balance between professional authority and society's well-being. Developmental theories have had a lot to say about where these individual differences originate.

A second way in which developmental theories focus on beliefs is how these nonmoral value systems influence choices and actions. These theorists suggest that nonmoral considerations tend to be less central to decision making as development proceeds. Thus, Kohlberg (1969) noted that emotions, attitudes, and situational considerations become less central to individuals who emphasize post-conventional interpretive strategies. This view has been supported in various professional settings. For instance, in-depth interviews with moral exemplars consistently note how ethical considerations begin to define the self and limit the role of other nonmoral beliefs and values on ethical action (e.g., Rule & Bebeau, 2005).

The developmental view holds that the understanding of beliefs changes across development and we should expect to find different understandings of what these beliefs mean and demand from the individual both across individuals at any given time and within the individual across time. That is, professionals do not learn their beliefs simply by direct exposure; they reflect on and modify their views as their conceptual strategies develop and change. Furthermore, changes in understandings and meanings of beliefs and values are viewed as patterned and predictable based on developmental transitions more generally.

Another way that a counselor develops ethical values or beliefs that are central to his or her professional ethical identity may be through principled ideology (Schlenker, 2008). Schlenker (2008) defined ethical ideology as "an integrated system of beliefs, values, standards, and self-images that define the individual's orientation toward matters of right or wrong" (p. 1079). Furthermore, Schlenker suggested that an ethical ideology involves a commitment to one's beliefs regardless of the circumstances and social influences on the person. Schlenker would likely be categorized as holding a moral absolutism view, compared to a moral relativism view. He differentiated a view of a principled ideology, which he supported, from a relativism view and called the principles based on the latter view "expedient ideologies." Ethical decisions based on expedient ideologies are based on context and not necessarily on principles that cut across situations. Conversely, he proposed that from a principled absolutism perspective, "commitment links the self-system to the ethical principles, producing an accompanying sense of obligation to perform consistently with those principles, an increased sense of responsibility for relevant actions, and a reluctance to condone and rationalize ethical transgressions" (p. 1080). In regard to counseling and therapy, his view would propose that motivation to act ethically is consistent across situations and is motivated based on the perspective of responsibility to behave ethically regardless of the context, that is, principled ideologies. Key in the definition of principled ideologies is the idea of commitment. Schlenker further noted when defining commitments,

> Commitments reflect a pledging or binding of the self to something else, such as a goal (e.g., to earn a college degree), a set of ideas (a particular ideology), another person (e.g., a marriage partner), or a group (social group or organization). To say that people have a commitment means that they have selected a particular set of prescriptions that they agree to follow and that can be used to evaluate and sanction their conduct. (p. 1080)

The idea of commitment to an organization for counselors and therapists may be interpreted as a commitment to a professional organization such as the American Counseling Association (ACA). ACA has developed codes of ethics that counselors/therapists should follow, so commitment to the organization denotes acceptance of the codes. Therefore, counselors/therapists should be motivated to adhere to these codes of ethics. Knowledge and complete comprehension of professional codes of ethics demonstrate the ideological commitment to the profession. The question for counselors in training is, How well do you know the professional codes of ethics? The motivation to adopt a professional ethical identity may be demonstrated in part through one's effort to fully know and understand professional codes of ethics. More concretely, this means becoming thoroughly familiar with professional codes and ensuring they are understood completely.

Schlenker's definition of principled ideology also proposed that commitments bind the individual to a set of ideas (a particular ideology), and this can be related to larger ethical theories such as utilitarian theory, virtue ethics, and so forth (we will discuss these theories later). A commitment to a larger ethical philosophical theory gives the counselor a broader framework than professional codes of ethics and theoretically can provide a broader perspective, an additional perspective to codes of ethics, to assist the counselor/therapist in making ethical decisions. Also, the ethical philosophical perspective can provide the counselor/therapist with the framework for commitment to such ideas and the motivation to maintain behaviors, feelings, and thoughts consistent with them. Such a commitment to philosophical theories also leads to a well-developed professional ethical identity. Similar to a well-developed understanding of professional codes of ethics, the counselor's/therapist's commitment to ethical philosophical theories is essential to developing a professional ethical identity.

Development of a strong principled professional ethical identity, including a strong commitment to being ethical, should produce significant motivation to act and behave ethically. Inherent in this state of principled professional ethical identity is the desire to continue professional ethical identity development. As we have noted, continued development does not stop but continues over one's professional life. Based on the perspective that one develops a strong central view of ethics (a hierarchy of ethical views and perspectives), and a principled ideology, is the relevance of gaining an internal frame of reference. An internal frame of reference based on a strong central principled view of ethics is a desirable goal in the process of developing a professional ethical identity. Counselors/therapists can use cognitive dissonance theory by attending to feelings or thoughts of incongruence between cognitions and behaviors. As with many aspects of counseling, self-reflection is a critical component of being an effective counselor/therapist. The specific focus needs to be on any incongruence between professional ethical identity and behaviors. This potentially could include incongruity between professional ethical identity and initial deliberations on courses of action prior to acting.

SOCIAL COMPARISON THEORY AND ETHICAL MOTIVATION

Another perspective in interpreting ethical motivation is a focus on social comparison (Brewer & Gardner, 1996; Kagan, 2005). Consistent with Kagan's (2005) interpretation that ethical or moral motivation concerns an effort to collect evidence about one's behaviors, thoughts, and feelings is an evaluation of appropriate professional counselor ethical actions and use of professional social comparisons. Conclusions about the efficacy of an ethical decision are based on what a reasonable person or counselor would do in such a situation or ethical dilemma, that is, social comparison. Also, it has been proposed that consulting with peers is important in good practice and in making ethical decisions (Corey, Corey, & Callanan, 2007; Houser, Wilczenski, & Ham, 2006). Festinger (1957) was the first to introduce the theory of social comparison. He proposed innovative elements of social comparison theory that included nine hypotheses to outline his theory, eight of which appear to apply to ethical motivation. One hypothesis is, "There exists, in the human organism, a drive to evaluate his opinions and his abilities" (Festinger, 1957, p. 117). This first hypothesis fits with Kagan's view of ethical motivation and suggests that there is an innate motivation to evaluate one's opinions (beliefs, values, and ethics). The evaluation may be anchored in comparison to others. In the case of counselors/therapists, the evaluation may be understood best through observation of and discussion with peers and supervisors. Also, professional codes provide a standard for evaluation. For example, the ACA's (1996) *ACA Code of Ethics;* Section A.5, Roles and Relationships With Clients; Subsection A.5.a, Current Clients, states, "Sexual or romantic counselor-client interactions or relationships with current clients, their romantic partners, or their family members are prohibited" (p. 5). A counselor may refer to the codes of ethics and compare his or her beliefs with the professional codes that have been developed by other counselors.

The second hypothesis that Festinger (1957) proposed in outlining social comparison theory stated, "To the extent that objective, non-social means are not available, people evaluate their opinions and abilities by comparison respectively with the opinions and abilities of others" (p. 118). This may seem to be in conflict with development of a principled view of ethics that is internal, but we view it as consistent and supplemental. A principled ethical ideology is important, but one should be careful not to conclude that he or she does not need to gather information from others in making ethical decisions. As has been noted earlier, consultation with peers and supervisors is an essential ingredient in developing a professional ethical identity but also can be used to critically evaluate one's set of ideas and beliefs so particular biases do not occur. Hearing other professional counselors' views on an ethical issue may serve as a motivation to explore further, change one's view, or strengthen the view. Ultimately the counselor/therapist must make an ethical decision that he or she feels comfortable with, maintaining consistency and avoiding cognitive dissonance—a decision that is founded on solid ethical thinking. Consultation and review of codes of ethics are not relevant in this hypothesis, because "non-social means" are indicated as not being available. Review of professional codes may result in inclusive evidence of which course of action the counselor/therapist may take, or it may not address the ethical dilemma at all.

Festinger's (1957) third hypothesis in explaining social comparison theory states, "The tendency to compare oneself with some other specific person decreases as the difference between his opinion or ability and one's own increases" (p. 120). This hypothesis may apply to ethical motivation through understanding whom to choose to compare oneself with when constructing a moral action. A good question here is, Whom do you choose as a mentor or model in seeking development of a professional ethical identity? In essence, this may be explained as seeking to identify an exemplary ethical counselor/therapist. What are his or her qualities, and how similar is he or she to you so you may develop into a professional ethical counselor? If you choose an ethical counselor who is distinctly different from yourself, you may not ever feel confident that you are ethical. You may feel unethical if the person is a counselor/therapist who has developed a sophisticated understanding of ethics that does not necessarily make sense to you (e.g., the person may be in a different stage of ethical development; Kohlberg, 1969). You may want to choose a mentor who is similar to you, who is possibly slightly more experienced, and who you (and others) perceive as an ethical counselor/therapist.

The fourth hypothesis defining the foundation of social comparison theory states, "There is a unidirectional drive upward in the case of abilities which is largely absent in opinions" (Festinger, 1957, p. 124). This hypothesis suggests that humans have a tendency to seek upward comparisons. Counselors/therapists may understand this hypothesis in terms of self-actualization; we seek to realize our potential and grow in a positive way. Ideally a counselor/therapist will seek to improve and choose a comparison that results in a higher level of professional ethical identity and ethical behavior. Concretely this means being motivated to seek a mentor who holds a slightly stronger professional ethical identity that can be used by the counselor/therapist to gage his or her own professional ethical identity. Discussions with supervisors and peers with a little more counseling/ therapy experience may be desirable. Such discussions should be viewed as opportunities to explore advancing one's professional ethical identity while maintaining the core principled ideology that has been developed (Schlenker, 2008). The actual process may involve discussions with and observations of the peer or supervisor to compare one's own views and choices of ethical actions. This process can lead to further development of a professional ethical identity.

A fifth hypothesis, according to Festinger (1957), states, "There are non-social restraints which make it difficult or even impossible to change one's ability. These non-social restraints are largely absent for opinions" (p. 125). This hypothesis may be applied to professional ethical identity through the particular stage of ethical or moral development of the counselor/therapist. If a counselor/therapist is in a particular stage of moral development, for example, Stage 4 (authority and social-order-maintaining orientation or a law-and-order level of morality), then ethical decisions that require a more abstract perspective, for example, Stage 6 (based on universal ethical principles or principled conscience), may not be possible. Motivation to act may be based in part on the stage of moral development. A counselor/therapist who does not understand a particular ethical reasoning is less likely to take any action. Concrete examples are when no professional codes of ethics can be applied to an ethical dilemma and when there are conflicting options and the counselor/therapist must consider ethical theories that require abstract interpretations. The problem with this particular issue is that if one cannot see higher levels of moral thinking, then he or she may not be aware of the abstract options that may resolve the dilemma.

Hypothesis 6 states, "The cessation of comparison with others is accompanied by hostility or derogation to the extent that continued comparison with those persons implies unpleasant consequence" (Festinger, 1957, p. 129). This hypothesis based on social comparison theory may be understood in counseling ethics as the counselor's/therapist's being exposed to a supervisor who presents a distinctly different perspective. It even may be categorized as the counselor's/therapist's being accused of being unethical by another counselor. The comparison that is being made places the counselor/therapist in a negative professional ethical identity and may challenge his or her identity. This experience also may be explained through cognitive dissonance theory and require confronting the counselor/therapist about his or her ethical behavior, which may be in conflict with the professional ethical identity. A counselor is likely influenced to reduce the dissonance, which acts as a motivation. Such information may be important for the counselor/therapist to consider in reflecting on choices and courses of ethical behavior. This does not mean that the person making the accusation is correct; it may be the feedback is based on personal reactions and is not an accurate assessment. However, it may be a reflection of an ethical problem and should be considered.

Hypothesis 7 is presented as, "Any factors which increase the importance of some particular group as a comparison group for some particular opinion or ability will increase the pressure toward uniformity concerning the ability or opinion within that group" (Festinger, 1957, p. 130). This hypothesis can be applied to specific disciplines in the helping professions such as counseling, social work, and clinical psychology. All of these professions have developed their own professional codes of ethics. Counselors adhering to the profession of counseling may be motivated to act based on codes of ethics due to a need to support and value the individual discipline. In addition to counseling (ACA), the specific counseling disciplines include school counseling (American School Counseling Association [ASCA]), mental health counseling (American Mental Health Counselors Association), rehabilitation counseling (Commission on Rehabilitation Counselor Certification), family therapy (American Association for Marriage and Family Therapy [AAMFT]), and career counseling (National Career Development Association). The codes of ethics within different counseling disciplines share similarities and differences. One of the issues that national accreditation organizations promote is the uniqueness of the discipline. For example, recently the accrediting body for counseling programs, the Council for Accreditation of Counseling and Related Educational Programs, included within its codes a requirement that future faculty in such programs must be graduates of Council for Accreditation of Counseling and Related Educational Programs programs. We can interpret this as fitting Festinger's (1957) seventh hypothesis and an effort to increase uniformity within the group. The intention is to develop a professional identity that is consistent with the discipline, and theoretically this includes a professional ethical identity. Students and practitioners in each discipline within counseling typically use the specific codes of ethics within each discipline. In practice, counselors/therapists want to use codes that are applicable to their disciplines because there are unique characteristics of ethical issues with each discipline. For example, in family therapy, the family is the client, not any particular individual. The limits of confidentiality may be slightly different. For example, the AAMFT codes state, "Marriage and family therapists have unique confidentiality concerns because the client in a therapeutic relationship may be more than one person. Therapists respect and guard the confidences of each individual client" (AAMFT, 2001). Counselors/therapists need to consider which professional code to use and most likely will use the specific discipline or the general code from ACA.

EMPATHY AS ETHICAL MOTIVATION

The idea of empathy as a motivation to behave ethically may be found in humans' capacity to comprehend and understand the emotions and feelings of others. Several definitions of empathy have been proposed (Ang & Goh, 2010; Besel & Yuille, 2010; Egan, 2009). Empathy is characterized as both a cognitive and an affective process. Affectively, empathy involves the sharing of emotions and feelings of others (Ang & Goh, 2010). Cognitively, empathy involves understanding the emotions of others. Both involve an ability to understand others through the empathic process. Humans have different levels of as well as abilities to have empathy for others (Besel & Yuille, 2010). It has been suggested that empathy involves taking the role or perspective of another (Day, Casey, & Gerace, 2010). This capacity to empathize with others seems to be a characteristic of most humans and typically can be seen developing in young children (Hoffman, 1975).

Staub (2005) suggested that motivations to help others originate from feelings related to empathy. He identified several motivations for helping others. These motivations include seeking approval from others for helping, avoiding punishment for not helping, expecting a benefit or reciprocal benefit, having an altruistic motivation or desire to reduce another's discomfort, and holding values that promote the welfare of others. Of these different sources of motivation to help others, altruistic motivation is closely associated with empathy. Staub linked altruistic motivation and empathy, stating,

> Altruistic motivation is likely to have at least two related but not identical roots. One is affective: empathy, or the vicarious experience of others' feelings. The kind of empathy that generates sympathy has been found especially important in motivating helpful action. (pp. 35–36)

There seems to be a strong connection between empathy and the motivation to help others and behave prosocially, an ethical principle.

Narvaez and Vaydich (2008) noted that an "Ethic of Engagement" involved emotional affiliation with others or an ethic of caring based on relationships. This type of engagement may be seen as empathy. Goetz, Keltner, and Simon-Thomas (2010) discussed how compassion or elements of empathy are evolutionary and have a biological basis of development. They defined compassion as "the feeling that arises in witnessing another's suffering and that motivates a subsequent desire to help" (p. 351). This definition of compassion fits with a definition of empathy, providing motivation to help on an ethical basis. Hoffman (2000) defined empathy as "the cognitive awareness of another person's internal states, that is, his thoughts, feelings, perceptions, and intentions" (p. 29). Humans seem to have the capacity to understand others' experiences, which frequently, although not always, motivates them to act. Empathy potentially involves one or more emotions. For example, one person may express anger and fear, and so the receiver of the information may feel empathy through understanding the fear and anger (Brener, 2008).

The act of empathizing with others appears to have a genetic and evolutionary link. Brener (2008) reviewed relevant evolutionary information addressing empathy. He cited, for example, the finding that humans and animals appear to have an empathy and social gene. Many species warn others of approaching danger. Brener, in describing the evolution of empathy, stated, "Without doubt individuals of many cultures today are far more humanistic, more empathetic, and more adept at communicating with and understanding others than are those cultures of earlier times" (p. 22). He concluded that the primary reason for changes in a humanistic orientation over the centuries is an increase in the development of empathy.

Goetz et al. (2010) discussed the evolutionary development of compassion. Compassion has been associated with empathy (Oveis, Horberg, & Keltner, 2010) and is linked to the ethical behavior of helping others. Goetz et al. concluded that the evolutionary development of compassion and subsequently empathy is associated with seeing suffering and seeking to alleviate the suffering. Observation of suffering leads to a motivation to act, ethically, and assist the person who is in distress. Researchers have identified the biochemical nature of empathy through neuroimaging (Decety, Michalska, & Akitsuki, 2008). Specifically, investigators have studied the similarity of brain processing in the experience of pain and the secondhand observation of pain. Decety et al. (2008) concluded that there have been consistent findings that secondhand observation of pain and empathy elicit activation of areas of the brain associated with affective and emotional arousal. How often have you come to a ridge while driving and seen another driver flash his or her headlights, warning you that a police officer is on the other side checking speeds. What motivates the person to share that information? Is it empathy and a desire to help? This may be an example of drivers' valuing the freedom to drive faster than the speed limit and violate the law. Another, law-abiding, example is the establishment of a neighborhood watch. Neighbors agree to watch and report any potential criminal activity to protect the community. This may be an example of empathy and humans' social nature, leading them to help others.

Hoffman (2000) suggested that empathy may be understood in terms of broader ethical principles such as caring (beneficence) and justice. Humans, in general, do value caring and helping others. There are many media stories citing how someone went beyond his or her moral duty to help another, such as a motorist who stops to help another motorist whose car is on fire, saving him or her. These are valued and celebrated events. Fairness and equal opportunities are important principles on which the United States was founded. Observing injustice appears to initiate empathic feelings. The U.S. Declaration of Independence states, "We hold these truths to be self-evident, that all men are created equal." The United States was founded in part on a belief in the importance of fairness, justice, and equality. Humans appear to have an empathic understanding of what is fair and just. Just talk to an adolescent who announces loudly, "That is not fair." Humans do seem to evaluate what is fair and just rather easily. Through empathy one can realize what may be unjust and unfair. Such empathy can be a signal or an awareness that a situation is unethical and is a motivation for a counselor to act ethically.

How does empathy affect counselors' motivation to act ethically? Some examples may help to further explain the use of empathy to monitor how motivation affects ethics. You most assuredly will discuss with clients circumstances that suggest child abuse (at least to you). You will likely use empathy to understand the child's perspective, but what about understanding the adult's perspective? Will your empathic understanding of the adult's reaction that led to what you might consider child abuse affect your ethical decision (the situation is not a cruel incident of child abuse)? Another, more severe example is the ability of a counselor to empathize with a murderer or a child abuser. The use of empathy, as hard as it may be, may help one avoid acting unethically in working with such an individual. For example, an attempt at empathic understanding (not accepting the illegal act) of a murderer or child abuser may preclude a counselor's acting unethically by showing disdain or transferring the client because of personal feelings. Empathy may interact with other ethical motivations such as centrality of values and beliefs. For example, priests' sexually abusing children may show that these priests lacked empathy with their victims. These priests likely held strong central values and beliefs, but something was missing, potentially empathy. Lacking empathy for victims allows the perpetrator to hurt others and depersonalize his or her actions, despite the perpetrator's holding central ethical beliefs. Another example may be found in war. Soldiers do not want to have empathy for the victims but simultaneously may hold strong central ethical beliefs.

The capacity for empathy is important; in addition, empathy is an important professional skill for the counselor to use in the counseling process (A. Clark, 2010; Egan, 2009; Ottens, Shank, & Long, 1995). This is not a profound statement, but it is important to understand that there are differences in how empathy skills develop. As with other types of development we have discussed, which demonstrate the complexity of ethical choices for the counselor, empathy involves different skill levels (Allen et al., 1995; Erdynast & Rapgay, 2009). Erdynast and Rapgay (2009) investigated how compassion, a component of empathy, related to ethical decisions involving different complexities of dilemmas. They found that more complex dilemmas were associated with higher levels of reasoning and more complex compassion responses. They suggested that the ability to understand more complex ethical dilemmas with higher stages of ethical reasoning (Kohlberg, 1969) was consistent with higher levels of complexity of compassion. Lafferty, Beutler, and Crago (1989) found that therapists who had lower levels of empathy were less effective. Allen et al. (1995) suggested that novice counselors/therapists were focused on conducting counseling the "right way" and consequently missed important deeper meanings. They stated,

> Compared with experienced counselors, novices may have difficulty deciding what use to make of incoming information (clues) about the client. Novices may lack the ability to judiciously select and process this information, manipulate it into patterns, focus on different case information, and apprehend different or more subtle problem features. (p. 200)

The focus of novice counselors/therapists is on using a linear model that does not allow for processing a multitude of information that potentially enhances advanced or complex empathy. Allen et al. proposed that novice counselors/therapists and those in training receive instruction in identifying relevant clues addressing ethical issues, practicing developing hypotheses about cases, developing and practicing nonlinear approaches to thinking (we will discuss the nonlinear hermeneutic model in Chapter 4), and developing skills in discovering hidden client meanings or deeper meaning issues (going beyond basic ethical issues presented). Clearly there is a benefit to developing advanced empathy skills to use in both the practice of counseling and being motivated to act ethically. Fully understanding issues through empathy helps the counselor/therapist identify relevant ethical issues and act on resolving them.

SUMMARY

The possible sources of motivation to behave ethically include centrality of ethical beliefs and congruency, comparison with others and professional standards, and empathy and social responsibility. Motivations for ethical behavior are complex and may involve one or more of these sources in practice. Also, the source of motivation may vary from situation to situation for each individual, and motivation may originate from several sources. Awareness of these possible motivations influencing ethical action may provide the counselor/therapist with knowledge of and sensitivity to an ethical issue. In addition, a counselor/therapist experiencing incongruence between professional ethical identity and experience may interpret the situation as needing attention to address potential ethical issues. Having the ability to empathize with others likely will improve the ethical behavior of the counselor and his or her understanding/prediction of the effects of a choice of action. Not considering the effects of ethical choices on others, through empathy, may result in unethical actions. An awareness of and sensitivity to ethical issues is a beginning step to acting ethically, but in addition one needs to be motivated to act ethically, and there are several sources that can contribute to developing this motivation.

CASE COUNSELOR AND ETHICS MOTIVATION

Anna is a student in a master's program in school counseling. She is in the second semester of her internship. Anna is of Mexican descent, a first-generation American. Her internship is in a high school in a suburban community, an upper-middle-class community. The community is primarily Caucasian, with an approximately 12% minority population. Anna has developed a good relationship with several 10th-grade girls who are in the top 10% of their class, academically. They all take advanced placement courses and rely on each other for support. They see Anna in a group on a weekly basis for career counseling. They want to enter more nontraditional science professions, and Anna thought it would be helpful to explore their options together in a group. The students meet with Anna during lunchtime in the school counseling office. Anna's supervisor is a Caucasian man, Robert, who has more than 10 years' experience in school counseling. He strictly adheres to school policies and consults ASCA codes of ethics when ethical situations arise. The school administration is very careful to follow local, state, and federal laws. The administration has demonstrated and communicated to staff the importance of informing parents of any problems or concerns with the children/adolescents.

Anna has held approximately 10 group sessions, and the students have begun describing cyberbullying actions they have engaged in against several other female students who are popular and are cheerleaders. The girls seem to enjoy attacking the other girls. Anna is troubled by the disclosure, and her initial reactions appear as intuitions about or gut reactions to the information. She saw teasing when she was younger, and she recognizes the cues that suggest unethical behavior. The cues for her from the environment are that these girls laugh at their activities and share reflections about how their efforts seem to hurt the feelings of the other girls. Anna experiences several gut reactions, including disgust and anger, directed at these students with whom she feels she has connected.

Anna is able to empathize with those who are being cyberbullied. She does not feel she understands the motivations and actions of the girls in her group, and she has difficulty empathizing with them on this particular issue. She is able to infer how the girls who are being cyberbullied feel based on the comments of the students in her group. They have described, with some glee, the anger and frustration of the girls they are bullying. Consequently, Anna is able to empathize with the bullied students, and this affects her and gives her a sense of need to act.

During her academic training, Anna had opportunities to identify ethical principles that were most important and central to her professional beliefs. Most important to her were the ethical principles of beneficence and autonomy. Beneficence concerns looking out for the welfare of others and acting in ways that promote the welfare of others. *Autonomy* may be defined as a right to self-determination and the freedom to choose a course of action. While Anna was growing up, her parents encouraged her to make personal choices and take responsibility for herself. She has transferred these beliefs to her work with clients. Her parents also encouraged her to assist others and promote the welfare of others. Despite her personal development and the influence of her parents, she has given thought to these values and believes they fit well with her professional ethical identity as a counselor/therapist. Reflecting on these values with the new information from the adolescent girls in her lunch group leads her to reason that she wants to encourage their autonomy and taking responsibility. However, she does not believe that they are being responsible. One aspect of being autonomous is the ability to make autonomous decisions; an adolescent is seen by society as not being fully developed and able to make independent choices, for example, parents have ultimate control over decisions for those younger than 18. Second, Anna is concerned about the welfare of the adolescents in her group but also about the adolescents they are cyberbullying. She does not believe the principles of either autonomy or beneficence are being fulfilled in this particular situation. Anna's decision to consider reporting the cyberbullying is motivation to act, focused on her cognitions of incongruency between her professional ethical identity and her actions. Anna sees herself as an ethical professional counselor/therapist who values clients' welfare and their autonomy. She feels anxious about not acting on what she learned in group because it would suggest she is not behaving ethically.

The third potential source of ethical motivation, social comparison, leads Anna to review the professional code of ethics of the ASCA. She finds several standards that may apply to the situation in her group. One standard that may apply concerns the primary obligation to the student or students in her case: Section A.1, Responsibilities to Students; Subsection a, Has primary obligation to the student who is treated with respect as a unique individual. Another standard that may apply addresses confidentiality: Section A.2, Confidentiality; Subsection b, Keeps information confidential unless disclosure is required to prevent clear and imminent danger to the student or others. Additional standards may concern confidentiality in groups, which notes the limitations of confidentiality in groups and danger to self or others. Anna attempts to compare her values and beliefs to the ASCA professional codes. In addition, she decides to consult a colleague who expresses concern that Anna should intervene, break confidentiality, and inform the students' parents. Her supervisor, as was noted earlier, adheres carefully to professional codes and school policies. Anna has strong motivations to act based on these sources.

Case Analysis and Reflection

Reflect on your personal and professional identity development, and consider how you would act in Anna's situation. Is your development different from or similar to Anna's? What impact do you think both your and Anna's development has on ethical choices?

Questions for Further Reflection

1. Reflect on cognitive dissonance you experienced around an ethical issue. Discuss with other students the dissonance and how it affected you and your actions.

2. Identify central values and beliefs you hold that may affect your counseling practice and your ethical decisions.

3. Recall situations that elicited strong intuitions or gut reactions such as disgust or anger. Discuss with other students whether your gut reactions provided insight into ethical issues and what were the outcomes.

4. Reflect on any situations wherein feelings of empathy were connected to ethical dilemmas and what you did based on your empathic understanding.

5. Discuss whether the four potential motivations identified here are adequate or there are other ethical motivations that influence action.

6. Identify a colleague who does not share your view of a particular ethical situation. Discuss the issue with him or her, and attempt to see his or her point of view.

7. Review a day in your life, and attempt to identify potential ethical issues. How significant are these issues, and do they reach a level of importance that warrants an ethical decision?

Additional Recommended Readings

Bebeau, M. (2002). The Defining Issues Test and the four component model: Contributions to professional education. *Journal of Moral Education, 31*(3), 271–295.

Bebeau, M., & Brabeck, M. (1994). Ethical sensitivity and moral reasoning among men and women in the professions. In B. Puka (Ed.), *Caring voices and women's moral frames: Gilligan's view* (pp. 240–259). New York, NY: Garland.

Brener, M. (2008). *Evolution and empathy.* Jefferson, NC: McFarland.

Chang, F. (1994). School teachers' moral reasoning. In J. Rest & D. Narvaez (Eds.), *Moral development in the professions: Psychology and applied ethics* (pp. 51–70). Hillsdale, NJ: Lawrence Erlbaum.

Decety, J., Michalska, K., & Akitsuki, Y. (2008). Who caused the pain? An fMRI investigation of empathy and intentionality in children. *Neuropsychologia, 46,* 2607–2614.

Haidt, J. (2001). The emotional dog and its rational tail: A social intuitionist approach to moral judgment. *Psychological Review, 108*(4), 814–834.

Hoffman, M. (1975). Developmental synthesis of affect and cognition and its implications for altruistic motivation. *Developmental Psychology, 11,* 607–622.

Hoffman, M. (2000). *Empathy and moral development.* Cambridge, UK: Cambridge University Press.

Kahneman, D., & Klein, G. (2009). Conditions for intuitive expertise. *American Psychologist, 64*(6), 515–526.

Koenigs, M., Young, L., Adolphs, R., Tranel, D., Cushman, F., Hauser, M., & Damasio, A. (2007). Damage to the prefrontal cortex increases utilitarian moral judgments. *Nature, 446*(7138), 908–911.

Oveis, C., Horberg, E., & Keltner, D. (2010). Compassion, pride, and social intuitions of self-other similarity. *Journal of Personality and Social Psychology, 98*(4), 618–630.

Rest, J. (1984). Research on moral development: Implications for training psychologists. *The Counseling Psychologist, 12,* 19–29.

Staub, E. (2005). The roots of goodness: The fulfillment of basic human needs and the development of caring, helping and nonaggression, inclusive caring, moral courage, active bystandership, and altruism born of suffering. In R. Dienstbier (Series Ed.), G. Carlo, & C. Edwards (Vol. Eds.), *Nebraska Symposium on Motivation: Vol. 51. Moral motivation through the life span: Theory, research, applications* (pp. 22–72). Lincoln: University of Nebraska Press.

Chapter 4

COGNITIONS AND REASONING/HERMENEUTICS

MORAL JUDGMENT

CHAPTER OBJECTIVES

- Acquire an understanding of the history of ethical reasoning
- Acquire an understanding of moral development and ethical development
- Develop an understanding of one's own moral development level and how it relates to ethical decision making
- Acquire an understanding of hermeneutic reasoning and how it can be used in ethical decision making
- Identity the relevant elements of the horizon based on a hermeneutic model of ethical decision making
- Learn how to apply the hermeneutic model of ethical decision making to counseling cases

Case

Jonathan is a counselor who lives in a rural community and has been working in a community agency for 5 years. Recently the agency signed a contract with the court to evaluate clients, including those accused of homicides. Some of these court-referred clients may be charged with crimes that could result in the death penalty. Jonathan realized during his graduate training, while taking an ethics course, that his professional ethical identity had developed, which included the perspective that he did not believe in killing. He recalled the development of his professional ethical identity and his personal development during the ethics course. He grew up hunting and fishing, which involved killing living things. At a point during young adulthood he stopped hunting and fishing because his own personal values and spiritual perspectives changed and he did not believe it was right to kill living things. Jonathan realizes his experiences influenced his own professional ethical development. He does not believe in capital punishment, and the current change in agency contacts poses a dilemma for Jonathan. He may be involved in evaluating these court-referred clients, but he does not want to support this activity by working in this agency. Jonathan has decided to leave the agency and start his own private practice.

He has had a goal of having a private practice since he entered his master's program more than 8 years ago. He feels he is knowledgeable, and he received his state license more than 2 years ago. The community in which he lives has only about 5,000 residents within a 30-mile range, and the pool of possible clients is limited, so he has decided to offer web-based counseling in addition to his office counseling services. Jonathan discussed setting up his online therapy with a colleague, Deborah, who lives in the same community, and the two have developed an online practice.

Jonathan decides to advertise online to recruit clients, and he has been contacted by Charini, a woman who grew up in India and is in her mid-40s. Charini has a background in software development, and she feels very comfortable communicating in an online format. She wants to pursue online therapy. Charini lives in an urban area in another state more than 2 hours away, so office visits are not acceptable to her. She is busy and does not feel seeing a local counselor in her city is acceptable. Charini states that she lost her son through death approximately 6 months ago. She reports feeling anxious and sad and crying frequently. The son was her only child, and he died in an automobile accident. Charini has been married for 25 years to Ashoka. Both Charini and Ashoka grew up in India and came to the United States to study software engineering; they remained after completing their education.

Jonathan and Charini initially speak by phone and agree to online therapy with a primary approach of using asynchronous e-mails. They begin online therapy and are in regular contact. Initially Charini reports benefiting from the therapy. She feels Jonathan understands her, she feels safe disclosing online, and she is able to be honest with her feelings. The therapy goes on for 3 months. Then abruptly Charini stops her e-mails, and Jonathan does not hear from Charini for a week. He attempts to contact Charini by phone but is unsuccessful. Finally Jonathan reaches her husband Ashoka, who informs Jonathan that Charini has been hospitalized for a suicide attempt. Jonathan is upset by the news, and he begins to reflect on his role in Charini's suicide attempt and whether he behaved in any way that contributed to the situation. Was he ethically at fault for his actions as a professional counselor?

Source: Adapted from Houser, Wilczenski, and Ham (2006). Reprinted with permission.

ETHICAL REASONING THEORY: HISTORY AND DEVELOPMENT

There are many theoretical approaches that help us understand how individuals come to understand and reason about ethical issues (Killen & Smetana, 2006; Rest, 1983). This focus is due in large part to the traditional view common in both philosophy and psychology that how one reasons about ethical issues is central to moral functioning (Rest & Narvaez, 1994). In this view, although one may be swayed by emotions, or influenced by competing claims on one's actions, one's conscious attempts to make sense of an ethical event are what make his or her resulting behavior moral. Without a cognitive focus, our actions are reactive, and although the result of these actions may have a moral result, they may be difficult to justify or communicate to others. Indeed, professionals are typically trained to focus on the quality of reasoning they bring to bear on moral situations because high-quality moral reasoning strategies are viewed as central to the competent professional (Bebeau, 2009).

What constitutes high-quality reasoning and where individuals learn these skills has been a central question within psychology for more than 50 years. Up until the late 1950s the prevailing view was that individuals learned about moral phenomena and how one responds through the socialization process. In this view, experience coupled with direct training is the mechanism by which we learn to adopt the dominant social views about what constitutes moral situations, how one should talk about them, and how one should respond. Given that the social norms might be different in various locations and subgroups within the population, this perspective suggested that ethical understandings and responses might vary from group to group and from culture to culture. At core, however, was the view that individuals are socialized to conform to the prevailing views of social and moral phenomena.

Beginning in the late 1950s this view was challenged by psychologists who claimed that the individual not simply was a passive recipient of moral knowledge but actively engaged the social world to develop a working understanding of ethical issues. Following Piaget (1932), Kohlberg (1969) championed a view that the individual engaged the social world in a very organized way that followed a developmental path. His famous six-stage model became the most influential perspective on how moral understanding was both cognitive and developmental.

At core, Kohlberg (1969) argued that with general social development, individuals form an understanding of cooperation. For children, cooperation is viewed in terms of avoiding punishment and later coordinating one's needs with those of others. An adolescent's cooperation focuses on maintaining positive regard with other people and groups. Later in youth and beyond, cooperation is understood in terms of social norms, laws, and religious prescriptions. These conventions are viewed as organizing cooperation at the societal level and must be adhered to to maintain social functioning. Finally, for some, cooperation is defined as the application of underlying foundational principles. Thus, to Kohlberg and his followers, moral understanding not simply is a steady accumulation of moral words and appropriate behaviors but includes a hierarchy of qualitatively different moral conceptions that represent how the individual views moral phenomena.

A second assumption embedded within the developmental model assumed by Kohlberg and his colleagues is the view that a sense of fairness is associated with each of the conceptions of cooperation. Thus, a child who is punished even though she didn't break a rule feels an injustice. Similarly, the individual who follows his part of the bargain but is denied the expected reward feels the situation is unfair. The adolescent who considers his friends' interests will feel it is wrong if his friends fail to do the same. So also the adult who follows the rules but sees others fail to do so will claim it is not fair. Finally, when the individual sees that the principle is not illuminated in practice, she will claim that the system is unfair. That is, the notion of fairness is part of the individual's understanding of cooperation and changes as the individual expands his or her notion of what defines cooperation.

Finally, the developmental model assumes that these conceptions of cooperation are interpretive structures that reside in our memory and are evoked when we recognize the situation as moral. These structures are helpful to us because they provide a system that allows us to problem solve by defining the important features of the situation: who has a stake in the situation and whose position ought to be considered and at what weight (see Rest, 1983, for a full discussion of these criteria).

The Kohlberg (1984b) model (see Chapter 2 for descriptions of developmental stages) in its various iterations became the dominant view in the field and is still influential today. The Kohlberg model was particularly important for professional ethics education in that it framed many of the objectives of these initiatives and also the methodology used to assess ethical development. However, the singular focus on reasoning generally and Kohlberg's stages in particular has declined during the past 20 years. One reason for this decline is captured by the four-component model (Rest, 1983) described earlier. As this model makes clear, research in moral psychology indicates that there is much more to ethical action than judgments of cooperation. Thus, professional ethics education needs to expand its focus and include instruction on moral sensitivity, moral motivation, and moral implementation, discussed in Chapter 3.

The focus on the quality of reasoning professionals use to attend to ethical issues remains a central feature of ethics education and theoretical concerns.

However, How best to capture ethical reasoning? is a more difficult question. Current trends suggest a broadening of the different perspectives, an openness to new perspectives. One relatively new approach is hermeneutics, which attends to the socialization process in helping to define the individual's current status within society and cognitive systems that help the individual understand and interpret moral phenomena.

HERMENEUTICS AND REASONING

There are several perspectives and theories of cognitions and reasoning with respect to ethics (Follesdal, 2001; Gadamer, 1975; Houser et al., 2006). One theory that seems especially suited for ethics and reasoning is a hermeneutic perspective. Follesdal (2001) described hermeneutics as "the study of interpretations" (p. 375). The term *hermeneutics* originates from the Greek word *hermeneno,* which means to interpret. The term was initially introduced in 1654 (Follesdal, 2001). Martin and Thompson (2003) described hermeneutics as "the art of interpretation" (p. 2). This art of interpretation is founded on a systematic approach that is nonlinear. It is a dynamic, evolving approach. Martin and Thompson observed that "human life involves a constant flow of interpretation and reinterpretation" (p. 2). Originally hermeneutics focused on interpreting text, but more recently it has been expanded to include understanding and interpretation of human behavior (Betan, 1997; Dilthey, 1978; Martin & Thompson, 2003). Several have proposed that hermeneutics is applicable to the counseling process (Chessick, 1990; Houser et al., 2006; Zeddies, 2002). A hermeneutic perspective requires a careful interpretation of all of the elements affecting an ethical dilemma, understanding the whole and its parts (Chessick, 1990). This dynamic interpretation consists of a circular process, including interaction between the whole and its parts. Chessick (1990) proposed the circular hermeneutic process as follows:

> Beginning with a preliminary notion of the whole, one then moves to an ever-more probing analysis and synthesis of the parts which in turn leads to an evolving ever-changing concept of the whole. This affords an increasingly internalized and thought-through understanding of the whole. (p. 257)

Follesdal (2001) explained the hermeneutic process as dynamic and stated,

> We revise our anticipation of what is expressed in the text, until we find an interpretation that seems to us to be true or at least reasonable. That is, we adjust our opinions until we find that we can agree with the text. (p. 377)

What this means is that humans seek to develop an understanding of texts or situations (hermeneutics may be applied beyond texts to human conditions or interactions) through continued redefinition and understanding until a reasonable picture or conclusion is reached. Key in the hermeneutic process is an analysis of the component parts and how they interact to form an understanding and picture of what is being interpreted or understood. As Chessick (1990) noted, a thought-through or reasoned approach is important in the hermeneutic process. Development of a reasoned view through hermeneutics is achieved in part with a beginning level of openness and awareness of what Follesdal (2001) called a "fore-meaning." He suggested that humans enter into an interpretation with preconceived or fore meanings that influence interpretations. It is essential (and is a condition of the counseling process) to enter into an interpretation, an ethical dilemma, with an open mind and an awareness of one's own preconceived and/or potentially biased views.

The criterion of understanding has been termed a "fusion of horizons" (Follesdal, 2001). Hathaway (2002) defined a horizon as "the range of possible meanings available to a person at their moment and place in history. It is composed of the dispositions the person brings to the present by virtue of their place in tradition(s) or culture" (p. 207). Horizons and fusions of horizons are essential concepts in hermeneutic theory. Fusion of horizons is the integration of multiple horizons. For example, if a counselor and a client identify a counseling goal, the understanding of what is needed to reach the goal may result in a fusion of horizons. The client and counselor enter the counseling relationship with preunderstandings based on their own histories, cultures, and traditions. Through interaction, they both change their original understandings of goal definition to a "fused" understanding. Another way to view this is the client and counselor seeing from a similar horizon (from the same point of view), a fused horizon, and focusing on similar aspects of the goal. Both the client and the counselor go beyond their own personal conceptions of the goal and develop a new revised view. Changing preunderstandings may be achieved through exposure to different sources of information, for example, each other's perspective. Also, because hermeneutics is circular, there may be dynamic change with the interaction of the preunderstandings, even ones that have been changed at one point by exposure to other horizons or information in a horizon. Gadamer (1984) proposed that preunderstandings may be altered through exposure to the horizon of a text or context. Chessick (1990) identified the development of the horizon and stated, "Meaning and understanding are subject to time and change. . . . We always survey the past from within our own horizon, a horizon which is always shifting" (p. 257). Important parts of the hermeneutic process are the meaning and interpretation, which are dynamic and change through interaction between parts and the whole. The moment in time and the context may alter the meaning of the situation. Chessick suggested that a horizon "involves the customs, institutions, and language of a given culture" (p. 259).

HERMENEUTIC MODEL OF ETHICAL DECISION MAKING/REASONING

Houser et al. (2006) identified a number of elements that constitute the horizon in counseling ethics based on a hermeneutics model. Figure 4.1 depicts the hermeneutic circle including the potential horizons in counseling ethics. Based on this model, the ethical dilemma is always located at the center, with component parts interacting dynamically with the dilemma. It is important to keep in mind that hermeneutics and the interaction between component parts and the whole affect each other in a continuous dynamic manner. In addition, the whole is the total horizon for a specific ethical dilemma. In the Houser et al. model, the interaction is between parts, for example, professional codes of ethics, and the ethical dilemma as well as the whole. The elements on the outer part of the circle influence the ethical dilemma, but the parts also influence each other. Houser et al. suggested that the hermeneutic model of ethical decision making is best represented by a sphere, a three-dimensional figure with the various components shown interacting simultaneously and influencing each other, as in Figure 4.1. For example, interpretation of professional codes is influenced by the professional ethical identity of the counselor, which may be influenced by the personal characteristics of the supervisor. The counselor may value autonomy as part of his or her professional identity, and how the counselor presents a dilemma to his or her supervisor will be influenced by what he or she hypothesizes about how the supervisor will respond. Another important consideration, the interpretation of the meaning of an ethical dilemma, is generally based on the time or historical context. There are several examples of the impact of the historical context. One example is the identification of child abuse. A second is posttraumatic stress disorder, and a third is an eating disorder. Fifty years ago all of these examples did not exist as problems as they currently do.

64è.
See pg. 82

HERMENEUTIC MODEL OF ETHICAL DECISION MAKING/REASONING IN COUNSELING

Houser et al. (2006) suggested that the horizon of ethical decision making, the whole, includes the following parts: an ethical dilemma in counseling, the

Figure 4.1 Hermeneutic Model of Counseling Ethical Decision Making/Reasoning

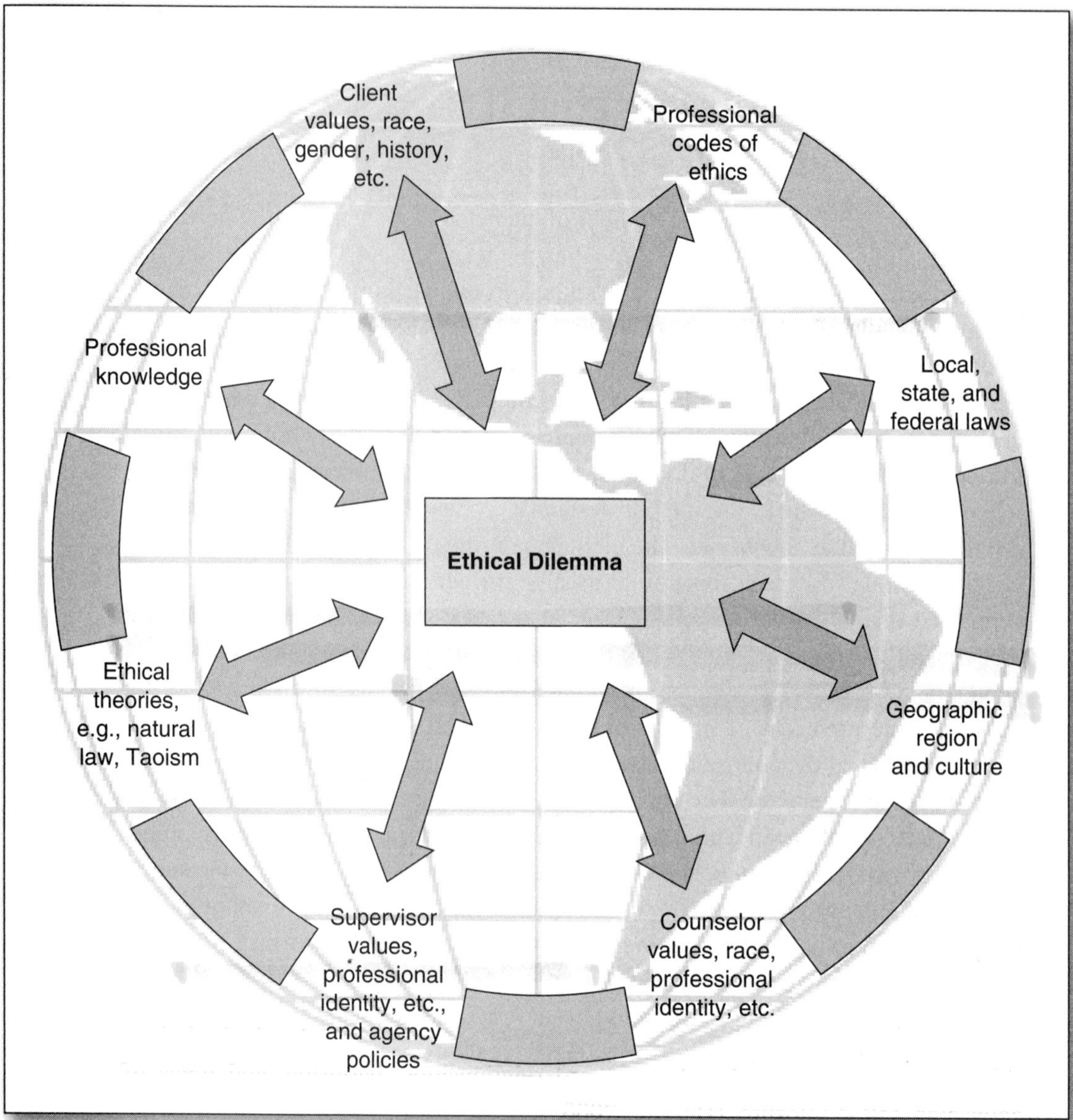

Client values, race, gender, history, etc.

Professional codes of ethics

Professional knowledge

Local, state, and federal laws

Ethical Dilemma

Ethical theories, e.g., natural law, Taoism

Geographic region and culture

Supervisor values, professional identity, etc., and agency policies

Counselor values, race, professional identity, etc.

Source: Adapted from Houser, Wilczenski, and Ham (2006).

counselor (his or her values, professional ethical identity, moral development level, race, gender, and personal history); the client (his or her values, race, gender, moral development level, and personal history); the supervisor (personal characteristics, professional ethical identity, moral development level, values, and agency policies); the geographic region and culture; local, state, and federal laws; professional codes of ethics; professional knowledge; and ethical theories (e.g., utilitarianism, Confucianism, or Latino ethics). We want to propose that ethical decision making/reasoning using a hermeneutic model can involve multiple ethical theories that may be relevant to consider primarily because we live in such a diverse society that requires an understanding of diverse views.

THE ETHICAL DILEMMA

According to Houser et al. (2006), the central part of the whole in the hermeneutic circle is the ethical dilemma itself. In their model, the ethical dilemma is shown as the innermost part of the reasoning process primarily because it is the focus of the decision making. Identifying the ethical dilemma is of significant importance (Corey, Corey, & Callanan, 2010; Welfel, 2009). Also, it is a significant step in ethical reasoning, according to Rest's (1983) four-component model. Several broad categories of ethical dilemmas may be identified. One source for identifying ethical dilemmas is complaints to state licensure boards, which can provide some insight into potential ethical dilemmas; however, it has been noted that not all ethical dilemmas come to the attention of such boards (Neukrug, Milliken, & Walden, 2001). In addition to those dilemmas culled from licensure board complaints, major ethical dilemmas that potentially confront practicing counselors have been identified by investigators (Bergeron & Gray, 2003; Merskey, 1996; Neukrug et al., 2001; Scott, 2000). Based on complaints to state licensure boards and information from professionals identifying ethical issues, a number of major ethical dilemmas can be addressed: boundaries, competence of the counselor, confidentiality, informed consent, multicultural competence, and professional demeanor.

Boundary Issues

There have been a number of boundary ethical issues that involve dual relationships: nonsexual, counselor-client sexual relationships, bartering, and types of counselor self-disclosure (Burien, 2000; Garrett, 2010; Lamb, Catanzaro, & Moorman, 2003). Burian proposed that dual social relationships can occur due to the loss of objectivity on the part of the counselor. Lamb and Catanzaro (1998) discovered that crossings of nonsexual boundaries were indicators to more serious problems such as sexual boundary violations. Somer (1999) proposed that boundary violations begin slowly and develop into more severe violations.

It has been found that the most frequent complaints made to state licensing boards are about violations involving dual, nonsexual relationships (Neukrug et al., 2001). An example of a dual relationship is counseling a friend, neighbor, or relative. Dual relationships also may involve receiving referrals from friends or coworkers who know the client and as a consequence may be aware of the counseling process. An example is a referral from a coworker who may have access to records. In circumstances in which a counselor has multiple roles with a client, there exists the possibility for an ethical dilemma of dual relationships. Rural areas have been found to have more possible problems because of smaller social networks, which result in dual relationships (Perkins, Hudson, Gray, & Stewart, 1998). Researchers have categorized dual relationships as ethical dilemmas and boundary issues (Corey et al., 2010; Okamoto, 2003).

Self-disclosure is another type of dual relationship involving boundary issues. An important question is, How much information should a counselor share with a client, and what types of self-disclosures might the counselor make (Kim, Hill, Gelso, Goates, Asay, & Harbin, 2003; Nyman & Daugherty, 2001)? Nyman and Daugherty (2001) pointed out that the professional literature suggests that a counselor's personal self-disclosure may be a burden to a client and possibly shift the focus away from client issues. For example, a counselor's discussing his or her own family history, issues, and problems with a client may be an ethical issue. This is particularly true if the talk time of the client is reduced by focusing on the counselor's issues. Shapiro and Ginsberg (2003) suggested that accepting referrals from current clients can create an ethical dilemma and can result in a boundary violation. The question that may arise is whether the counselor achieves personal financial gain and is almost using clients as sources of referrals. Another example of a boundary issue involves socializing with a client outside of the counseling session (Corey et al., 2010). This might involve attending the wedding of a client. Finally, the use of bartering with a client to exchange services for goods can result in a boundary problem. An example is exchanging counseling sessions for new tires if they happen to fit your car.

Counselor Competence

A second type of ethical dilemma in counseling is counselor competence. Graduate-level training and professional credentials are methods to increase the level of competence, but they do not guarantee effective practice of counseling techniques. Neukrug et al. (2001) found the second-most-common complaint to state licensure boards against counselors involved competence. An important question is, How do counselors develop and maintain counseling skills and competence? There are several important questions to address when considering counselor competence. One question is, What level of professional training is necessary to be effective? A related question is, What is competence, and what level of skill is necessary? McLeod (1992) stated there is "an expectation that counselors will possess qualifications and certificates which validate their capacity to practice effectively" (p. 359). Researchers have identified a relationship between counselor effectiveness and client satisfaction (Constantine, 2002; W. Jones & Markos, 1997). There may be questions about whether it is unethical for a counselor to read a book about an intervention such as hypnosis and then begin using the technique with clients without receiving any formal training. The counselor who reads about hypnosis does not have the expertise necessary to provide such a counseling service. A second important ethical issue around counselor competence concerns continued updating of the counselor's skills after completion of formal graduate training. A third major area of competence involves the use of assessments by the counselor. One of the ethical issues involving assessment includes the use of diagnostic tools such as the *Diagnostic and Statistical Manual of Mental Disorders*. An ethical problem with using the *Diagnostic and Statistical Manual* may involve making accurate diagnoses if one has adequate experience and holds appropriate qualifications.

Houser et al. (2006) suggested that another relevant question to address when considering counselor competence is, What level and type of continued training or updating is adequate to prepare the counselor for continued effective practice? State licensure and national certifications require continuing education for counselors to maintain licensure and certification. Do taking a course online and learning a new counseling technique qualify as the necessary level of competence?

Confidentiality

Another important ethical dilemma concerns confidentiality. Isaacs and Stone (2001) stated, "Confidentiality is one of the most critical aspects of any counseling relationship" (p. 342). Confidentiality involves maintaining privacy and not disclosing information to those outside the counseling relationship unless there is consent by the client. Clients enter into the counseling relationship with strong expectations that what is discussed will be maintained in confidence. Neukrug et al. (2001) found, in reviewing state licensure complaints, that violations of confidentiality were frequently reported against counselors to state licensing boards. Confidentiality is not absolute, and there are conditions under which counseling session information may be disclosed (Isaacs & Stone, 2001; Kermani & Drob, 1987). Clinical judgment is required to assess the possible ethical issues regarding confidentiality. Confidentiality may be broken in the treatment of minors, when there are indications of harm (harm to a client who is considering suicide or a client who is expressing thoughts of harming others), in the treatment of court-involved clients, when the mandated reporting of child abuse is appropriate, and in the treatment of clients with medical conditions such as HIV who may be determined to be engaging in dangerous acts related to their condition, for example, spreading contagious diseases. Confidentiality is viewed as an important issue, and federal legislation, the Health Insurance Portability and Accountability Act (HIPAA; U.S. Department of Health & Human Services, 2003), was passed to improve the confidentiality of patient records.

Autonomy

Autonomy is another important issue in ethical decision making for counselors (Houser et al., 2006). There are two elements that constitute autonomy: freedom to choose a course of action and competence to make an informed choice. Beauchamp and Childress (2001) proposed that informed consent is predicated on full disclosure of information. An informed choice can be made through voluntary choice of a course of action and with competence to understand the choices. Competence involves the capacity—intellectual and emotional—to make informed decisions and choices. An individual who is impaired cognitively may not be able to make an informed choice, and an individual with a significant mental illness may not be thinking clearly enough to make an informed choice. However, for a person to be determined not competent to make an informed choice, there needs to be a judicially determined decision. An example is someone who is severely depressed and who is expressing thoughts of suicide. The ethical dilemma may be whether to pursue hospitalization against the person's will to protect him or her. Autonomy may be taken away in this example if the client is hospitalized. A psychiatrist or physician makes such a determination about the person's competence to make informed decisions and legally has the person detained until an assessment can be completed.

The concept of empowerment has been associated with autonomy in counseling, and it has become more of a concern during the past 20 years (Banja, 1990; C. Clark & Krupa, 2002; Fawcett et al., 1994; Houser, Hampton, & Carriker, 2000; Ozer & Bandura, 1990). Fawcett et al. (1994) offered the following definition of empowerment: "the process of gaining some control over events, outcomes, and resources of importance to an individual or group" (p. 472). The empowerment concept is similar to the view of autonomy and ethical issues of autonomy in counseling.

Multicultural Competency

It has been suggested that multicultural competency is an ethical issue in counseling (Bellini, 2002; Constantine, 2002; Houser et al., 2006; Kim & Lyons,

2003), and multicultural competency has been differentiated from general counselor competence in importance (Constantine, 2002). *Multicultural competency* refers to the counselor's having the necessary awareness, knowledge, and skills to work with groups diverse in terms of race, disability, gender, and so forth (Constantine, 2002; Pedersen, 2007; Sue, Arredondo, & McDavis, 1992). Sue et al. (1992) proposed that multicultural competence includes three general dimensions: being aware of one's own values, biases, and preconceived beliefs about culturally diverse groups; actively trying to understand the worldview and experiences of culturally diverse group members; and developing counseling skills appropriate for culturally diverse clients. Sue et al. further proposed that not having these competencies is unethical: "A serious moral vacuum exists in the delivery of cross-cultural counseling and therapy services because the values of the dominant culture have been imposed on the culturally different consumer" (p. 68). There have been numerous efforts to define multicultural counseling competencies (Fuertes, 2001; Fuertes & Brobst, 2002; Kocarek, Talbot, Batka, & Anderson, 2001). There is some lack of clarity about competencies, which potentially creates ethical dilemmas for counselors who work with culturally diverse populations. An important question for counselors is, What is the level of competence necessary before a counselor can ethically work with diverse populations? An improvement in graduate-level training in this area has been suggested, but this does not guarantee the necessary level of competence (Constantine, 2002).

Professional Demeanor

We have discussed the development of professional identity and professional ethical identity (Houser et al., 2006). One area that is consistent with the development of a professional identity is professional demeanor. Professional demeanor has not been a particularly significant focus of research in regard to ethics in counseling. However, there are discussions about this issue in the professional literature (Scheffler, Garrett, Zarin, & Pincus, 2000). One dilemma that potentially falls under professional demeanor is fees for counseling services (Wolfson, 1999). Lanza (2001) concluded, "Money is a taboo subject for many people" (p. 69). She proposed that because of attitudes toward quantifying personal worth, counseling fees are generally difficult for counselors to discuss. The counselor may avoid discussing rates with clients and simply set the fees, possibly either too high or too low. Wolfson (1999) concluded that "the fee is likely to evoke a range of ethical-clinical tensions and dilemmas for practitioners in private and agency practice settings insofar as it represents the practitioner's or the agency's income" (p. 270). Scheffler et al. (2000) suggested that another issue with fees originates with managed care. Lakin (1988) noted that reducing fees and making inappropriate diagnoses to gain access to services are potentially significant problems confronting counselors in managed care.

Houser et al. (2006) suggested that counselor dress can affect the client in a positive or negative way. Researchers have studied the impact of counselor dress on client outcomes (Littrell & Littrell, 1982). Littrell and Littrell (1982) investigated the perceptions of Native American adolescents; they wanted to understand how dress affected their counselor preference. They discovered that counselor dress actually did affect clients' perceptions. They found that counselors who were dressed more fashionably were preferred by adolescent clients. Houser et al. suggested several questions for counselors in regard to dress:

> Do counselors have a responsibility to dress more currently, particularly with certain populations such as adolescents who may prefer to work with such a counselor? Do they have an ethical responsibility to be fashionable and dress a certain way so that clients are more receptive? (p. 110)

Houser et al. cited another issue concerning counselor dress: whether counselors have any responsibility to avoid dressing provocatively. "What impact may counselors who dress more sexually provocatively have on their clients and what are any ethical issues?" (p. 110).

Hite and Fraser (1988) noted that another potential ethical dilemma related to counselor demeanor is the question of whether professionals should advertise their services. Hite and Fraser noted that "advertising by professionals was restricted by professional associations. In the late 1970s, key rulings by the Supreme Court forced relaxation of historic advertising bans by professional associations" (p. 95). The major problem with advertising by professionals is the maintenance of credibility and dignity. One can see less than attractive commercials on television, such as those with car salespeople screaming at the camera, which are not the professional presentation that counselors should employ. Counseling, particularly in a private practice, is a business. How should professional counselors seek referrals and business for their practices? What methods of advertisement are acceptable and still maintain dignity?

THE COUNSELOR: PERSONAL VALUES, PROFESSIONAL ETHICAL IDENTITY, RACE, GENDER, AND PERSONAL HISTORY—COMPONENTS OF COUNSELING ETHICAL HORIZON

Counselors' values, race, gender, professional ethical identity, moral/ethical development, and personal history are parts of the whole on the horizon of the hermeneutic circle (see Figure 4.1). Corey et al. (2010) identified potential ethical concerns involving counselors. The level of the counselor's self-awareness is critical (Corey et al., 2010). Unresolved personal issues are one example of how a counselor may affect the counseling process beyond what is expected from the professional relationship.

Countertransference is another possible concern in this element of the hermeneutic circle, the counselor. Houser et al. (2006) noted that "in the twenty-first century, we need to be aware that counseling involves two dissimilar participants in a therapeutic encounter" (p. 111). Counselors often work with diverse populations and need to identify their own uniqueness in an effort to be accepting within the therapeutic relationship. Counselors are influenced by numerous factors such as their cultural heritage(s) and various aspects of identity, including ethnic and racial identity, gender socialization, socioeconomic experiences, and other aspects of identity that lead to certain biases and assumptions about themselves and others. It is not possible for counselors to remain neutral to differences, and counselors are not immune from their own cultural biases and the impact they have. Houser et al. (2006) noted that "while counselors will need to be culturally aware and knowledgeable about their clients' worldviews, it is equally important that they be informed about themselves. Ethical dilemmas arise when counselors' own personal values affect the treatment of clients" (p. 112).

There are other countertransference issues that potentially affect the counseling relationship; one is the counselor's personal need to be a caretaker. In addition, the counselor may have a need to receive reinforcement and recognition by the client (Houser et al., 2006). Last, the counselor's potential need for power is an issue that most in counseling do not care to acknowledge because of the negative perceptions of seeking power (Bargh & Avarez, 2001; Duncan, 2003). Clients are generally very vulnerable and open to influence. A counselor who has a high need for power may influence a client to do things that is not in his or her best interests.

We have discussed the professional ethical identity of the counselor in previous chapters. One of the purposes of this text is to promote the development of counselor professional ethical identity. Hendricks (2008) provided a specific connection between professional identity and professional ethical identity. He stated,

> What role do ethics play in our development of a "professional identity?" The answer is rather simple. Our ethics code are integral to our process of defining ourselves as a profession in a changing world because they unify us, give us methodologies for practice, and point us to a more unified profession. (p. 259)

Ponton and Duba (2009) suggested that the counseling profession is still developing. As a consequence, the professional ethical identity of a counselor is still developing too, it is hoped along with the growth of counseling as a profession.

A counselor's awareness of his or her own ethical/moral development is helpful in understanding and using decision making in a professional relationship, for example, a counselor-client relationship. A counselor who functions primarily in a postconventional stage of moral development may interpret an ethical dilemma differently than one who functions in a conventional stage (see Chapter 2 for stages of development). For example, a counselor hears an adolescent state she has been hit by her mother. A counselor functioning in the conventional stage, following rules, would immediately contact social services. A counselor in the postconventional moral development stage might gather more information from the adolescent and find out that she was mad at her mother and wanted to get her in trouble. The postconventional counselor might seek out universal principals to guide his or her actions and seek to understand deeper issues versus just adhering to what initially appeared to be a legal issue. We as humans have a tendency to interpret information based on our developmental perspective and what makes sense to us. An awareness of our ethical developmental level can help us understand ethical issues and monitor how it may affect decisions. Think about your own ethical developmental level (consult your results from the Defining Issues Test; see http://www.ethicaldevelopment.ua.edu/), how you might respond to a situation such as suspected child abuse, and what can be done to ensure that you do not let your own personal developmental level hinder ethical decision making.

THE CLIENT: PERSONAL VALUES, RACE, GENDER, AND PERSONAL HISTORY

Currently there is considerable controversy about how we should acknowledge differences. There are social, financial, and political perspectives that affect how counselors may think about client diversity. Despite these negative views of whether we should acknowledge diversity, there is a major shift anticipated in U.S. demographics (U.S. Census Bureau, 2004). The U.S. Census Bureau (2004) estimates that if demographic data follow recent trends, during the period of 2000 to 2050, the outcome will be that the White population will be the slowest growing racial group and will be reduced by 10% overall in total population by 2050. The Hispanic population will be a major factor in population growth and will reach 24% of the total population by 2050 (U.S. Census Bureau, 2004). The Hispanic population is projected to be the largest minority group. The Black and/or African American population will grow at a little more than twice the annual rate of change for the White population; the African American population will increase by about 2% of the total population. The Asian and Pacific Islander populations are projected through the year 2050 to continue to be the fastest growing races or ethnic groups; Asian growth rates are projected to increase to 8% of the total population. The issue for counselors based on these anticipated changes lies in the divergent sets of philosophical assumptions and worldviews that these clients will bring to the therapeutic relationship. A counselor's response to a client could be problematic because of lack of understanding of clients who are diverse and potentially considerably different from the counselor. As counselors, we are encouraged to adopt the ethical codes and the philosophical frameworks developed in our professional training programs and that are founded on Western views. By not examining the philosophical assumptions of the current ethical codes, we may unwittingly accept the perspective of the dominant culture and possibly minimize or trivialize the role of culture in ethical decision making (Ibrahim, 1996). Also, using solely Western ethical theories in making decisions limits our understanding of the diversity of our clients, but most important, it is disrespectful of the clients' views.

Values have been defined as beliefs that guide actions across various situations (Connor & Becker, 2003). Vashon and Agresti (1992) suggested that the personal values of a client affect the counseling relationship. Researchers have discovered that client outcomes in counseling are related to the similarity between client and counselor values (Arizmendi, Beutler, Shandfield, Crago, & Hagaman, 1985). Houser et al. (2006) posed several questions that are important ethical issues in changing client values:

> How similar do the client's values have to be to the counselor's for counseling to be successful? Also, another dilemma is whether promoting similarity between the client and counselor is ethical and best for the client. For the profession as a whole, the question becomes: Do counselors use those moral and ethical frameworks presented by their training programs—which reflect society's norms—as the sole basis for their ethical decision-making? Or can counselors come to an ethical decision while considering the values, morals, and ethical positions of their diverse client population? (p. 112)

There are other influences on the development of a client's values. A client may enter counseling with certain values that may be in conflict with community values. An example is a client who has a sexual orientation that conflicts with the community's values, for example, a gay or lesbian sexual orientation. Today this is influenced significantly by geographical location, with many states passing same-sex marriage laws. A second example of client values that potentially conflict with community values is child-rearing practices. A family, based on cultural or geographical background, may see value in corporal punishment, whereas the community may define it as child abuse.

Clients may be seen through specific characteristics such as race, ethnicity, gender, and disabilities to the process of ethical decision making; the cultural environment in which clients have lived is very influential in their construction of moral reasoning. Ethical dilemmas develop when the dissonance between clients' and counselors' experiences, interpretations, and analyses are not acknowledged.

SUPERVISOR VALUES AND AGENCY POLICIES

Supervisors' values and personal characteristics, as well as agency policies, constitute another major element of the horizon for ethical decision making for counselors (see Figure 4.1; Houser et al., 2006). As has been suggested from a review of ethical decision-making models, it is an important step that supervisees consult with supervisors about ethical dilemmas (Herlihy, Gray, & McCollum, 2002; Welfel, 2009). Supervisors, like counselors and clients, enter into discussions of ethical dilemmas with their own personal values that affect the decision-making process (Bucky, Marques, Daly, Alley, & Karp, 2010). What impact do supervisor personal values have for the counselor attempting to make an ethical decision? Two examples of supervisor values are helpful in understanding this issue. The two are multicultural sensitivity to clients and supervisor sensitivity to multicultural perspectives of counselors (Ladany, Lehman-Waterman, Molinaro, & Wolgast, 1999). As we have discussed, multicultural sensitivity concerns sensitivity to and understanding of issues of gender, race, culture, sexual orientation, disability, and so forth. The counselor can increase his or her effective use of supervision through awareness and understanding of the supervisor's personal values.

Ladany et al. (1999) proposed that the expertise of the supervisor with the ethical issue addressed is important. Counselors should continually seek out professional development activities; supervisors also should update their knowledge with participation in continuing education (Wheeler & King, 2000). Supervisors should be aware of and acknowledge their limitations and their responsibly to pursue information addressing the ethical dilemma. Many supervisors do not realize that they may be held responsible for the actions of their supervisees (Herlihy et al., 2002). One aspect of this responsibility is to be knowledgeable in the area of the ethical dilemma. When one is not, he or she should refer the counselor/supervisee to someone who is (Magnuson, Norem, & Wilcoxon, 2000).

The counselor may at times be supervised by a professional who received training in social work, psychology, or psychiatry. The ethical codes adhered to by the supervisor and the counselor may be different, and it has been noted that not all professional codes share the same views on various ethical issues. Perhaps the counselor follows the American Counseling Association (ACA) code of ethics, and the supervisor, who trained in counseling psychology, follows the codes of the American Psychological Association. The ACA has a section addressing confidentiality that allows for disclosure of information to a third party, breaking confidentiality, if the ethical issue involves protecting him or her from a contagious fatal disease. The American Psychological Association codes do not have a standard for such a disclosure. Which professional code should be followed in such an example, the counselor's or the supervisor's?

Agency policies and values influence the supervisor and how he or she interprets ethical dilemmas (Linzer, 1992; Watkins, 1989). The agency may follow policies and practices that are not compatible with the counselor's code of ethics, values, or professional ethical identity. One example is a social service agency funded by a religious organization where there may be differences of opinion between the counselor and supervisor/agency around the sexual behavior of clients. Another example of how agency policies may affect a counselor's ethical decision making is diagnosing clients for eligibility of services. A counselor may be encouraged to use a more severe diagnosis in an effort to increase income for the agency. Managed care, it has been noted, is a source of ethical dilemmas for the counselor (C. Cooper & Gottlieb, 2000).

PROFESSIONAL CODES OF ETHICS

Houser et al. (2006) noted that professional codes are also a consideration in ethical decision making and on the horizon for the counselor (see Figure 4.1). Different professional codes have been developed for the various counseling professions, such as school counseling, mental health counseling, rehabilitation counseling, career counseling, pastoral counseling, family therapy, and counseling (ACA, 2005; American Association for Marriage and Family Therapy, 2001; American Association of Pastoral Counselors, 2010; American Mental Health Counseling Association, 2010; Commission on Rehabilitation Counselor Certification, 2010; National Career Development Association, 2007). Professional codes are only relatively recent additions to the profession and practice of counseling, first introduced 40 years ago compared to the older codes of other professions such as law, medicine, and psychology (Neukrug & Lowell, 1996). Generally ethical codes were developed based on certain Western ethical theories such as utilitarianism, virtue ethics, and respect for persons (Kantian ethics; C. E. Harris, 2002; Henry, 1996).

The strengths and limitations of professional codes of ethics have been identified by various authors addressing counseling ethics (Hadjistavropoulos, Malloy, Sharpe, Green, & Fuchs-Lacelle, 2002; Neukrug & Lowell, 1996). Some of the benefits or strengths that have been cited are standards that protect consumers, a framework for ethical decision making, and a reference for defense in judicial proceedings. Neukrug and Lowell (1996) provided additional insight into why ethical decision making is problematic when only professional codes are employed. The limitations they cited include concerns that many ethical dilemmas are not addressed by professional codes, the client's view is not considered, and conflicts exist among different professional codes (Hadjistavropoulos et al., 2002; Neukrug & Lowell, 1996).

PROFESSIONAL KNOWLEDGE

Another element to review on the ethical decision-making horizon is the professional knowledge of the counselor (Houser et al., 2006; see Figure 4.1). A counselor's professional knowledge base requires commitment, understanding, and competent practice (Houser et al., 2006). A counselor should acquire a professional ethical identity that encompasses all aspects of counselor roles and functions, including knowing standards for ethical practice and knowing the latest research findings for an evidence-based practice. It is important for counselors to understand the cultural contexts of relationships, issues, and trends in a multicultural and diverse society. Consideration of factors such as culture, ethnicity, nationality, age, gender, sexual orientation, mental and physical characteristics, education, family values, religious and spiritual values, and socioeconomic status, as well as the unique characteristics of individuals, couples, families, ethnic groups, and communities, is important. It is helpful for counselors to be aware of the nature and needs of humans at all developmental levels and be knowledgeable about career development and other work-related life factors. Counselors should be competent in individual counseling, consultation, and helping processes as well as in the theory and process of group work. They should have basic understanding of measurement concepts, norm and criterion-referenced testing, and individual and group assessment skills. Counselors should also acquire research skills to evaluate the effectiveness of counseling (Council for Accreditation of Counseling and Related Educational Programs, 2009). A review of these necessary skills in counseling demonstrates the complexity and knowledge required to be an ethical and effective counselor.

Counselors are required to engage in continuing professional development to update skills and keep abreast of new developments in the field. One area of increasing importance is knowledge of psychopharmacology as it relates to treatment of mental health problems. In the past, mental and emotional disorders were conceptualized as psychogenic, with treatment consisting of counseling and psychotherapy. Today, however, the biological bases of behavior are emphasized more and more, with treatment including drug treatments. Ingersoll (2000) suggested that counselors have at least an introduction to psychopharmacology. It is helpful for counselors to know how medications may affect a client's functioning and progress in counseling.

GEOGRAPHIC REGION AND CULTURE

According to Houser et al. (2006), geographic region and culture are other relevant variables to consider on the horizon of ethical decision making for counselors (Baca, Alverson, Manuel, & Blackwell, 2007; Sue et al., 1992; Welfel, 2009). Geographic region issues typically involve discussion of rural versus urban counseling practice (Baca et al., 2007; C. Campbell & Fox, 2003; Schank & Skovholt, 1997). However, geographic regions such as the North, South, West, and East can potentially influence counseling practice. Those practicing in rural settings are faced with issues of dual relationships and have more frequent contact outside of counseling, such as in a grocery store or a health club. Seeing a client outside of counseling potentially creates dual relationships. For example, one problem can be trust in such a dual relationship. Does the client question whether the counselor shares information about his or her sessions with others in the health club? C. Campbell and Fox (2003) suggested that one problem is bias in the counselor's objectivity by having close associations with those in his or her community.

Geographic region may involve different physical regions of the country. Various regions of the country may in general hold specific values and beliefs. We mentioned earlier an example of reporting child abuse when corporal punishment is used. There is considerable variability in values and beliefs about the use of corporal punishment.

Recently there have been significant changes in the location where counseling takes place (Ganote, 1990; Kuntze, Stoermer, Mueller-Spahn, & Bullinger, 2002). Kuntze et al. (2002) noted that there has been a significant increase in offering counseling online or virtually, and several ethical concerns arise out of online counseling. When the state licenses qualified professionals, who monitors the counselors' action? Another issue concerns the possibility that someone can hack into electronic files and access client information with online counseling, creating new issues of confidentiality (see Chapter 9).

There are other nontraditional counseling settings that may create ethical concerns, including long-term care facilities (Ganote, 1990), correctional settings, and client homes (home-based counseling; Evans et al., 2003; M. Harris & Mertlich, 2003). Each of these settings provides additional issues for the counselor. For example, what level of confidentiality is available in a correctional setting? There may be problems with privacy in all of these types of settings.

Culture is another issue that may be included in this part of the horizon of ethical decision making (Houser et al., 2006). Ruggiero (2004) suggested several important questions to consider when thinking about culture and ethics. He proposed that choosing a reliable standard of ethical judgment requires review of several questions: (a) Are moral judgments accurate and ethical outside of one's own culture? (b) How does one understand differences between moral standards of one's own culture and another? and (c) Are there common values, morals, and ethics across different cultures? As clinicians, our experiences with diverse clients often expose our own confusion and tension when we are confronted with norms and values for living that may be contradictory to those principles and values from our prevailing society. How counselors incorporate such information in ethical decision making is significant and affects choice of actions.

LOCAL, STATE, AND FEDERAL LAWS

State, local, and federal laws are important issues in counselor ethical decision making and, as Houser et al. (2006) noted, are another issue on the ethical horizon as depicted in Figure 4.1. It is important for counselors to be aware of legislation that governs their practices. For example, there are statutes that address issues such as child and elder abuse that vary from state to state. Also, many states have mandated reporting abuse of those with disabilities. However, reporting abuse of children, the elderly, or persons with disabilities may violate a professional code of maintaining confidentiality and create an ethical dilemma.

There are a number of laws and court decisions that affect the practice of counseling. Confidentiality is an essential element in all counseling professions. It is the basis of trust, which is a key element in the counseling relationship. Counselors attempt to maintain confidential information to protect the rights of clients and promote trust. There are both state and federal laws that affect the maintenance of confidentiality. The first national standards to protect individuals' medical records (electronic) and other personal health information was introduced with HIPAA. HIPAA requires a patient's specific permission to release sensitive information.

Kermani and Drob (1987) suggested there are exceptions to maintaining confidentiality. One example is the *Tarasoff* decision, which established the legal foundation for requiring counselors to warn intended targets of potentially homicidal clients. *Tarasoff* does not apply universally, because some states have laws that are in conflict with this court decision (see Chapter 12). Another example of differences in laws by state is found in situations wherein minors seek abortions without parental consent (Lawrence & Robinson Kurpius, 2000). The legal right of the minor client to seek an abortion may conflict with the personal values of the counselor who believes parents have a right to know and should be included in such an important decision. The counselor may want to breach confidentiality and inform the parents.

Counselors may be confronted with an ethical issue in following professional codes of ethics and the law; there may be times they are in conflict (see Chapter 12). There are common circumstances in which any of these (laws, codes, values) conflict and the counselor is left to consider the ethical course of action. For example, a counselor may want to follow professional codes, disclose a client has a communicable disease, and seek to inform possible partners when state law prohibits such a disclosure.

ETHICAL THEORIES

As was noted earlier, we live in a diverse society that is becoming more diverse each year. Houser et al. (2006) suggested that due to the increasing diversity in our society, ethical theories used in ethical decision making must reflect this diversity. Consequently another element of the horizon for ethical decision making should include ethical theories representative of various groups and not just Western perspectives. Cottone and Claus (2000) criticized the lack of inclusion of major philosophical and ethical theories in ethical decision-making models. They stated that "it was surprising to find the number of practice-based models developed apparently without attention to underlying philosophical or theoretical tenets" (p. 281). Hare (1991) and Rest (1984) also recommended including major philosophical theories in developing ethical decision-making models. As stated previously, all of the professional codes are based on Western ethics, specifically virtue ethics and natural law (Freeman, 2000).

Shanahan and Wang (2003) reviewed a number of ethical theories and concluded that "if you look around the world, what you see is not moral unity but rather moral diversity. Each culture has its own peculiar (and sometimes very peculiar) moral perspective on the world, and these different moral perspectives frequently clash" (p. 12). The hermeneutic model proposed by Houser et al. (2006) is based on fusion of horizons (perspectives of the client, counselor, supervisor, community, and agency) and includes consideration of such things as the cultural and ethical philosophies of those affected by an ethical dilemma. An understanding and consideration of a wide range of ethical philosophies and theories is critical for counselors, and such an understanding is consistent with multicultural competence (Bryan & Lyons, 2003). A counselor interpreting the fusion of horizons may consider one or several ethical theories as part of the decision-making process. An example is a counselor's choosing to use a theory that is consistent with his or her own views and a theory that is consistent with the client's views and values or those of the community. He or she is open to fusing both counselor and client horizons in an effort to make the best ethical decision. Chapter 13 ("Western Theories of Ethics"), Chapter 14 ("Eastern Theories of Ethics"), Chapter 15 ("Middle Eastern Ethical Theories"), and Chapter 16 ("Native American, Hispanic/Latino, and African Ethics") provide information relevant to understanding different ethical perspectives relevant to interpreting the ethical horizon.

SUMMARY

We are suggesting using an ethical decision-making model that is dynamic and involves a comprehensive understanding of ethical dilemmas facing counselors: a hermeneutic model. Hermeneutics is the accurate interpretation of a situation, and seeking the best ethical understanding is key in counselor ethical behavior. Effective use of a hermeneutic ethical decision-making model is identification, understanding, and application of relevant elements of the horizon. We agree with Houser et al. (2006) that the whole horizon of ethical decision making includes the following parts, and we expand the counselor element to include professional ethical identity:

- an ethical dilemma;
- the counselor and his or her values, professional ethical identity, moral development stage, race, gender, personal history, and so forth;
- the client and his or her values, race, gender, personal history, and so forth;
- the supervisor's personal characteristics, professional identity, moral development stage, values, agency policies, and so forth;
- the geographic region and culture;
- local, state, and federal laws;
- professional codes of ethics;
- professional knowledge; and
- ethical theories.

We believe that an element of the horizon, ethical theories, involves the selection of context-relevant ethical theories that are consistent with the fusion of horizons, such as those of the counselor, the client, and the supervisor. This may involve a horizon that is dynamic and responsive to the circumstances of the ethical dilemma.

APPLICATION OF THE HERMENEUTIC MODEL

A key consideration in applying the hermeneutic ethical decision-making model is the identification and selection of relevant elements of the horizon, including use of various ethical theories. The practical application of a hermeneutic ethical decision-making model potentially involves the use of several ethical theories relevant to the situation along with other components of the horizon. We will use the case of Jonathan to illustrate the application of a hermeneutic model. Reread the case at the beginning of the chapter.

A month after hearing from the spouse of Charini that she had been hospitalized for the suicide attempt, Jonathan received a letter from the licensing board in the state of Ohio where Charini lived. The board stated the spouse, Ashoka, had made a formal complaint to the licensure board. The board stated that Jonathan had not fulfilled the requirements for providing counseling in the state as Jonathan was not licensed by the state. The complaint by the spouse was that Jonathan provided online therapy and opened up strong emotions in Charini without providing any intervention or procedures to address associated crises. Ashoka was alleging unprofessional conduct, violation of competence, and not having a license to practice in Ohio.

Jonathan was upset by the charges, and he wanted to attend an interview and explain his side; so Jonathan agreed to a meeting time with licensure board members. Jonathan had an initial meeting with the licensure board to discuss the review process. The licensure board and Jonathan agreed to use a hermeneutic ethical decision-making model. They identified the elements of the horizon relevant to the case of Charini. The elements of the horizon in this hermeneutical model include the ethical dilemma; the counselor's values, race, gender, professional ethical identity, moral development level, personal history, and so forth; the client's values, race, gender, personal history, and so forth; the supervisor's (in this case the consultant's; see below) values, professional identity, moral development level, race, gender, personal history, and so forth as well as counseling agency policies; applicable local, state, and federal laws; professional knowledge; geographic region; professional codes of ethics; and the ethical theories of Buddhism and virtue ethics. They decided to use Buddhism because they were aware that Charini was a practicing Buddhist. They also decided to use virtue ethics because many of the professional codes were based on virtue ethics.

CASE OF JONATHAN: ONLINE THERAPY[1]

| Figure 4.2 | Hermeneutic Model of Integrating Theories in Ethical Decision Making |

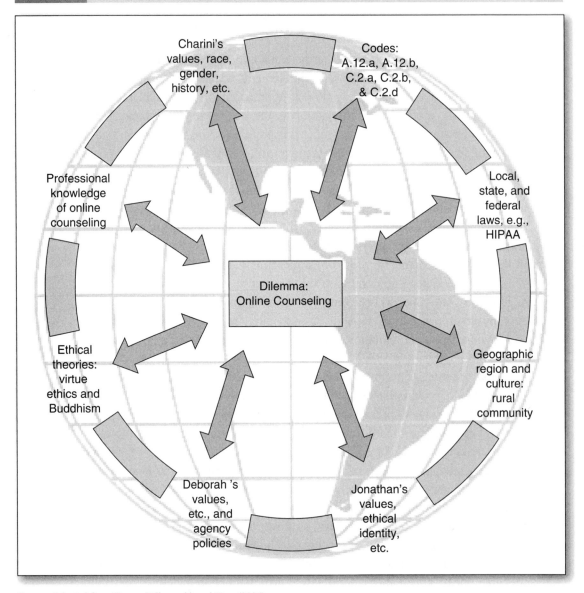

Source: Adapted from Houser, Wilczenski, and Ham (2006).

Note: HIPAA = Health Insurance Portability and Accountability Act.

---

[1] Adapted from Houser, Wilczenski, and Ham (2006). Reprinted with permission.

Ethical Dilemma

Jonathan decided to open a practice after 5 years of working in a counseling agency. He is licensed in his state and has received the appropriate supervision during his agency work. He consulted with a former colleague, Deborah, who has a successful online therapy practice. Jonathan met with Deborah for a couple of hours and discussed how he could set up his online practice. Deborah shared her experiences. Jonathan accepted Charini as a client, and both agreed on using asynchronous communication through e-mails. He informed Charini of HIPAA guidelines, and Charini acknowledged she understood them. Jonathan acknowledged that he had not informed Charini that he was her first online client, nor did he indicate he was not licensed to practice counseling in Ohio. Jonathan made an assumption that because he was licensed in his state, he could practice in other states online (see Figure 4.2).

First, the licensure board noted he was not licensed in Ohio to practice counseling. Second, it noted he had not met with the client in person for the first session, which is a requirement of Ohio standards of practice for counseling. The face-to-face session may be done using video electronically, but Jonathan had not completed such an interview. The licensure board also noted that Jonathan failed to establish a method to assess the severity of his client's problems and failed to have a procedure for monitoring his client's mental status. He failed to provide a format for accessing crisis services for his client. The licensure board wanted to discuss these violations with Jonathan and determine if they were true.

Jonathan: The Counselor's Personal Values, Professional Ethical Identity, Moral Development Level, Race, Gender, and Personal History

Jonathan grew up in the rural community in which he currently resides. He attended college at a university more than 60 miles away, and he also completed his master's degree in counseling there. His family members were long-time residents of the area; both his mother and his father grew up there and operated a small grocery store. He has an older brother who did move away from the area and now lives in a large urban area, 45 minutes from Jonathan's home. Jonathan grew up with traditional rural values of hard work and a strong sense of community. As was stated in the earlier description of the case (at the beginning of the chapter), Jonathan developed a professional ethical identity that valued living things and human life. He was disturbed by the killing and death of living things. He saw himself as someone who would make every effort to avoid harming an individual, including avoiding engaging in professional activities that may involve the death of a client.

Jonathan lives with his spouse, whom he married after completing his undergraduate degree. They met in high school, and both attended the same college. She is a teacher in the local high school. They have two young children, both boys.

After graduating with his master's degree, Jonathan took a job as a counselor in a counseling center in a medium-size town of 50,000. He did not enjoy the long-distance drive each day to work and back and felt it necessary to reach his goal of opening a private practice close to home. He also did not agree with the recent change in services provided to the local courts, evaluating clients for competency and possible eligibility for the death penalty.

Charini: The Client's Personal Values, Race, Moral Development Level, Gender, and Personal History

Charini is a 45-year-old woman who was born in Nepal, India. She immigrated to the United States when she was in her late teens. She was educated as a software engineer and stayed in the United States after her training. She worked for more than 20 years as a software engineer in an urban area in Ohio. Her company had offices in the community. She met and married another software engineer. Charini saw herself as a practicing Buddhist, and she valued living things, but she also believed in a more liberal perspective, that those in pain may take their own lives. Jonathan, over several asynchronous sessions, concluded that Charini demonstrated a conventional moral development level. She believed in following rules, and her time working in the software industry reinforced the importance of following procedures and rules.

Charini and her spouse had one child, a boy who died in a car accident when he was 19 years old. Charini was raised as a Buddhist, and she actively practices this religion. Her family also practices Buddhism. Charini's son died suddenly in an automobile accident 6 months prior to her seeking online counseling. She continued working for a short time after her son's death but decided to quit her job because she felt she was not performing well. She decided to set up a private consulting software firm. She contacted Jonathan after her spouse encouraged her to seek counseling. Charini was embarrassed to seek counseling in her community and felt online counseling would allow her to maintain her privacy. Also, she was busy setting up her consulting software business, and she did not feel she could take time to go to an office for counseling.

Deborah: The Supervisor's/Consultant's Personal Values, Moral Development Level, Race, Gender, and Personal History

Deborah is more of a consultant than a supervisor in this case. She is a 40-year-old White woman. Deborah lives in the same town as Jonathan. Deborah, similar to Jonathan, worked in a community counseling center to gain the appropriate experience and supervision to achieve licensure. She has been licensed for 10 years and has established a private practice including an online practice. Deborah has attended a few workshops at professional conferences addressing online therapy. However, when she established her practice online she did not seek out supervision. Deborah has had positive experiences with online therapy and generally has 5 to 10 online clients at any one time as part of her practice. Deborah met with Jonathan for a few hours before Jonathan started his online practice. They discussed how to set up an online practice and some of the clinical issues. Deborah volunteered to be available to answer questions as they arose. Jonathan did contact Deborah to update her about his success and stated things were going well. Deborah provided no further consultation. Deborah describes herself as highly ethical and could not imagine herself violating major ethical codes or state laws. She demonstrated a conventional moral development level, following rules and ethical codes.

Professional Codes

The following ACA (2005) professional codes appeared to be relevant:

A.12.a Technology applications: Benefits and limitations—Counselors inform clients of the benefits and limitations of using information technology applications in the counseling process and in business/billing procedures. Such technologies include but are not limited to computer hardware and software, telephones, the World Wide Web, the Internet, online assessment instruments and other communication devices.

A.12.b Technology applications: Technology-assisted service—When providing technology-assisted distance counseling services, counselors determine that clients are intellectually, emotionally, and physically capable of using the application and that the application is appropriate for the needs of clients.

A.12.c Technology applications: Inappropriate services—When technology-assisted distance counseling services are deemed inappropriate by the counselor or client, counselors consider delivering services face to face.

C.2.a Professional competence: Boundaries of competence—Counselors practice only within the boundaries of their competence, based on their education, training, supervised experience, state and national professional credentials, and appropriate professional experience. Counselors gain knowledge, personal awareness, sensitivity, and skills pertinent to working with a diverse client population.

C.2.b Professional competence: New specialty areas of practice—Counselors practice in specialty areas new to them only after appropriate education, training, and supervised experience. While developing skills in new specialty areas, counselors take steps to ensure the competence of their work and to protect others from possible harm.

C.2.d Professional competence: Monitor effectiveness—Counselors continually monitor their effectiveness as professionals and take steps to improve when necessary. Counselors in private practice take reasonable steps to seek peer supervision as needed to evaluate their efficacy as counselors.

An important question for Jonathan and the licensure board is whether Charini was an appropriate client for online therapy. What effort did Jonathan take to assess whether Charini was appropriate for this medium of counseling (ACA Code A.12.a)? The second question concerns whether Jonathan clearly and adequately explained the strengths and limitations of online therapy (Code A.12.b). A third issue is whether Jonathan is competent in providing therapy via an online format (Code C.2.a). Jonathan was trained in traditional person-to-person counseling. He had consulted with a colleague who was practicing online therapy, but does this constitute adequate training and competence for conducting online therapy? A related code addresses the counselor's responsibility to develop procedures to ensure adequate care for the client and protection for the client while the counselor is developing expertise in a new specialty area (Code C.2.b). Jonathan was developing skills in a new area, but he appears not to have developed procedures to ensure protection of his client, particularly in regard to any crisis and emergency needs. Another important issue is that Jonathan does not have a license to practice in the state of Ohio. ACA standards that apply concern professional qualifications, specifically "claiming" credentials that a counselor currently has (Code C.4.b). Jonathan did not claim he was licensed in Ohio, just that he was licensed, in this case in another state. The last issue, and the professional code that may apply, is the importance of appropriate supervision (Code C.2.d). Jonathan did not seek out supervision necessary to monitor his effectiveness in this new intervention format.

Professional Knowledge

Jonathan reviewed the professional literature addressing online therapy before going to the hearing so he would have a good background to talk about the current literature addressing online counseling. He discovered that online clinical therapy is growing (Elleven & Allen, 2004; G. Jones & Stokes, 2009; Rassau & Arco, 2003; Rochlen, Zack, & Speyer, 2004) and potentially includes telepsychology and online therapy. Maheu (2003) defined online clinical practice as "the use of any technology to deliver therapeutic dialogue at a distance, whether conducted over a direct video link (e.g., telepsychology or telepsychiatry) or over a network such as the Internet (e.g., therapy online)" (p. 20). Rochlen, Zack, et al. (2004) defined Internet therapy "as any type of professional interaction that makes use of the Internet to connect qualified mental health professionals and their clients" (p. 270). Online therapy can be asynchronous or synchronous. Asynchronous online therapy is generally conducted via e-mail. Synchronous online therapy employs chat-based formats conducted in real time (Rochlen, Zack, et al., 2004). The vast majority of online therapy is conducted asynchronously through e-mails (Elleven & Allen, 2004).

Jonathan discovered the benefits of online therapy cited in the professional literature (Haberstroh, Duff, Evans, Gee, & Trepal, 2007; G. Jones & Stokes, 2009; Mantovani, Castelnuovo, Gaggiioli, & Riva, 2003; Rochlen, Zack, et al., 2004). Benefits of online therapy include convenience and increased access to counseling services, disinhibition in expressing emotions, and the positive effects of writing (e-mails) as a therapeutic intervention. Limitations of online therapy include the absence of nonverbal cues, which have been a foundation of counseling theory and intervention (Rochlen, Zack, et al., 2004). Another limitation is decreased ability to identify and address crises because the majority of online therapy takes place through e-mails, through which depression and suicidal behaviors may be less visible than in face-to-face counseling (Maheu, 2003; Rochlen, Zack, et al., 2004).

There has been minimal research addressing online therapy, primarily because it is a new modality for providing counseling (T. Chang & Yeh, 2003; Haberstroh et al., 2007; Lange & Rietdijk, 2003; Rochlen, Land, & Wong, 2004). Research supports the effectiveness of online therapy. For example, Rochlen, Land, et al. (2004) studied counseling with males both online and in person, and there were essentially no differences in preferences for both modalities. Lange and Rietdijk (2003) studied online therapy in the treatment of posttraumatic stress and found positive outcomes. However, because of the limited amount of research, researchers note the preliminary nature of the results (Rochlen, Land, et al., 2004).

Jonathan reviewed the professional literature for ethical concerns cited about online counseling (Fisher & Fried, 2003; Maheu, 2003; Ragusea & VandeCreek, 2003; Skarderud, 2003). Fisher and Fried (2003) stated,

> Questions about validity, efficacy, and safety of different Internet-mediated techniques for psychological assessment and therapy remain largely unanswered as the field rapidly evolves. Frequent innovation in telehealth continues to outpace the development of specific guidelines for the delivery of services. (p. 103)

Specific ethical concerns evolve around counselor competence in using online therapy and around protection of confidentiality (Barnett & Scheetz, 2003; Fisher & Fried, 2003). Fisher and Fried noted the importance of having appropriate training and supervision in providing online therapy. The question for Jonathan is whether he had received enough training and supervision in providing online therapy. Fisher and Fried also stated, "Harm to Internet clients/patients may be incurred when psychologists fail to appropriately diagnose a disorder, fail to identify suicidal or homicidal ideation, or reinforce maladaptive behavior" (p. 104). Another question is whether Jonathan caused harm to his client by not detecting suicidal ideation. Maheu (2003) proposed that counselors need to establish adequate crisis procedures prior to beginning online therapy. Also, Jonathan did not know the laws in Ohio, and he was not licensed as he needed to be to practice online counseling in this case.

Geographic Region and Culture

Jonathan lives in a rural community, and Charini lives in an urban community. They have limited access to each other in a face-to-face format; they live more than 2 hours away from each other. Consequently they agree on counseling via the Internet. Both have access to e-mail and know how to use it. E-mail, which is an asynchronous interaction, has been found to be the primary format used in online therapy (Elleven & Allen, 2004).

Researchers have found that Asian Americans generally underutilize counseling services (Atkinson & Lowe, 1995; Chang & Yeh, 2003), and Charini's seeking out counseling took a significant effort on her part. Some have proposed that online counseling provides move confidentiality than face-to-face counseling and results in less of the stigma associated with mental illness (Ragusea & VandeCreek, 2003). This level of confidentiality may have been a contributing factor to Charini's seeking out this modality of counseling.

Local, State, and Federal Laws

Ohio Statute 4757-5-13, Standards of Practice and Professional Conduct: Electronic Service Delivery (Internet, Email, Teleconference, etc.), requires that "all practitioners providing counseling, social work or marriage and family therapy via electronic service delivery to Ohio citizens shall be licensed in Ohio." Clearly Jonathan did not meet this requirement, and he was in violation of this statute. Also, the statute requires that the online counselor provide the client with local assistance and crisis intervention if necessary. Jonathan did not have any identified qualified professionals in Ohio to help with crisis intervention, nor did he provide information about a crisis hotline to Charini.

A federal law that addresses the handling of health information electronically, HIPAA, applies in this case. The intent of this legislation, as described in Chapter 12, is to protect and limit the disclosure of an individual's health care information, particularly electronic disclosure (Office of Civil Rights, 2003). Disclosure is permitted only with the fully informed consent of a client or patient. The question here is whether Jonathan sought informed consent from Charini and explained the limitations of protecting privacy on the Internet (Fisher & Fried, 2003; Ragusea & VandeCreek, 2003). Ragusea and VandeCreek (2003) proposed methods for protecting confidentiality when using the Internet, such as employing firewalls.

Ethical Theories: Virtue Ethics and Buddhism

Jonathan and the licensure board agreed to use virtue ethics and Buddhism in attempting to make an ethical decision based on this case. It was determined that four primary ethical principles of virtue ethics apply to this case: nonmaleficence (the duty to do no harm), beneficence (the duty to do good or help), fidelity (the duty to be truthful and to honor others, their rights, and their responsibilities), and autonomy (the duty to maximize the individual's right to make decisions).

Nonmaleficence applies because the licensure board questioned whether Jonathan should have known to establish a crisis procedure. Setting up crisis procedures locally is required by Ohio statute in conducting online counseling from a distance. The fact that he established his online therapy service without a clear, well-thought-out procedure for dealing with crises is the result of his lack of awareness of Ohio law. Beneficence applies as in most counseling relationships. The question becomes, What does the counselor do to promote the welfare of the client? Did Jonathan act with beneficence in providing online therapy to Charini, or was his interest in establishing his business? Another possible virtue ethic that applies is fidelity, and the issue here is whether Jonathan clearly informed Charini of the dangers and limitations of online therapy. Was he truthful in informing Charini of such risks? The last principle that applies in this case is autonomy. Charini is an adult and should have the right to make autonomous decisions about her psychological care. If this is true, then Charini was free to choose to pursue online counseling, but the associated risks must have been clearly stated to her by Jonathan.

Jonathan and the licensure board also applied concepts from Buddhism (see Chapter 14) in an effort to understand the ethical issues in this case. The board discovered that Buddhism in general did not support a practice of suicide; there may be rare circumstances such as severe illness in which suicide is considered acceptable, but the circumstances are rare when most Buddhists would support such a choice (Keown, 2005). The board and Jonathan also discovered that the concepts of the Noble Eightfold Path applied. The specific concepts that applied included right understanding, right thought, right livelihood, and right effort. Right understanding according to Buddhism refers to an accurate perception of the world and an understanding of suffering. Did Jonathan have right understanding of Charini's suffering? Could he have done anything to improve right understanding such as meeting with her face to face, at least in the beginning? Right thought concerns thoughts of compassion and unselfishness. Did Jonathan have such thoughts, or did he care about starting his online business and not have compassion? Another Buddhist concept that applies is right livelihood, and this concerns pursuing a job that does not harm others. The question here is whether Jonathan pursued a job and an activity that caused harm to others. His apparent intention in taking on this job was to help others. The final concept that applies is right effort, which concerns the use of mental discipline to promote good (potentially similar to beneficence). The issue for Jonathan and the licensure board is, What effort did Jonathan take to promote the welfare and good of Charini? Was the online counseling adequate and helpful to Charini? Could Jonathan have done more to help Charini?

HERMENEUTIC ETHICAL DECISION MAKING

The licensure board and Jonathan met and reviewed the elements of the horizon for this ethical dilemma. Jonathan explained to the board that he was highly motivated to pursue the use of online therapy to maintain his rural lifestyle. Charini came from a culture that typically underutilizes counseling services and may prefer the more confidential and anonymous counseling format that online therapy provides. The board noted that Jonathan had consulted with Deborah, who also values living in a rural community. They shared this value and shared a goal of establishing online therapy services.

Jonathan did not meet with Charini face to face to assess her mental health issues. He violated his own professional codes and did not comply with state law in representing his license, nor did he develop procedures to ensure adequate care for and protection of the client (ACA Code C.2.b). Jonathan acknowledged to the licensure board that he did not provide information to Charini about any limitations of computer technology, for example, the extra effort needed to monitor nonverbal cues that might not be revealed in online therapy, such as depression (Code A.12.b).

The ACA code addresses the issue of counselors' practicing outside the boundaries of their competence. Jonathan did meet with Deborah, who had started her own online therapy business; however, Jonathan did not establish a continuous long-term supervisory relationship to gain feedback and improve his skills. The licensure board concluded that Jonathan violated this particular professional code (ACA Code C.2.a). Another code concerns counselors' practicing in new areas after receiving appropriate training and supervision (Code C.2.b). Jonathan made minimal effort to gain additional skills in online therapy through further training or ongoing supervision. Jonathan did not seek appropriate supervision (Code C.2.d), and Charini was hospitalized for a suicide attempt. This may have been avoided if Jonathan had been receiving supervision and had received feedback about and monitoring of Charini's progress. Last, Jonathan did not appropriately represent his professional qualifications. He inferred he was licensed in Ohio when he was not, but he was licensed in another state (Code C.4.b).

Researchers have noted the importance of having well-defined crisis intervention procedures in place prior to beginning online therapy (Fisher & Fried, 2003; Maheu, 2003). Jonathan and the licensure board agreed that Jonathan should have established crisis intervention procedures locally and informed Charini of what they were and how to use them. The professional literature also notes the importance of appropriate supervision, particularly with such a new form of counseling. Jonathan did provide Charini with a written statement describing how to contact him in the case of an emergency.

The licensure board and Jonathan discussed the application of both virtue ethics and Buddhism to this case. The first concept that possibly applied from virtue ethics is nonmaleficence; Jonathan explained to the licensure board that he intended to help Charini. Jonathan acknowledged he was naïve about the complexity of providing online counseling and neglected to set up crisis procedures and comply with Ohio standards. The board concluded that Jonathan did violate the ethic of nonmaleficence because he was not adequately prepared to provide this new method of counseling, online counseling. Another concept from virtue ethics that applies is beneficence. Charini reported early in her treatment that she was benefiting from the online counseling. However, beneficence requires an analysis of benefit versus risk or harm. The counseling provided by Jonathan helped initially but not later in treatment. Jonathan was not monitoring treatment as closely as he should have. Another component of beneficence is the ability and knowledge necessary to provide the help. Jonathan did not have the skills he needed, nor did he seek supervision to ensure effective online counseling. The board determined that Jonathan violated the concept or principle of beneficence.

A third principle that applies in this case is fidelity. Jonathan did not inform Charini that she was his first online client, nor did he clearly communicate that he was not licensed in Ohio as a counselor. Jonathan acknowledged he did not want Charini to know he was just beginning his practice in online counseling. The last principle that possibly applies is autonomy. Jonathan did provide Charini with information about online counseling and encouraged her to make a free choice in seeking counseling.

Jonathan and the licensure board discussed Buddhist concepts that apply to this case. Charini's choice of seeking to end her life is not consistent with Buddhist practices. Jonathan did not demonstrate right understanding of his client's suffering; this became evident when Charini attempted to commit suicide. Jonathan acknowledged he did not initially meet with Charini in person to assess her symptoms before starting the online therapy. Jonathan did demonstrate right thought with his compassion early in treatment, and Charini felt she was understood. The question is whether Jonathan entered into online counseling before he was fully prepared, which may be interpreted as selfish and not focused on the needs of Charini. Engaging in self-focus violates the concept of right thought. Right livelihood is the last Buddhist concept that applies. Preliminary research suggests that online counseling is effective. So Jonathan did not engage in a violation of right livelihood. If the research had demonstrated that harm results from online counseling, then he may have been considered in violation of this concept.

SUMMARY

The licensure board concluded that Jonathan violated Ohio standards for the practice of counseling. First, he was not licensed to practice in Ohio as a counselor. Second, he violated the Ohio standard of meeting face to face at the initial interview and conducting an assessment. The board concluded that Jonathan engaged in unprofessional conduct and was in violation of expected levels of competence.

The licensure board considered the following disciplinary actions: (a) contacting his state licensure board, informing them of the circumstances, and recommending revocation of his license; (b) imposing a fine; and/or (c) reprimanding him and requiring additional ethics education.

The board and Jonathan recognized the complexity of using a hermeneutic approach in reviewing this case, but ultimately they concluded that it provided the most comprehensive view of the ethical dilemma. In addition, Jonathan concluded he had a much better understanding of how to go about making ethical decisions. The easy, simple solution is not always the most effective or the most useful.

Questions for Further Reflection

1. Do you agree with the board's recommendations, or would you change some or add recommendations?

2. Can you identify elements of the horizon that were not discussed?

3. How would the board's conclusions be different if it had used only virtue ethics or only Buddhist ethics?

4. How did Jonathan's professional ethical identity influence his actions? Was he consistent with his professional ethical identity?

Additional Recommended Readings

Baca, C., Alverson, D., Manuel, J., & Blackwell, G. (2007). Telecounseling in rural areas for alcohol problems. *Alcoholism Treatment Quarterly, 25*(4), 31–44.

Bucky, S., Marques, S., Daly, J., Alley, J., & Karp, A. (2010). Supervision characteristics related to the supervisory working alliance as rated by doctoral-level supervisees. *Clinical Supervisor, 29,* 149–163.

Garrett, T. (2010). The prevalence of boundaries violations between mental health professionals and their clients. In F. Subotsky, S. Bewley, & M. Crow (Eds.), *Abuse of the doctor-patient relationship* (pp. 51–63). London, UK: RCPsych.

Hendricks, C. (2008). Introduction: Who are we? The role of ethics in shaping counselor identity. *Family Journal: Counseling and Therapy for Couples and Families, 16*(3), 258–260.

Larin, H., Geddes, E., & Eva, K. (2009). Measuring moral judgment in physical therapy students from different cultures: A dilemma. *Learning and Health in Social Care, 9*(2), 103–113.

Ponton, R., & Duba, J. (2009). The ACA code of ethics: Articulating counseling's professional covenant. *Journal of Counseling & Development, 87,* 117–121.

SECTION II

ETHICAL ISSUES IN COUNSELING

Chapter 5

CLIENT AUTONOMY AND CLIENT RIGHTS

CHAPTER OBJECTIVES

- Acquire an understanding of informed consent and the importance of informed consent in the counseling process
- Develop an understanding of the concepts of autonomy, beneficence, and fidelity and how they apply in counseling practice
- Develop an understanding of the importance of informed consent and the best methods of obtaining written informed consent
- Develop an understanding of the differences between consent and assent and how they apply to adults and children
- Acquire an understanding of client empowerment and how counselors can actively promote client empowerment
- Develop an understanding of client-counselor complementary relationships that promote client autonomy and self-control

---

Case

Wilma is a 17-year-old Latina who is living at home with her family of five. She is the middle child in the family, with an older sister (age 19) and a younger brother (age 12). She has been referred for counseling by the school nurse. She comes in for the first session to see Jeremy, a school counselor, who is in his late 20s and has been a counselor for 5 years. Jeremy likes working with adolescents and is happy to share his knowledge and experience. Wilma has been dating a Caucasian male for a year, and she comes into the session upset and crying. She states she is pregnant, that she confirmed it with a home pregnancy test. She tells Jeremy that she knows her family will be upset, particularly her mother. She is adamant that she cannot tell her parents. She is considering an abortion and wants a chance to discuss this decision. She knows that the state in which she lives allows adolescents older than 16 to seek a court approval for the abortion without parental approval. The school where Jeremy works promotes a policy of informing parents when students have significant issues such as drug use and pregnancy. Jeremy, on self-reflection, knows he likes to act with a nurturing approach in working with the adolescents in his school. The question is whether this is the correct ethical perspective to take with Wilma.

INTRODUCTION

Individual choice seems to be an important issue, particularly for those from Western countries such as the United States (Savani, Markus, Naidu, Kumar, & Berlia, 2010). Savani et al. (2010) studied perceptions of the importance of individual choice in the United States and India. They found that Americans construed their perceptions of actions as personal choices versus Indians who did not see many actions as personal choice. In another study on choice, Stephens, Markus, and Townsend (2007) found that socioeconomic status played a role in choice perceptions. Those from middle-class families valued personal choice more than those from working-class families. Personal choice is an underlying principle of client autonomy and client rights. There seems to be particularly a significant Western value of personal choice and control. Counselors acting ethically probably should recognize and promote such personal choice.

A discussion of clients' rights may begin with an overview of the philosophical considerations and concepts that apply, such as autonomy, beneficence, and fidelity. Certainly perspectives of client rights can be traced initially to medical treatment and then transferred to psychological and counseling treatment. What are issues that may be included under these philosophical perspectives? Autonomy may include such client rights as informed consent, use of restraints, forced medication compliance, and active participation in treatment planning. Beneficence may include the right to competent treatment, an obligation to help, and a balance between autonomy and beneficence. Fidelity may involve client rights of confidentiality and keeping promises or contracts (treatment plan contracts). Counselor personal needs play a role in the promotion or hindrance of client rights. Understanding one's personal needs, particularly the need for control, is important for acting ethically and fostering client rights.

HISTORY OF INFORMED CONSENT

You may find a historical review of informed consent not overly interesting; however, you may have heard the statement "Those who do not remember history are condemned to repeat it." This statement was a rephrase from American philosopher George Santayana, who stated, "Those who cannot remember the past are condemned to repeat it." We want to review the history of informed consent so, we hope, earlier views that were not based on autonomy are not repeated and implemented today. The history of consent is not just a recent phenomenon (Dalla-Vorgia, Lascaratos, Skiadas, & Garanis-Papadatos, 2001; Faden, Beauchamp, & King, 1986). Consent and informed consent originated within medicine, and therefore they have a relatively long history. One can trace the history of consent back to ancient Greece and Plato. Dalla-Vorgia et al. (2001) described how Plato acknowledged consent before the medical treatment of those who were free, not slaves. Plato would not treat a patient until he had consent from the person. However, Plato did see that his job, in part, was to persuade the patient to participate through providing information about the treatment. Despite believing that he had a responsibility to persuade the client to pursue treatment, Plato did believe that the best course was to obtain client consent prior to treatment. Dalla-Vorgia et al. made the following interpretation of Plato's philosophy: "Knowledge of good is inherent in every human being. . . . The patient knows what is good for him" (p. 59). Treatment after Plato included aspects of consent. For example, there are specific historical examples wherein physicians sought consent to protect themselves from liability in providing medical treatment (Dalla-Vorgia et al., 2001). For example, physicians carefully considered providing medical treatment to leaders of significant stature such as Alexander the Great (300 BCE) and Justin II (mid 500 AD) for fear of retribution if the patient died as part of the medical treatment. Dalla-Vorgia et al. gave an account of how a physician cautiously provided treatment through patient consent. They described how consent was viewed and stated that "the scalpel for the operation should be given to them by the emperor's own hand. That would be a gesture which declared his own free will for the surgical intervention" (p. 60). These early efforts at providing consent and informed consent were based on protection and not necessarily a perspective that patients/clients had rights. The physicians were attempting to protect themselves. More recent history of informed consent may be traced to England in the middle 1700s (Welfel, 1998). Historically the medical profession held a paternalistic attitude based on the view that the patient was not smart enough to make decisions. Henkelman and Everall (2001) noted that a paternalistic view included the following perspectives: information is provided to the patient/client only if it is determined to be necessary, obtaining informed consent is simply pro forma and not a benefit to the patient/client, and too much patient/client knowledge can impede the treatment.

Faden et al. (1986) noted that providing consent and informed consent prior to the 1900s was based on an attempt to obtain compliance, not based on patient rights. It was not until the 20th century that a shift in emphasis was felt in recognizing patient rights as the foundation for ethical action. One of the early judicial decisions promoting consumer rights in the early 1900s was in *Schloendorff v. the Society of the New York Hospital,* which focused on a patient's not giving consent for treatment but treatment's still being provided (http://www.lawandbioethics .com/demo/Main/LegalResources/C5/Schloendorff.htm). Consumer rights were slow to pick up as a practice. The medical profession maintained a paternalistic practice for a long time, until the 1970s. The problem with others' taking responsibility is based on several issues: Patients do not take responsibility for the outcome, and patients may be exploited.

A major impetus for change occurred with medical malpractice. Other influences were medical abuses such as the Nazis' medical experiments and the Tuskegee syphilis study. A number of incidents have contributed to recognition of the importance of providing informed consent during the past century. One of the major contributors was the treatment of patients by the Germans, the Nazis in particular (retrieved from the National Institutes of Health Office of Extramural Research, http://phrp.nihtraining.com/). The Nuremberg War Crimes Tribunal of 1946 provided insight into the importance of providing informed consent prior to participating in medical procedures. The tribunal found 16 German physicians guilty of crimes against humanity. Much of their misconduct was a consequence of not providing informed consent and autonomy to choose to receive treatment. Another medical treatment that contributed to increased monitoring of informed consent concerned the Tuskegee syphilis study, which started in 1932 and ended in 1972. The study initially involved an intention to study 600 African American men, 400 with syphilis and 200 without syphilis. The primary purpose was to study the natural course of syphilis—despite the fact that this information was obtained several years earlier with Caucasian participants. E. Brussgaard (Harrison, 1956) studied untreated syphilis in Caucasians and published his results in 1929 (3 years before the Tuskegee study started). Another study that affected the development of federal guidelines requiring informed consent was the Stanley Milgram study on obedience. The study involved requesting that a participant teach another, a research confederate, and use shock as a negative reinforcement if the learner (research confederate) responded incorrectly (which he or she was instructed to do). The study participant was presented with increasingly higher voltage in shocking the learner. Despite the danger noted in the increasing voltage, many followed the researcher's instructions to continue. When debriefed, these participants were upset that they would be so obedient and potentially harm others.

The medical profession has led the way in promoting informed consent, which has affected how informed consent has been implemented in counseling. By the 1960s, case law was established that gave the right to make informed decisions about patient care. The major case law was *Canterbury v. Spence* (1972). The court concluded that "the duty to disclose is more than a call to speak merely on the patient's request, or merely to answer the patient's questions; it is the duty to volunteer, if necessary, information a patient needs to make an intelligent decision" (http://www.lawandbioethics.com/demo/Main/LegalResources/C5/background01.htm). In 1980 a California court concluded and expanded the case law to state that "informed refusal refers to the physician's obligation to explain medical consequences if patients refuse treatment" (*Truman v. Thomas,* 1980).

There have been several judicial decisions ruling that patients/clients need to be informed particularly about risks of interventions, such as *Leyson v. Steuermann* (1985; http://www.lawandbioethics.com/demo/Main/LegalResources/C5/Leyson.htm) and *Catalano v. Moreland* (2002), which provided a decision on the need for informed consent despite institutional procedures that may be contradictory (http://www.lawandbioethics.com/demo/Main/LegalResources/C5/Catalano.htm). There are exceptions to informed consent, for example, if the patient or client expresses no interest in obtaining information, then the professional is bound to provide it (*Henderson v. Milobsky,* 1978; http://www.lawandbioethics.com/demo/Main/LegalResources/C5/Catalano.htm). Most recently, the Health Insurance Portability and Accountability Act of 1996 provided opportunities for patients to decide whether to disclose health insurance information; this is accomplished through informed consent. We will discuss the Health Insurance Portability and Accountability Act in a later chapter in more detail.

Recently the concept of informed consent has been more clearly defined. Henkelman and Everall (2001) suggested that consent consists of three important components: demonstrated competence for decision making, voluntariness, and understanding. They defined competence as "the ability to decide whether or not to participate in treatment, to withdraw, or continue during the process of treatment" (p. 111). They defined a voluntary decision as "an absence of coercion, either implied or actual" (p. 111). Last, understanding is the "person's degree of discernment regarding the process and ramifications of the treatment being presented" (p. 111). All three elements are necessary in considering the use and application of informed consent.

AUTONOMY

The concept of autonomy may be traced back to Greek terms of self-rule (Beauchamp & Childress, 2008). Beauchamp and Childress (2008) described autonomy as including the following: "self-governance, liberty, rights, privacy, individual choice, liberty to follow one's will, causing one's own behavior, and being one's own person" (pp. 67–68). Autonomy as it relates to informed consent is founded in part on virtue ethical theories. Beauchamp and Childress (2001) also suggested that informed consent is founded on respect for persons and utilitarian theories. Respect for persons (Kantian ethics) suggests that humans are bound by certain duties. In the case of informed consent, professionals are duty bound to openly share information so clients can make informed choices. Whatever duty is demanded of reasonable persons is expected of all. Kant believed that humans should be self-governing and should be able to act autonomously. Utilitarian theory concludes that each person should be able to pursue his or her own interests as long as they do not interfere with others' pursuit of their own interests.

BENEFICENCE

Beneficence is a term as well as a goal that is a foundation of counseling: helping others. The concept of beneficence is defined in terms of looking out for the welfare of others, showing kindness and charity (Beauchamp & Childress, 2008). Tjeltveit (2006) described the central value of beneficence in counseling, stating, "Beneficence is, for many, crucial for professional ethics and, indeed, for the very concept of the profession" (p. 187). An important consideration of beneficence in counseling is the emphasis placed on client needs versus the personal needs of counselors (Tjeltveit, 2006). The counseling profession is based on a view that first and foremost is the welfare of the client; it is the counselor's primary responsibility. The first code in the *ACA Code of Ethics* (American Counseling Association, 2005) states, "The primary responsibility of counselors is to respect the dignity and to promote the welfare of clients" (Section A.1.a, Primary Responsibility).

Beneficence requires that one help if one sees another in distress. Also, the person helping must possess the abilities and skills to help. For example, seeing someone drowning meets the first requirement of having a responsibility to help. However, if one cannot swim, jumping in will only exacerbate the situation by placing more people at risk. Consequently, beneficence must include both conditions: (a) a need for help where there is an obligation to help and (b) an ability to help.

FIDELITY

Fidelity involves keeping a promise or being faithful. Maintaining fidelity with respect to professional activities concerns the types of promises made (Beauchamp & Childress, 2008). In essence, one makes promises that are consistent with the actions and services that are expected of one in that profession. If a counselor promised to bake a cake for a client, the promise would not fall under fidelity. If a counselor did promise to bake a cake and forgot, it would not be an ethical violation because it is not part of his or her occupational services. Fidelity is based on keeping promises around counseling services and not on other, unrelated actions.

WRITTEN INFORMED CONSENT

We have discussed the importance of informed consent, but what is the best approach to use to ensure consent is communicated and understood? Some have suggested that a written statement of informed consent is the best way (Remley & Herlihy, 2005). A related question is, What should be included in providing informed consent? The American Counseling Association's (2005) *ACA Code of Ethics* suggests the following types of information is necessary: (a) the nature of the services; (b) the purpose of the counseling; (c) the goals, techniques, and procedures provided; (d) limitations and possible risks of the services; (e) potential benefits of the services; (f) qualifications and credentials of the counselor; (g) explanation of rights of confidentiality and limitations of confidentiality; (h) fees; and (i) the freedom to participate in counseling.

Fisher and Oransky (2008) proposed several important elements of ensuring an ethical process in providing informed consent and specifically in the case presented here, written informed consent. One consideration is that the written informed consent should be presented in a culturally sensitive manner. This may involve using language that is easily comprehended by the client. In addition, it may mean providing a written consent in the client's native language. The intention is to ensure that the client fully understands and comprehends the extent of the consent. A second consideration is the capacity of the client to give informed consent, specifically with certain populations such as children (Alkhatib, Regan, & Jackson, 2008). Alkhatib et al. (2008) suggested that professionals take extra care to obtain consent (assent) from children and explain the relevant information in providing professional services. For example, they noted that many professionals attempt to pressure a child into agreeing to services once parental consent has been obtained. A challenge for counselors is to encourage a child/adolescent to participate freely. There are circumstances in which an adult with a particular disability does not have the ability or capacity to give informed consent, such as when an adult has a developmental disability or a severe mental illness.

INFORMED CONSENT/ASSENT WITH CHILDREN

Henkelman and Everall (2001) acknowledged that children are not given autonomy because of a perception about their ability to make reasoned decisions. Whereas adults are initially assumed to be competent and able to make reasoned decisions, children and adolescents are assumed to not have such a capacity. Henkelman and Everall described the argument as to why children are not considered competent to make autonomous decisions and stated, "Children have limited cognitive understanding and lack of experience" (p. 111). Recall that one of the key elements of participation in informed consent is competence to give informed consent and give permission to participate. There also is a legal issue around informed consent; children in most states are not able to legally give informed consent before the age of 18. Generally it is accepted that children give assent, which does not carry legal status but recognizes the rights of everyone, including children and adolescents, to agree to participate in treatment. According to *Merriam-Webster's Dictionary* assent may be defined as "agreeing to something after thoughtful consideration" (http://www.merriam-webster.com/dictionary/assent). Assent does not hold the same legal status as consent. The ethical dilemma for counselors is how far to push a child or adolescent in participation in counseling when the parent has given full legal consent. If a parent gives legal consent and a child does not give assent, how should a counselor proceed?

Drotar (2008) suggested that children and adolescents do want information about treatment before making a decision to participate. Vitiello (2008) made the following recommendations for use when considering both informed consent for parents and assent for children/adolescents: (a) review the parent consent and adolescent assent information for length and similarity of information, and ensure understandability; (b) test out the understanding of the adolescent; (c) use assent procedures that promote the relationship; and (d) develop an assent process, and revise it over time based on feedback.

AUTONOMY AND USE OF RESTRAINT: PHYSICAL AND CHEMICAL RESTRAINTS

Those working with individuals with mental illnesses, particularly severe mental illnesses, may be involved in working with clients who experience physical or chemical restraint (Herrera, 2006; Johansson & Lundman, 2002; Webb, 2008).

Certainly, the use of either physical or chemical restraint takes away autonomy of the client; it takes away free will. Johansson and Lundman (2002) concluded that "being treated involuntarily in psychiatric care is a threat to integrity of the patient and this way of treating the patient is one of the worst" (p. 646). Specifically they refer to the use of a four-point restraint. A client experiences four-point restraint as having both wrists and both ankles restrained by leather straps attached to a bed, which is attached to a floor. In addition, the client may be restrained with a strap across his or her chest. This type of treatment is typically done in a secure hospital setting where a client is in danger of injuring himself or herself or injuring others. It has been suggested that the use of four-point restraints affects the client and results in humiliation. One is at the mercy of the medical staff, who make a determination as to when the restraints come off. Investigators have attempted to determine whether coercive treatments such as forced hospitalization have negative impacts such as posttraumatic stress disorder (Meyer, Taiminen, Vuori, Aijala, & Helenius, 1999). Meyer et al. (1999) investigated whether hospitalization resulted in posttraumatic stress disorder. They found that psychotic symptoms themselves actually had more negative impact on the patient than did the hospitalization.

Despite the findings that the symptoms themselves may be more traumatic than being restrained, a question remains as to how much loss of autonomy is ethical in the treatment of those who are experiencing significant mental health problems such as psychosis. Herrera (2006) proposed that whenever possible, advance directives be obtained for treatments such as four-point restraints or forceful use of medication. Obtaining advance directives provides the client with a chance to provide a more reasoned informed consent versus attempting to reason at a time when the client is experiencing significant mental health problems and potentially a psychotic episode. Certainly, the individual may indicate he or she wants to rescind the advance directive, but this can be written into the directive (options to either go ahead or stop the treatment).

EMPOWERMENT AND CLIENT RIGHTS

An underlying theoretical principle that can play an important role in client rights is empowerment. The concept of empowerment has been around for a few decades, and it fits well within the ethical principles of autonomy, beneficence, and fidelity. Empowerment is inherent in the promotion of autonomy. Empowerment is primarily concerned with gaining personal control or power (autonomy; Cattaneo & Chapman, 2010). Cattaneo and Chapman (2010) defined *empowerment* as

> an iterative process in which a person who lacks power sets a personally meaningful goal oriented towards increasing power, takes action toward that goal, and observes and reflects on the impact of this action, drawing on his or her evolving self-efficacy, knowledge, and competence related to the goal. (p. 647)

The ethical behavior of a counselor is to engage in client empowerment and promote the client's personal rights. Consistent with empowerment is the pursuit of client goals and increasing the client's feeling of self-control and impact. A barrier to treatment in counseling may be a client's permanently taking on the sick role, which encourages compliance and is based more on a paternalistic perspective. Using the empowerment process can help to promote client rights. Cattaneo and Chapman proposed an empowerment process. It starts with the client's setting meaningful power-focused goals. This may involve making decisions about treatment choices and plans for future treatment such as advance directives. A second part of the process is changing human interactions that promote power in relationships. Specifically this involves changing the individual's internal frame of reference or how he or she thinks about himself or herself. Changing intrapersonal feelings about power and influence is part of acting ethically and promoting client rights. The last step in the process is carrying out actions and movement toward goals. A concrete example is a client's seeking to make choices in his or her treatment: client rights. Key is the client's being fully informed and the counselor's maintaining commitment to following through.

COUNSELOR NEEDS

The importance of counselor awareness of personal needs and how they affect the counseling process, counseling relationship, and client rights is noted as an important issue in ethical practice (Corey, Corey, & Callanan, 2007; Remley & Herlihy, 2005). A number of issues and needs have been identified that may affect the counseling relationship. These include counselor personal values such as proabortion or antiabortion views. Other counselor values affecting decisions and actions toward clients' rights include values about assisted suicide, criminal behavior such as pedophilia, rape, and sexual orientation. A counselor potentially may lead the flow of the counseling session to support or encourage a change in client attitudes to those that are more consistent with the counselor's own views. This may meet the counselor's need to influence others and in essence control the relationship. Awareness of and reflection on personal needs is a critical step in acting ethically. Unawareness may lead to overt and covert unethical acts.

Need for Control and Affiliation

A recent model of interpersonal interaction is the interpersonal circumplex model, and the structural analysis of social behavior (SASB) model may provide a clear understanding of counselor need for control and affiliation and the ethical issues connected to client autonomy and client rights (Benjamin, 1994; Gurtman

& Lee, 2009; Horowitz et al., 2006; Kiesler, 1983; Markey & Markey, 2010). A primary underlying assumption of both models is that interactions are symmetrical and asymmetrical. The models are based in part on reciprocal emotion. For example, Kiesler (1983), in describing the interpersonal circumplex model, stated, "A person's interpersonal actions tend (with a possibility significantly greater than chance) to initiate, or evoke from the interactant complementary responses that lead to a repetition of the person's original actions" (pp. 200–201).

The interpersonal circumplex model is based on two dimensions and polar opposites. The two dimensions are dominance and affiliation. The poles are dominance-submission and affiliation (friendly)–hostility (aggression). The dominance-submission dimension is on a continuum with dominance at the top of the circle, the y-axis, and submission at the bottom. The friendly-hostile dimension is presented as hostile on the left side of the x-axis and friendly on the right side of the x-axis. Kiesler (1983) associated certain characteristics with each dimension. For example, dominance is associated with controlling, leading, influencing, and taking charge. The opposite pole, submission, is associated with following/complying, being passive, and obeying. Kiesler describes the characteristics on the horizontal dimension of friendly as trusting, generous, warm, and gentle. Characteristics on the opposite pole, aggression, are defined as cold, mistrusting, harsh, and antagonistic.

Horowitz et al. (2006) offered several postulates of the interpersonal circumplex model that are relevant to counselors. One postulate states, "Interpersonal motives may be organized hierarchically" (p. 68). This means that an individual may, for example, emphasize power over friendliness or some other configuration. A second postulate is that "the first expression of communal and agentic motivation appear [*sic*] early in infancy" (p. 69). Horowitz et al. used the term *communal* to refer to the pole of friendly. Also, agentic is consistent with the pole of controlling or an emphasis on the individual's having personal influence. It is interesting that Horowitz et al. postulated that these personality characteristics develop early, during infancy. These characteristics are learned early and carry over into later life. Family dynamics and relationships influence the development of these characteristics. A family that is supportive and provides a child with opportunities to explore likely is promoting agentic feelings, or feelings of control. Another relevant postulate for counselors is the following: "The complement of a behavior is the reaction that would satisfy the motive behind it" (p. 73). An example is a client with a motivation to be cared for who seeks a counselor to act agentic or controlling. The client's passive behavior and motivation are complemented by a counselor's acting strong and influential, meeting the client's needs.

The SASB model (Benjamin, 1994) is an extension of the interpersonal circumplex model and is based on a depiction of three surfaces: interpersonal other, interpersonal self, and intrapsychic. The interpersonal surfaces apply easily to understanding client rights and ethics (see Figure 5.1).

| Figure 5.1 | Structural Analysis of Social Behavior Surfaces |

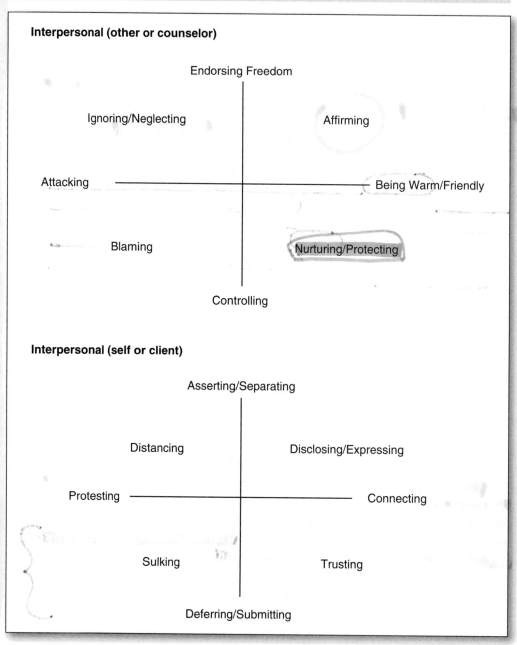

Source: Benjamin (1994).

The SASB model provides a format for thinking about an ethical relationship between the counselor and client. Reflection on how you, as a counselor, fit on the interpersonal (other or counselor) grid can provide direction for ethical behavior. A counselor falling in the upper left part of the grid would be a problem. This type of counselor would be ignoring and neglecting. He or she may simply go through the motions if sessions were scheduled and appear to be uninterested. Such behavior could harm the client and even turn him or her away from pursuing counseling. Also, a counselor acting within this part of the grid may replicate prior relationships, for example, one with a neglectful parent. A counselor acting within the blaming quadrant could be experienced by the client as critical and could blame the client for his or her situation. A counselor acting within the affirming quadrant of the grid (upper right quadrant) could be acting more to promote autonomy and care for a client. The client is likely to experience the counselor as empathic and caring. Ultimately this is the quadrant the counselor wants to reach in the counselor-client relationship because it is theoretically the quadrant that is consistent with the professional orientation and identity of a counselor. Client rights are emphasized the most in this quadrant. Such an orientation may be associated with the person-centered approach of a counselor who recognizes client autonomy and acts in a supportive communal fashion. A counselor's acting within the lower right quadrant, nurturing/protecting, could be a necessary approach early in the counseling relationship for several reasons. A client could need such support because of the intensity of his or her problems. However, a long-term counseling relationship within this section of the grid could promote dependence and hinder client rights.

We mentioned earlier that the SASB is a complementary model, and a counselor-client relationship may be understood within this view. For example, a counselor acting within the nurturing/protecting quadrant in the lower right would be complementary to a client seeking trust and submission. In essence, the client may seek out a relationship in which someone takes care of him or her. Acting ethically and emphasizing client rights and autonomy may not happen as much in the beginning of the counseling relationship, although it can. The counselor may need to be supportive and nurturing and over time encourage more autonomy and freedom within the client. Unfortunately, many counseling relationships end with the counselor's and client's remaining in complementary quadrants of nurturing (counseling) and trusting (client). Such a complementary relationship maintains a dependent relationship style, hindering client autonomy. Also, the counselor is almost guaranteed a client will remain in counseling, a financial benefit, if he or she remains in the lower quadrant of submission. Remember, the goal of counseling from the first session is successful termination; the counselor and client are working to terminate the relationship.

CASE ANALYSIS AND REFLECTION

Reread the case at the beginning of the chapter. Based on what you have read and what you believe to be ethical, what are your thoughts about Jeremy's actions or intended actions? What would you likely do if you were Jeremy? In which quadrant would your actions be displayed on the counselor section of the SASB model?

Questions for Further Reflection

1. Based on personal reflection, which quadrant of the SASB model do you most value and prefer?

2. Which counselor perspective in the SASB model would be most helpful to Wilma in addressing her problem?

3. Which actions do you think the counselor would take if he considered all four quadrants, one at a time, of the other or counselor section of the SASB model? Which response would the client express based on the quadrants of the self or client section of the SASB model?

4. Which of your personal values would potentially affect your counseling (e.g., proabortion, antiabortion, pro–death penalty views)?

Additional Recommended Readings

Cattaneo, L., & Chapman, A. (2010). The process of empowerment. *American Psychologist,* *65*(7), 646–659.

Faden, R., Beauchamp, T., & King, N. (1986). *History and theory of informed consent.* Oxford, UK: Oxford University Press.

Harrison, L. (1956). The Oslo study of untreated syphilis: Review and commentary. *British Journal of Venereal Diseases, 32,* 70–79.

Herrera, C. (2006). Restraint use and autonomy in psychiatric care. *Journal of Ethics in Mental Health, 1*(1), 1–4.

Kiesler, D. (1983). The 1982 interpersonal circle: A taxonomy for complementarity in human transactions. *Psychological Review, 90*(3), 185–212.

Savani, K., Markus, H., Naidu, N., Kumar, S., & Berlia, N. (2010). What counts as a choice? U.S. Americans are more likely than Indians to construe actions as choice. *Psychological Science, 21*(3), 391–398.

Stephens, N., Markus, H., & Townsend, S. (2007). Choice as an act of meaning: The case of social class. *Journal of Personality and Social Psychology, 93*(5), 814–830.

Vitiello, B. (2008). Effectively obtaining informed consent for child and adolescent participation in mental health research. *Ethics & Behavior, 18*(2/3), 182–198.

Chapter 6

DUAL RELATIONSHIPS

BOUNDARY ISSUES

CHAPTER OBJECTIVES

- Acquire knowledge of theories of social roles and how they relate to dual relationships and boundary issues in counseling
- Develop an understanding of psychological, financial, and physical boundaries in counseling and the ethical issues that can arise

---

Case

Carol is a counselor who has a private practice working primarily with adolescent girls who have eating disorders. Carol grew up in a middle-class family. She was diagnosed with anorexia nervosa at the age of 15. She struggled for 2 years with the condition, and she received treatment. Carol returned to a normal weight, and she received counseling that helped her resolve several personal issues.

She lives in a small rural community of about 7,000. Consequently everyone knows everyone else. Carol set up her office in her home; the entrance to her office is separate from the entrance to her primary residence. Carol has a master's degree in clinical mental health counseling, and she completed a course in professional ethics. She graduated 4 years ago, and she has been in private practice for 2 years. Carol is married, and she has a 3-year-old daughter. She lives in a comfortable home in a middle-class community.

Carol recently began counseling with two adolescent girls who are 16 years old. The girls are friends, and both have been diagnosed with an eating disorder, anorexia nervosa. One adolescent, Susan, lives a few blocks from Carol. The second adolescent, Brenda, lives more than a mile from Carol's office.

Carol shops at one of the two major grocery stores, and she has seen both adolescents with their families in the stores. One day when Carol is shopping, she has a large bag of potato chips in her shopping cart. She has several bags of candy and cookies too. One of her 16-year-old clients, Susan, comes by with her mother. She clearly looks into the cart and most likely sees the potato chips, candy, and cookies. Carol and the client exchange greetings and continue shopping. In addition, Carol has an account on Facebook, and she has posted pictures of family events including picnics and large gatherings. Some of the pictures show large amounts of food on tables for the events. One of these two adolescent clients is a friend of a relative, and she has gained access to Carol's Facebook page.

There are several potential ethical boundaries that arise in Carol's counseling with these two adolescents. Social boundaries are a potential ethical issue simply because Carol lives in a small community and she likely will see clients in the community. In this case Carol did come across one of her adolescent clients in a grocery store, and Carol's role as a shopper was the primary relationship in her interaction with the client, Susan. Carol's use of electronic communications (specifically Facebook) opens up another potential ethical issue and boundary problem (a social boundary). Her postings about family outings, particularly those involving food, may initiate a boundary ethical issue with these particular adolescents. What should Carol do in the next counseling sessions with her adolescents who likely may have questions about the new information they have come across in her different social roles as a shopper and Facebook participant? She has several options. She can ignore the issue and hope that Susan and Brenda do not bring up what they know from these other roles. The problem is that both adolescents may lose confidence in her and question her understanding and empathizing with them. Carol can bring up the two role conflicts and discuss with the adolescents how they may affect their relationships. She can discuss what the adolescents saw through the social roles, the food that the adolescents possibly find excessive and in direct conflict with their food intake. She actually may use the exchange to discuss alternative diets and what it means for others. Experiences with crossing these boundaries may be used in counseling to directly address issues; however, one has to be careful not to create such dissonance more directly because a client may perceive this as manipulation. Other options for Carol are more future oriented and involve changing access to her clients within these boundaries. Carol could limit or shut down her Facebook account, and she could find another grocery store in which to do her shopping.

Carol has not disclosed her own personal experience with an eating disorder to either Susan or Brenda. She has been considering sharing the information but wanted to be sure that the disclosure would be helpful to the adolescents. She is wondering whether now is the time to disclose that she had an eating disorder given the recent social boundary disclosures. The question is whether this is a good time or whether it would further the development of dual relationships and complicate the counseling relationship. Carol needs to consider all the information in making decisions about the impact of these cross-boundary dilemmas, which potentially change the clients' view of her in the role of counselor. What are relevant issues for Carol to consider in pursuing ethical professional actions?

INTRODUCTION TO DUAL RELATIONSHIPS

Boundaries of the counselor potentially affect the counseling relationship and may result in ethical problems. These boundaries may include not just physical boundaries that are commonly associated with ethical violations such as sexual contact between counselor and client. Counselor boundaries that potentially affect ethical behaviors, in addition to physical boundaries, include psychological, financial, and social boundaries. Having dual or multiple relationships with clients may or may not be a problem; however, the potential for problems increases (Gabriel, 2005; Zur, 2007). Zur (2007) noted that one problem with dual relationships between client and counselor is the power differential. Inherent in counselors' professional role is their increased level of power and influence. Clients look to counselors for assistance to address significant problems. This power differential creates the risk that a counselor will take advantage of a client, particularly when there are dual relationships. The easiest dual relationship to understand, based on the power differential, is a professional relationship and a sexual relationship. A client, who typically comes into counseling vulnerable and open to influence, may readily agree to more than a professional relationship because he or she wants to be accepted by the counselor. Consequently, a relationship initially based on a professional role may come to include an additional relationship due to the strong influence of the counselor. Essentially the counselor, knowingly or unknowingly, may enter into a sexual relationship based on his or her personal influence on a client; this sets up a significant potential to harm a client.

Zur (2007) noted that one potential source of counselor effectiveness is the power he or she holds as part of his or her role and status. Alternatively, the counselor's power and influence can be used to harm a client, whether or not the counselor knows it. A professional and sexual relationship is only one example of a dual relationship that can harm a client.

The American Counseling Association ([ACA] 2005), in its *ACA Code of Ethics,* and the American Psychological Association (2010), in its *Ethical*

Principles of Psychologists and Code of Conduct, provide insight and direction concerning dual relationships. The ACA codes include standards addressing duals relationships under Section A.5, Roles and Relationships With Clients. Standards cover issues such as sexual relationships and nonsexual relationships. Additional standards address changes in role and the professional relationship. Bartering and fees are covered in Standard A.10. The guidelines developed are designed to reduce harm to the client. Dual relationships may potentially harm a client, but not always (Zur, 2007). Certainly a dual relationship adds concern and potential for harm. Consequently an awareness of and opportunity to avoid dual relationships is desirable. The reality is that avoiding dual relationships in certain circumstances may not be possible. We will discuss other dual relationships and how they can harm a client.

COUNSELOR ROLES

A boundary is based in part on the role the person plays. Social role theory provides insight into how boundaries may be understood (Eagley, 1987). Social role theory initially focused on roles related to gender and position. A basic premise is that people behave differently based on the social role that is currently played. Turner (1990) defined social roles as "a comprehensive pattern of behavior and attitudes, constituting a strategy for coping with a recurrent set of situations, which is socially identified more or less clearly as an entity" (p. 87). Gabriel (2005) defined dual relationships as consisting of those where a counselor has two or more types of relationships with a client concurrently.

Cognitive schemas are associated with social roles (Bussey & Bandura, 1999). Once a counselor walks into his or her office, a cognitive schema should kick in that is characteristic of the behaviors he or she should demonstrate as a professional counselor. Even a hello to another staff member is expressed from a professional perspective. Pearson and Piazza (1997) provided an interesting way to interpret how contexts influence social roles. They identified several types of relationships that affect professionals: circumstantial multiple roles, structured multiple roles, shifts in professional roles, and personal and professional role conflicts. Circumstantial multiple roles occur when the professional and a client meet in an unstructured social setting such as a store. Structured multiple roles can occur in a training setting. Training setting relationships include the relationship between the teacher and student, the role each plays in the relationship. A third possible relationship is a shift in professional roles (Gabriel, 2005). For example, a counselor may change roles by becoming a supervisor. This shift in roles may affect the counselor-client relationship, reducing contact or time spent with a client. A fourth type of relationship is personal and professional role conflicts. This type of conflict may occur in a rural community where personal contact is more likely outside the professional relationship. Seeing a client in a church to which one belongs can create conflict with the professional role: How does the counselor greet the client/church member? Greeting a client in a public setting may unintentionally break confidentiality. For example, a counselor's saying hello to a client at church may prompt a family member to ask the counselor how he or she knows the individual.

Zur (2007) offered another perspective on defining boundaries; he suggested one can differentiate boundaries into two categories: structural elements of the relationship or role and acceptable behavior. Structural elements include boundaries set up through the legal system and professional organizations. Legally counselors are bound, through boundaries, to maintain a relationship that is characterized by activities such as doing no harm, maintaining confidentiality (in compliance with the Health Insurance Portability and Accountability Act), following acceptable billing practices, and so forth. Professional organizations, through ethical codes, provide additional information about boundaries such as confidentiality and the use of informed consent. Acceptable counselor behavior is expected and may include maintaining boundaries around avoiding visiting a client at home (under most circumstances, unless the person is not able to come to an office, e.g., the elderly) or inviting a client into your home. Other examples may include not attending parties with clients. How does one interact with a client in such a setting, in the counselor role or in the personal role as another party attendee? The important question in considering the counselor social role and boundaries is, What should they be?

COUNSELOR SOCIAL BOUNDARIES

Pipes, Holstein, and Aguirre (2005) noted the importance of differentiating professional boundaries from personal boundaries. They cited how professional codes explicitly describe the difference between professional and personal boundaries. Codes can provide guidance around relationships such as those between former clients, students, and employees. For example, personal relationships with such individuals create ethical problems and need to be carefully considered. The *ACA Code of Ethics* (ACA, 2005), states that sexual relationships with former clients or their family members are prohibited for a period of 5 years after the cessation of counseling. The code further provides guidance about personal relationships between counselor supervisors and students (Section F.3.a, Relationship Boundaries With Supervisees), stating, "Counseling supervisors avoid nonprofessional relationships with current supervisees." All of these are examples of potential nonprofessional relationships that could create ethical dilemmas for counselors.

Other counselor social boundaries involve social contact outside the counseling office, in the community, and at activities in public arenas such as the Internet. Living in the community where contact with clients may occur on a frequent basis may create ethical dilemmas. Casual contact at a grocery store or department store is more likely to occur in rural areas or small communities. Such contact can hardly be avoided. However, attending the same health club and belonging to similar community organizations, where there may be ongoing interactions, may create ethical dilemmas because the counselor has intimate knowledge of a client's issues and illustrations of such issues may arise in these community activities. What does the counselor do to avoid letting the information from the counseling session affect what he or she does as a participant in these community organizations? The counselor has a choice of continuing participation, stopping participation, or carefully monitoring his or her reaction to the client in these settings so as not to impart information that is confidential, including even the fact that a client is in counseling.

Another potential ethical concern with social boundaries—boundaries between clients and counselors—can be found in recent advances in technology and ways we now communicate. The use of social networking sites potentially creates ethical issues for counselors (L. Taylor, McMinn, Bufford, & Chang, 2010). L. Taylor et al. (2010) noted the potential for use of a social network that may result in considerable self-disclosure. Self-disclosure on electronic sources may involve extremely personal information such as family information, vacation activities, and even sometimes questionable practices via photos of drinking or other private personal activities. The counselor needs to carefully monitor the use of such electronic mediums to avoid disclosing information that potentially interferes with the counseling process. Such consideration involves a reflection on and assessment of how a client may react to seeing personal information about a counselor such as that showing intimate relationships or recreational activities, including drinking alcoholic beverages.

In regard to counselor and supervisor relationships, several issues may arise. All of the potential ethical issues center on dual relationships. One type of dual relationship that may occur is where the counselor and supervisor interact around roles of counselor and clinical supervisor or counselor and administrative supervisor (Tromski-Klingshirm & Davis, 2007). Tromski-Klingshirm and Davis (2007) suggested that whenever possible supervisors should separate clinical supervision from administrative supervision because of the potential ethical issues with a dual relationship. The dual relationship in providing clinical and administrative supervision arises out of these two distinct roles. Clinical supervision may involve exploration into the counselor's personal issues that interfere with the client-counselor relationship. A supervisor's having such information may create problems if the supervisor serves in a dual role and conducts administrative and evaluative supervision. An evaluation based on personal conflicts disclosed in a different role introduces ethical concerns into the evaluation: Is it a fair evaluation? Tromski-Klingshirm and Davis proposed that the level of trust needed in clinical supervision may be affected if there is such a dual relationship. The solution is to avoid such dual relationships, but if this is not possible, the supervisor needs to be careful and aware of the potential impact of hearing personal information that may affect an administrative evaluation.

PSYCHOLOGICAL BOUNDARIES

Counselor self-disclosure, it has been noted, is a potential problem; it has been defined in terms of boundary violations (Nyman & Daugherty, 2001; Zur, 2007). There have been mixed results with counselors' making self-disclosures in counseling sessions. Those who practice a psychodynamic approach have historically recommended against the use of self-disclosures in counseling or therapy. Freud was an early opponent of counselor or therapist self-disclosure. He believed the counselor should maintain a blank screen to encourage client transference. The more the counselor self-discloses, the greater is the interference in developing the transference, which is a key ingredient in treatment. Another major concern for psychodynamic theorists is that when counselors self-disclose they likely are sharing unresolved issues. Consequently a counselor who shares unresolved issues runs the risk of shifting the focus of counseling from the client to the counselor. In essence the counselor is using the session for his or her own personal therapy and as a chance to address his or her own needs.

Counselor self-disclosure has been defined in various ways. Thomas, Veach, and LeRoy (2006) described counselor self-disclosure as "the act of revealing information about one's self to another individual" (p. 163). Myers and Hayes (2006) defined self-disclosure as "statements that the therapist makes that reveal something personal about the therapist" (p. 174). There have been additional efforts to define and characterize counselor self-disclosure into more specific types (Kim, Hill, Gelso, Goates, Asay, & Harbin, 2003). Cashwell, Shcherbakova, and Cashwell (2003) proposed that two common ways of interpreting counselor self-disclosure are as either a self-disclosing statement or a self-involving statement. Self-disclosing statements are more consistent with the common definition of self-disclosure and involve disclosing facts about the counselor's past and experiences. Self-involving statements refer to a counselor's sharing of cognitions and feelings related to a client, for example, "Hearing your difficult life story makes me feel sad." Counselor self-involving statements have been found to increase client perceptions of expertness and trustworthiness (Danish, D'Augelli, & Hauer, 1980; McCarthy, 1982). Counselor self-disclosure—sharing past experiences and facts—has had mixed results (Barrett & Berman, 2001; Kim et al., 2003).

It has been noted frequently that research into counselor self-disclosure is inconsistent (Nyman & Daugherty, 2001; Thomas et al., 2006). T. Wells (1994) proposed that counselor self-disclosure may burden the client. Clients may feel that they need to help the counselor, who is expressing potentially difficult personal experiences. Consequently the counseling shifts from a focus on the client's needs to a focus on those of the counselor. Wells proposed that counselor self-disclosure may be an attempt to obtain approval from the client. Such efforts may interfere with the client's confidence in the counselor's ability to help. Wells, in a study with participants who had been in counseling/therapy, found that counselor self-disclosure that was based on the counselor's personal history resulted in the client's having questions about the professional abilities of the counselor. There have been other studies that have found the opposite—that counselor self-disclosure increases client perceptions of and confidence in the counselor's expertise. McCarthy (1982) found that counselor self-disclosure using self-involving and self-disclosing statements increased client confidence in the expertise of the counselor.

There clearly are no definitive findings on the impact of counselor self-disclosure and the benefits or harm associated with such self-disclosures. Consequently, counselors need to consider carefully the use of self-disclosures. Guidelines for counselor self-disclosure have been proposed (Mahalik, Van Ormer, & Simi, 2000; Myers & Hayes, 2006). The first guideline is that any counselor self-disclosure should be made with the intent of facilitating the counselor-client relationship. Second, the counselor should reflect and determine whether the disclosure would be made to meet his or her needs versus the client's. Last, the self-disclosure should address the client's needs and the focus of the treatment. These guidelines are a good source for determining when and if to make disclosures to clients. Awareness of the relevance of counselor-client relationships in terms of boundaries is an important consideration in acting ethically.

FINANCIAL BOUNDARIES

There are several issues related to financial boundaries: bartering, fee arrangements, and time management (Woody, 1998; Zur, 2007). Bartering has a long history in human civilization (Zur, 2007); however, the use of state-supported monetary systems has replaced this practice. Zur (2007) defined bartering as "the exchange of goods and services" (p. 90). Bartering in counseling may be an ethical issue because one moves from a professional counseling relationship to a financial one. Setting up a barter based on a service, for example, may create a situation in which the counselor becomes a manager of services (evaluating the quality of the service). This can change the relationship and may affect the counselor's feelings toward the client; he or she may become angry if the service is not performed to his or her expectations (Zur, 2007). One example is providing the service of cleaning the counselor's office in exchange for counseling. The client may not perform the cleaning well, and this may create a problem in the relationship. Another type of bartering may involve the exchange of goods for counseling. The problem still may be a change in the relationship and role (a financial role). There may be a question about the fairness of the exchange. The counselor's status creates an imbalance of power, and the client may feel he or she cannot fairly negotiate a reasonable price for a particular good that is being considered in exchange for counseling. For example, the counselor needs a set of specialty tires, and the client has them. How can there be a fair decision about the number of sessions and the value of the tires? This is an important question and is not easy to determine. Here again, the counselor acts outside his or her role (i.e., dual role and relationship) and becomes an expert on tires.

The *ACA Code of Ethics* (ACA, 2005) states that the counselor may engage in bartering only if the relationship is not exploitive and does not give the counselor an unfair advantage. The dilemma for the counselor is how not to exploit the client when a dual relationship occurs as a consequence of engaging in bartering. One solution is to engage another party who negotiates the terms of the bartering and takes on the financial role.

Another financial ethical issue with dual relationships concerns loaning clients money. One can see that loaning clients money creates a dual relationship (counselor and a loan officer?). There are several problems that may occur. One is that the client may feel indebted to the counselor, and this may affect the client's decision to continue counseling (Zur, 2007). The client may continue in counseling even though he or she is not receiving a benefit because he or she feels this debt. Another issue is a client's not paying back the loan and the problems that this creates for the client. A possible outcome of the client's not having the money to pay back the loan is the client's disappearing and not returning to counseling for fear of retribution from the counselor.

COUNSELOR PHYSICAL BOUNDARIES

Physical boundaries in counseling most frequently are identified as those involving the most severe types of violations such as a sexual relationship between a client and counselor. There are several other types of physical boundaries that are relevant to note when considering ethical issues in counseling. These include the use of nonsexual touch in counseling and the physical space where counseling occurs (Zur, 2007).

Zur (2007) suggested that physical touch in counseling between the client and counselor is quickly associated with sexual contact. He stated, "Touch in therapy has probably been the most controversial of all boundary crossings because of the cultural and professional associations of touch and sexuality" (p. 167). He noted that culture plays a role in the interpretation and implications of touch in counseling/therapy. Compared to other boundaries, touch involves a clear boundary, the body. Zur suggested that there has been debate about what constitutes sexual and nonsexual touch. For example, one interpretation regards the location of the touch, and another concerns the intent of arousal in sexual touch. There are treatments in therapy and counseling that involve touch, such as Reichian therapy. The approach is based on a holistic view and a connection between the body and the mind. Zur provided a detailed differentiation of nonsexual touch (pp. 173–174):

- ritualistic gestures such as handshaking;
- conversational markers that may be expressed through a touch on the arm or shoulder to make a point;
- consolatory touch that may involve touching/holding the hand or touching the arm/shoulder to console the person;
- reassuring touch involving a touch to reaffirm the person and encourage him or her, possibly on the arm or shoulder;
- playful touch involving touch with a child or adolescent while playing a game;
- grounding or orienting touch, which refers to touch on the arm or hand to assist the client in reducing anxiety or affirming the here and now; and
- task-oriented touch involving assistance in getting up from a chair or preventing the client from falling.

Researchers have noted the importance of touch for humans, and it has been found to be associated with attachment (Bowlby, 1969; Harlow, 1958). Research supports the inherent need of humans to have touch and contact with other humans. However, Zur (2007) noted that culture plays an important role in how touch is expressed. He noted that North Americans are somewhat hesitant in the use of touch. Zur proposed that Americans tend to avoid touch because there can be easy misunderstandings of the intent of touch, for example, sexual intentions.

The important question is, What do the research and attitudes toward touch suggest for counselors and the maintenance of boundaries in counseling? Zur (2007) noted that touch can best be understood and interpreted based on the context. For example, categorizing touch based on nonsexual touch (e.g., reassuring touch, task-oriented touch) can provide the counselor with guidelines for determining the boundaries associated with touch between a counselor and client. Certainly ritualistic touching such as handshaking at the beginning of a counseling session is appropriate. However, handshakes between male counselors and female clients or female counselors and male clients who are Hassidic Jews would be inappropriate (men and women do not shake hands due to the belief that the body is sacred and not open to touching). Playful touch in counseling may be rarely used. Playful touch may involve hitting another on the arm or a giving a high five. Such actions are not generally within the role of a professional counselor. Task-oriented touch may be appropriate, for example, when assisting someone who is blind or visually impaired, one may act as a guide and provide the person/client with one's arm/elbow. Touch may be easily misunderstood, and use of touch in a counseling session should be done with caution. Counselor awareness of and attention to timing and cultural views about touch should be considered when establishing such boundaries.

Another type of physical boundary is the space that is used for counseling (Schlachter, 1975). Schlachter (1975) noted benefits of and issues with home counseling visits. Certainly observing a client in the home provides information about the interactions within a family, which may be beneficial in understanding potential issues to address in counseling. However, caution should be taken to reduce the impact of being perceived in other roles such as a visiting friend rather than a counselor. Visiting a client's home may encourage the feeling that the relationship is more like a friendship than a professional relationship between a client and counselor. The benefits include the following: The counselor can see the environment where the client lives, the client may be more comfortable, and assessment of the family in a natural environment can be made. Furthermore, Schlachter cited the following issues: There is a reduction in client privacy, the counselor's arriving on time may be difficult with traffic congestion, and frequent interruptions can occur outside a controlled environment. The traditional office space in a professional building provides the clearest boundary, for example, the focus is on counseling and the professional relationship. However, other counseling space can include a counselor's home office, home visits to a client's residence, and community space such as a park or coffee shop. The use of a home office creates an opportunity for the client to see the counselor in another environment that may open up conversations unrelated to counseling and the professional

WARNING

relationship. Counselors who have home office space without direct access to the office from the outside potentially open up opportunities for clients to ask questions about family and other aspects of a counselor's life. Some may question why this is a problem, but the lifestyle of the counselor may provide the client with information that creates either positive or negative feelings toward the counselor that are unrelated to the counseling relationship, for example, opulent furnishings. Also, the tidiness of the home may give the client further information that may affect the counseling relationship. Others may argue that such sharing of private counselor information shows the professional in a more genuine light. If the counselor chooses to set up a home office, awareness of such issues should be considered, and an awareness of the potential impact on the counseling relationship should be reviewed.

Seeing clients in other public spaces, such as coffee shops, opens up issues of confidentiality and privacy. A counselor's seeing a client in a coffee shop may open up the possibility that others who know the client or the counselor may enter the coffee shop and start up a conversation. The problem occurs when there is an expectation communicated that the counselor or client be introduced to the third party. How are introductions made? How do they know each other? Another issue is one of confidentiality and talking in an open environment like a coffee shop. A coffee shop opens up opportunities for others to hear confidential information. Also, the client may express intense emotions, and this may create problems; the client may be angry at being vulnerable in a public setting.

A formal office space limits ethical problems and reduces the chances that dual relationships will occur. However, there are circumstances wherein meetings in the community or the client home are the most practical. A client may not be able to get to the office due to transportation issues. A client may have a disorder such as an anxiety disorder that makes coming to an office too stressful. Adolescents may not particularly like coming to a counseling office, so providing an alternative site such as a park or a coffee shop in the community may address this population's needs. Providing counseling in a space other than an office (separate from a counselor's home) shows the counselor has reflected on and is aware of how dual relationships may create ethical dilemmas and how best to reduce the impact.

SUMMARY

Boundaries and dual relationships pose potential ethical dilemmas for counselors. We can insert understanding of boundaries in the hermeneutic model in the counselor, client, and supervisor elements (see Figure 4.1 in Chapter 4). Each has specified social roles and expectations about boundaries and dual relationships.

There are several counselor boundaries that potentially affect ethical behaviors: physical, psychological, financial, and social boundaries. Understanding the professional counselor role is the first step in addressing possible ethical issues with dual roles and boundary issues. Counselors are entrusted through the public, licensure laws, and professional organizations to act professionally and behave according to a counselor role that is founded on doing no harm, maintaining confidentiality (in compliance with the Health Insurance Portability and Accountability Act), following acceptable billing practices, and so forth. Social boundaries that the counselor wants to monitor include social contact outside the counseling office, contact in the community, and contact through activities in public arenas such as the Internet. A psychological boundary and dual relationship may involve counselor self-disclosure. There are two ways of interpreting counselor self-disclosure: as a self-disclosing statement or a self-involving statement. Self-disclosing statements are defined as more consistent with the common definition of self-disclosure and involve disclosing facts about the counselor's past and experiences. Self-involving statements are the counselor's sharing of cognitions and feelings related to a client—here-and-now statements. Such self-disclosures create boundary issues and dual relationships, and the counselor may become the client by addressing his or her own personal issues. Carefully monitoring and reflecting on the use of self-disclosure is necessary to avoid ethical issues and problems. What impact will the disclosure have, and what is the intent of the disclosure?

Case Analysis and Reflection

Reread the case at the beginning of the chapter. What are your thoughts about Carol's disclosing her personal history with an eating disorder? Are there really any major concerns with violating psychological boundaries such as those presented in this case? If there are boundary issues in this case, what can be done to reduce any negative impact?

Questions for Further Reflection

1. Which social roles that you value and engage in, such as the use of electronic communications (e.g., Facebook), do you think may affect your counseling relationship? Do you consider such relationships dual relationships?

2. What is your definition of the counselor role, and what are the parameters/ boundaries of the counselor role?

3. What would you be willing to self-disclose? What are your psychological boundaries in terms of disclosure of personal experiences in a counseling session? What might be the psychological circumstances of the self-disclosure?

4. What are your boundaries around physical touch? What roles do age, gender and/or race/ethnicity play in the use of physical touch?

Additional Recommended Readings

Barrett, M., & Berman, J. (2001). Is psychotherapy more effective when therapists disclose information about themselves? *Journal of Consulting and Clinical Psychology, 69*(4), 597–603.

Cashwell, C., Shcherbakova, J., & Cashwell, T. (2003). Effect of client and counselor ethnicity on preference for counselor self disclosure. *Journal of Counseling & Development, 81,* 196–201.

Eagley, A. (1987). *Sex differences in social behavior: A social-role interpretation.* Hillsdale, NJ: Lawrence Erlbaum.

Gabriel, L. (2005). *Speaking the unspeakable: The ethics of dual relationships in Counselling and psychotherapy.* New York, NY: Routledge.

Kim, B., Hill, C., Gelso, C., Goates, M., Asay, P., & Harbin, J. (2001). Counselor self-disclosure, East Asian American client adherence to Asian cultural values and counseling process. *Journal of Counseling Psychology, 50*(3), 324–332.

McCarthy, P. (1982). Differential effects of counselor self-referent responses and counselor status. *Journal of Counseling Psychology, 29*(2), 125–131.

Myers, D., & Hayes, J. (2006). Effects of therapist general self-disclosure and countertransference disclosure on ratings of the therapist and session. *Psychotherapy: Theory, Research, Practice, Training, 45*(2), 173–185.

Nyman, S., & Daugherty, T. (2001). Congruence of counselor self-disclosure and perceived effectiveness. *Journal of Psychology, 135*(3), 269–276.

Taylor, L., McMinn, M. R., Bufford, R., & Chang, K. (2010). Psychologists' attitudes and ethical concerns regarding the use of social networking web sites. *Professional Psychology: Research & Practice, 41*(20), 153–159.

Thomas, B., Veach, P. M., & LeRoy, B. (2006). Is self-disclosure part of the genetic counselor's clinical role? *Journal of Genetic Counseling, 15*(3), 163–177.

Tromski-Klingshirm, D., & Davis, T. (2007). Supervisees' perceptions of their clinical experience: A study of the dual role of clinical and administrative supervision. *Counselor Education & Supervision, 46,* 294–304.

Turner, R. (1990). Role change. *Annual Review of Sociology, 16,* 87–110.

Woody, R. (1998). Bartering for psychological services. *Professional Psychology: Research and Practice, 29*(2), 174–178.

Zur, O. (2007). *Boundaries in psychotherapy: Ethical and clinical explorations.* Washington, DC: American Psychological Association.

Chapter 7

COUNSELOR COMPETENCE

CHAPTER OBJECTIVES

- Develop an understanding of the components of counselor competence such as functional and foundational competence
- Develop an understanding of how to monitor possible counselor impairment
- Acquire an understanding of the developmental stages of counselor competence
- Acquire an understanding of the importance of continuing education and continued professional development

---

Case

John is a 2nd-year master's student in a rehabilitation counseling program. He wants to work in the state vocational rehabilitation system when he graduates. John has started an internship at a state vocational rehabilitation office. His supervisor, Dave, has 3 years of experience, and he is about the same age as John. Although Dave has only 3 years of experience, he presents as very confident and somewhat brash. He does not speak well of his colleagues in the office, and he suggests they are not as competent as he. The state has purchased a new caseload-monitoring software program to assist the counselors in tracking client progress. Dave has discounted the importance of using this new system, stating that he does not need a computer to help him know what his clients are doing. Other rehabilitation counselors in the office have embraced the new software system, and they are using it regularly. John feels he will lose out if he does not have an opportunity to learn such software programs, particularly because he wants to work in the system after graduation.

John is assigned several clients, and he wants to begin entering information into the software system, but Dave does not take the time to teach him the new system. John decides to talk with another rehabilitation counselor who is the most expert at using the software program; Dave observes their interaction. Dave chides John about working with this "geek" counselor. He asks John if he has difficulty with his memory and cannot track clients the old-fashioned way. John does not want to alienate his supervisor, but he realizes he needs to acquire skill in using the caseload-tracking program. The question for John is whether to possibly alienate his supervisor to obtain necessary and important competence in the use of technology so he can provide the best services for clients or to learn the software just through trial and error without learning the necessary skills.

INTRODUCTION

Competence is certainly a critical consideration in the practice of a profession such as counseling, and there are ethical issues that are associated with counselor competence. Counselor competence fits within the hermeneutic model of ethical decision making on the "Counselor values, race, professional identity, etc." element (see Chapter 4, Figure 4.1). There are several ways to define and consider competence. In addition, competence may be understood in terms of those in training and those in practice. One perspective on competence was provided by Rodolfa et al. (2005), who stated, "Competency is generally understood to mean that a professional is qualified, capable, and able to understand and do certain things in an appropriate and effective manner" (p. 348). Simply acquiring or having the characteristics of being qualified, capable, and so forth does not guarantee competence, because the professional must act or carry out competent behavior. Acting competently includes having the capacities of critical thinking and good decision making (Rodolfa et al., 2005). R. Epstein and Hundert (2002) defined *competence* as "the habitual and judicious use of communication, knowledge, technical skills, clinical reasoning, emotions, values, and reflections in daily practice for the benefit of the individual and community being served" (p. 227). Both definitions of *competence* are founded on the belief that competence is developmental and is continuous. Epstein and Hundert incorporated the foundational components proposed by Rodolfa et al. (2005), for example, the relevance of reflections and the use of clinical reasoning.

M. Roberts, Borden, Christiansen, and Lopez (2005) noted the importance of beginning professionals' embracing a culture of competence based initially on self-assessment and self-reflection. A culture of competence is founded on a view of developing a routine and systematic approach to ensuring a high level of quality and effectiveness. Such a culture of competence is one that is developmental and continuous from the beginning of training until the professional retires or leaves counseling practice. There need to be multiple levels of assessment beginning with counselors who are training and extending to seasoned professionals and practitioners (M. Roberts et al., 2005). The multiple levels of assessment need to include self-assessment, supervisor assessment, peer assessment, and for those in training, faculty assessment. All of these methods of assessment should begin during the professional training.

Professional codes of ethics describe the importance of an overall level of competence for a particular counseling position. Code D.1.c of the Commission on Rehabilitation Counselor Certification ([CRCC] 2009) states, "Rehabilitation counselors accept employment for positions for which they are qualified by education, training, supervised experience, professional credentials and appropriate professional experience." The American Counseling Association's ([ACA's] 2005) *ACA Code of Ethics,* Standard C.2.c, Qualified for Employment, states, "Counselors accept employment only for positions for which they are qualified by education, training, supervised experience, state and national professional credentials and appropriate experience." The standards are essentially the same and note the importance of accepting employment for which one is qualified.

Rodolfa et al. (2005) offered a systematic method of thinking about competence and suggested a "cube model" of competence. This model incorporates several functional competency domains that are relevant in understanding counselors' competency activities: assessment/diagnosis, intervention, consultation, research/ evaluation, supervision/teaching, and management/administration. Functional competencies concern what the counselor may do or how he or she may act in practice. They also proposed several foundational competencies that are relevant for counseling: ethical/legal understanding, cultural diversity, and reflective practice. Foundational competencies concern the development of certain attitudes or internal frames of reference or understanding by the counselor: professional identity and professional ethical identity.

FOUNDATIONAL COMPETENCE

Self-Reflection

Belar et al. (2001) suggested relevant questions for self-reflection on competence. Examples of relevant questions for beginning counselors to consider in regard to competence are the following (adapted from Belar et al., 2001):

- Do I have knowledge of the problem?
- Do I have knowledge of how to assess the problem?

- Do I have the skills and knowledge to implement interventions?
- Do I have the knowledge of any ethical or legal issues in regard to the problem?
- Do I understand the problem in relation to the environment, including family issues?

As has been noted above, the following are foundational competencies that are relevant for counseling: ethical/legal understanding, cultural diversity, and reflective practice. There are other considerations in foundational competence and self-awareness such as counselor wellness or impairment. A counselor needs to be aware of any personal issues or problems that may affect or impair his or her level of competence. Professional codes of ethics offer guidelines for self-awareness of impairment. The *ACA Code of Ethics*'s Standard C.2.g states,

> Counselors are alert to the signs of impairment from their own physical, mental, or emotional problems and refrain from offering or providing professional services when such impairment is likely to harm a client or others. They seek assistance for problems that reach the level of professional impairment, and, if necessary, they limit, suspend, or terminate their professional responsibilities until such time it is determined that they may safely resume their work. (ACA, 2005)

American Association for Marriage and Family Therapy ([AAMFT] 2001) Standard 3.3 states, "Marriage and family therapists seek appropriate professional assistance for their personal problems or conflicts that may impair work performance or clinical judgment." American School Counselor Association Standard E.1.b addresses self-awareness and states, "Monitor emotional and physical health and practice wellness to ensure optimal effectiveness. Seek physical or mental health referrals when needed to ensure competence at all times" (2010). CRCC (2009) Standard D.3, Functional Competence, Subsection a, Impairment, states, "Rehabilitation counselors are alert to the signs of impairment from their own physical, mental or emotional problems."

Counselor burnout and counselor impairment certainly can affect counselor competence. Several definitions of *counselor burnout* have been offered (Maslach & Jackson, 1981; Maslach, Schaufeli, & Leiter, 2001; Osborn, 2004). Osborn (2004) defined *counselor burnout* as "the process of physical and emotional depletion resulting from conditions at work or, more concisely, prolonged job stress" (p. 319). Maslach et al. (2001) described *job burnout* as "a psychological syndrome in response to chronic interpersonal stressors on the job. Three key dimensions of this response are an overwhelming exhaustion, feelings of cynicism and detachment from the job, and a sense of ineffectiveness and lack of accomplishment" (p. 399). One can see that a counselor's having any of these three symptoms of burnout can significantly affect his or her competence. A counselor who is exhausted is not able to perform basic counseling functions. A related concept is counselor fatigue (Stebnicki, 2008). Stebnicki (2008) described counselor fatigue as "a state of psychological, emotional, mental, physical, spiritual, and occupational exhaustion" (p. 3; see Table 7.1). Counseling requires great concentration and focus, and a counselor who is not able to attend because of exhaustion is not going to be effective or competent. Also, a counselor who is cynical or detached from completing job tasks will perform ineffectively and not perform competently; the basic skills of communicating empathy require a connection with a client. Finally, a counselor who feels incompetent may show little motivation for working with a client and attempting to help and bring about change. He or she may just go through the motions and perform minimally the essential functions of counseling. The professional counselor needs to monitor and develop a sensitivity to all three symptoms if they arise. As noted in the *ACA Code of Ethics* (ACA, 2005), if a counselor experiences such impairment, he or she needs to terminate treatment with clients until receiving his or her own tre atment and recovering from any significant personal impairments.

Another issue under counselor self-awareness is counselor professional presentation. Counselor presentation includes how the counselor dresses. This may seem to be an unusual area to include under self-awareness, but physical presentation has been connected to perceptions of competence (Johnson, Podratz, Dipboye, &

Table 7.1 Characteristics of Counselors Who Experience Burnout

Counseling Conditions	Characteristics
Crisis counseling	Counselors who engage in crisis counseling services are at a higher risk for burnout and counselor fatigue syndrome. Symptoms include mood disorders, substance abuse, and marital problems.
Client satisfaction	Higher levels of client satisfaction are related to lower levels of counselor burnout/counselor fatigue syndrome.
Supervision	Counselors who report good supervision indicate they have lower levels of counselor burnout/counselor fatigue syndrome.
Counselor ego development	Counselors who have higher levels or ego development or feelings of self-efficacy report lower levels of counselor burnout/counselor fatigue syndrome.

Source: Adapted from Stebnicki (2008).

Gibbons, 2010). The appearance of the counselor potentially provides information to the client about the competence of the counselor. A counselor who presents as well dressed may communicate to the client a level of competence and expertness. On the contrary, a counselor who dresses poorly may communicate less competence. The context or setting in which the counselor works provides a good reference for how the counselor may best present as competent. Work in a substance abuse residential facility may involve less formal dress, whereas an outpatient counseling center may expect more formal dress. In addition to formal and informal dress, there is the issue of presenting as competent when one dresses more provocatively. Self-awareness of personal dress and what is communicated to a client is important in presenting and acting competently.

FUNCTIONAL COMPETENCE

Assessment

Assessment is a first step in the counseling process. One needs to have a good understanding of the problem(s) that the client brings into sessions. There is a range of assessments that may be used to develop an understanding of a client's problems. The various types of assessment require different skills and knowledge. Some require significant advanced, graduate-level training whereas the administration of others is not as complex. Krishnamurthy et al. (2004) noted the complexity of completing psychological assessment. These authors conceptualized assessment as a problem-solving process and not just a technical administration of assessment instruments. Consequently, a counselor's competence in administering assessments involves the development of complex decision-making skills. Krishnamurthy et al. identified the key competencies in assessment. These include a basic understanding of psychometric theory; the ability to assess outcomes of treatment or interventions; an understanding of the connection between assessment, interventions, and treatment planning; and technical skills such as case conceptualization, communication of findings, and data collection.

Professional ethics codes provide further direction for acting ethically and competently in using assessments. The *ACA Code of Ethics* (ACA, 2005) includes a standard focused on competence and assessment. Standard E.2.a, Limits of Competence, states, "Counselors utilize only those testing and assessment services for which they have been trained and are competent." Another professional code, the *Code of Professional Ethics for Rehabilitation Counselors* (CRCC, 2009), notes the importance of competence in using assessments. Code G.4, Limits of Competence, states, "Rehabilitation counselors utilize only those testing and assessment services for which they have been trained and are competent." The

AAMFT (2001) provides guidelines for family therapists around assessment: Standard 3.11 states, "Marriage and family therapists do not diagnose, treat or advise on problems outside the recognized boundaries of their competencies." All professional counseling ethical standards provide clear direction and note the importance of using assessments only when one is trained and competent to administer.

Interventions

Functional competence with interventions concerns the counselor's selecting, using, and implementing counseling strategies/interventions. Spruill et al. (2004) suggested a developmental model of using and selecting interventions; they proposed significant differences in definitions of levels of competence. A novice counselor who is completing an initial practicum clearly does not have advanced skills and knowledge in implementing interventions compared to a seasoned counselor with decades of experience. Spruill et al. (2004) described how a beginner or novice who has limited knowledge of counseling strategies/interventions uses basic principles and techniques that are "rule bound" and not flexible or based on clinical judgment (see Table 7.2). Advanced beginning counselors begin to recognize patterns of behavior beyond basic principles and begin to generalize to new situations (Spruill et al., 2004). A third developmental stage is when the counselor is able to see long-term goals and how to design interventions to reach these goals. A fourth developmental stage is when the counselor uses a holistic approach and demonstrates a good understanding of the principles and interventions that are appropriate. At this level of development the counselor is able to train and impart information to others. The last stage of development, the expert level, is where the counselor has an intuitive understanding of the problem, assessing the situation quickly and beginning appropriate interventions. Needed changes are made easily and quickly to adjust to the situation.

Spruill et al. (2004) described how the selection of an intervention is closely linked to competence. Selection of an intervention that is matched to the assessment and problems identified is an important skill. The counselor develops treatment plans based on identified goals and objectives. The competence of the counselor is in developing appropriate treatment plans, goals, and objectives and in matching goals and objectives to assessments and problems identified. Another aspect of competence in completing an intervention is the communication of the theories and techniques to the client (Spruill et al., 2004).

Professional codes of ethics, such as the *ACA Code of Ethics* (ACA, 2005), provide specific guidelines concerning counselor competence. Standard C.2.a, Professional Competence, states that "counselors practice only within the boundaries

Table 7.2	Counselor Skill Development Stages

Counselor Stage of Development	Characteristics and Skill Acquisition
Novice or beginner stage	The beginning counselor has limited knowledge and understanding of the analysis of client problems.
Advanced beginner stage	The advanced beginner counselor has acquired the knowledge, skills, and experience to begin recognizing patterns of behavior in a single situation but is not able to generalize to new situations.
Competence stage	The counselor is aware of long-term goals for the client and is able to adapt interventions to meet the plans/goals.
Proficient counselor stage	The counselor has a clear understanding of client problems and how interventions may be applied. The counselor also has an understanding of subtle issues in applying counseling interventions.
Expert-level counselor stage	The counselor has an intuitive understanding of each client situation and case. He or she can quickly assess the problem and develop appropriate interventions. He or she is able to adapt and alter interventions as needed.

Source: Adapted from Spruill et al. (2004).

of their competence, based on their education, training, supervised experience, state and national professional credentials, and appropriate professional experience." Important elements relevant in determining competence are types of training and supervised experience. These are key in determining competence. Accredited counseling programs seek to provide counseling students with systematic training through coursework followed by intense supervision. Professional counselors who no longer are in graduate programs may still obtain needed supervision when learning new skills and techniques. It is important to note that the professional counselor should seek appropriate supervision until both the supervisor and the counselor are confident that the counselor has acquired the necessary competence to practice.

It is clear that beginning counselors do not have the advanced skills of more seasoned counselors in selecting and implementing interventions. Does this mean that beginning counselors are acting unethically because they are not demonstrating advanced competence in implementing interventions? One cannot expect a beginning counselor to have the same skills as a seasoned counselor. Providing appropriate supervision to beginning counselors is necessary to ensure appropriate levels of competence. There is a discussion of the relevance of using and providing competent supervision in Chapter 10. Both training models and licensure/certification procedures are founded on receiving necessary supervision to ensure appropriate levels of competence. It is the responsibility of the counselor (including the beginning counselor, midlevel experienced counselor, and experienced counselor) to obtain and use supervision as is developmentally appropriate.

Consultation

Consultation is another functional type of competence, and professional associations have indicated that it is an essential function of counseling. *ACA Code of Ethics* (ACA, 2005) Standard D.2.a, Consultation competency, states, "Counselors take reasonable steps to ensure that they have the appropriate resources and competencies when providing consultation services. Counselors provide appropriate referral resources when requested or needed." Definitions of *consultation* vary and are somewhat specific to different counseling professions. CRCC defined *consultation* as "the application of scientific principles and procedures in counseling and human development to provide assistance in understanding and solving problems that the consultee may have in relation to a third party, be it individual, group or organization" (CRCC, 2009, p. 2). Consultation involves interaction with other professionals or family members to identify solutions to problems. The counselor is the expert who is sharing his or her knowledge with others to help in the treatment of an identified client. Competencies in consultation involve knowledge of different models such as mental health, behavior, organization, and so forth (Hall & Lin, 1994). Also, the consultant must have knowledge of the issue that has arisen and is identified. A client issue of substance abuse requires that the consultant is in essence an expert in the area. Generally the consultant interacts with the consultee based on an equal professional relationship. The counselor-client relationship is hierarchical, but the consultant-consultee relationship is an egalitarian one. Consequently, there is a different type of interaction that occurs; it is more of a collaborative relationship in problem solving. Competence involves an understanding of developing a collaborative relationship in problem solving around an area of counseling in which the counselor is an expert.

MAINTAINING KNOWLEDGE AND SKILLS: CONTINUING EDUCATION

You likely have a primary care physician and a general practice dentist. You may have a lawyer you use. An assumption you make about these professionals is that they maintain their knowledge and skills and are most current in their practice. Certainly you do not want to see a professional who is not competent, and one consideration of competence is that the professional maintains his or her knowledge and skills. The same is true for professional counselors. The *ACA Code of Ethics* (ACA, 2005) states,

> Counselors recognize the need for continuing education to acquire and maintain a reasonable level of awareness of current scientific and professional information in their fields of activity. They take steps to maintain competence in the skills they use, are open to new procedures, and keep current with their diverse populations and specific populations with whom they work.

The CRCC (2009) code of ethics describes the importance of continuing education; Standard D.1.e, Continuing Education, states, "Rehabilitation counselors recognize the need for continuing education to acquire and maintain a reasonable level of awareness of current scientific and professional information in their fields of activity." AAMFT's (2001) Standard 3.1 states, "Marriage and family therapists pursue knowledge of new developments and maintain competence in marriage and family therapy through education, training, or supervised experience."

Fifty states plus the District of Columbia and Puerto Rico have counselor licensure laws. Each has a requirement of continuing education to maintain a license. There is variation in the number of continuing education units required during a specified period of time before renewal of a license. Consequently there is a mandatory requirement for maintaining one's counseling skills. The question for counselors is, What types of continuing education are most appropriate and helpful to maintain one's skills and knowledge (Neimeyer, Taylor, & Wear, 2010)? Wilcoxon and Hawk (1990) stated that continuing education includes activities such as attending workshops, brief presentations, and formal courses. There are numerous opportunities for continuing education (through the ACA, etc.), and the counselor should consider which skills and what knowledge he or she wants to maintain or improve. Taking graduate-level classes is another way to accomplish advancement of knowledge and skills and can serve as continuing education.

An important consideration is the development of new skills and techniques. New fads and approaches are developed and proposed, and counselors need to be cautious about jumping on the bandwagon of such fads. One example in counseling that resulted in problems was the introduction of recovered memory interventions (S. Smith et al., 2003). Counselors, psychologists, and social workers developed techniques, mostly using regressive hypnosis, to "recover" memories of abuse that adults supposedly had during childhood. There has been considerable debate about and identification of problems with such techniques; clients were highly suggestible and the techniques produced many false memories (Meyersburg,

Bogdan, Gallo, & McNally, 2009; S. Smith et al., 2003). When considering new interventions, key in the practice of counseling is the use of evidence-based research (Houser, 2009). Houser provided a description of evidence-based practice and stated that it is about "the best available research and thoughtfulness in selecting practices to be used" (p. 82). Mayer (2004) identified six steps in implementing evidence-based practice. The steps include the following:

1. development of a question that needs to be addressed,

2. a careful review of the professional literature,

3. identification of the study and methods that are similar to what the counselor wants to implement,

4. careful analysis and critique of the identified study to be sure it applies,

5. determination of how the study findings can apply, and

6. evaluation of the results once the new approach is implemented.

There is pressure on professionals to demonstrate the effectiveness of their practice from society and insurance companies funding these services. Simply a statement or conclusion that one is having a positive impact because of one's positive intentions is not adequate to address such expectations. It is to the benefit of professional counselors and their clients to engage in evidence-based practice.

SUMMARY

Counselor competence is an important component of acting ethically as a counselor. Competence includes functional and foundational competencies. Functional competencies concern what the counselor may do or how he or she may behave in practice. Foundational competencies that are relevant for counseling are ethical/legal understanding, cultural diversity, and reflective practice. Functional competency domains are assessment/diagnosis, intervention, consultation, research/evaluation, supervision/teaching, and management/administration. Developing a culture of competence in which the beginning counselor engages early in self-assessment and self-awareness is an important first step in this development process. Monitoring and maintaining competence is a career-long process. One can link this culture of competence to professional ethical identity and how one sees oneself. It is easy to be focused on learning the skills and knowledge of counseling as a beginning counselor and miss the importance of identifying the levels of competence one needs to perform well as a counselor.

Case Analysis and Reflection

Reread the case at the beginning of the chapter. What are the possible courses of action for John? How does his counselor developmental stage influence his actions? What impact may one's ethical development have on his or her ethical choices and actions? What would you do in this situation?

Questions for Further Reflection

1. What may be personal issues that affect your competence in performing counseling assessment, interventions, and so forth?

2. Developing a plan for continued learning and professional development is a good strategy. What are potential sources of future professional development?

3. Can you identify situations in which you or others dressed incongruously with a context or situation?

4. What is your current counselor developmental stage?

Additional Recommended Readings

Fall, M. (1995). Planning for consultation: An aid for the elementary school counselor. *School Counselor, 43*(2), 151–156.

Hall, A., & Lin, M. (1994). An integrative consultation framework: A practical tool for elementary school counselors. *Elementary School Guidance & Counseling, 29*(1), 16–27.

Houser, R. (2009). *Counseling and educational research: Evaluation and application.* Thousand Oaks, CA: Sage.

Johnson, S., Podratz, K., Dipboye, R., & Gibbons, E. (2010). Physical attractiveness biases in ratings of employment suitability: Tracking down the "beauty is beastly" effect. *Journal of Social Psychology, 15*(3), 301–318.

Krishnamurthy, R., VandeCreek, L., Kaslow, N., Tazeau, Y., Miville, M., Kerns, R., . . . Benton, S. (2004). Achieving competency in psychological assessment: Directions for education and training. *Journal of Clinical Psychology, 60*(7), 725–739.

Maslach, C., & Jackson, S. (1981). The measurement of experienced burnout. *Journal of Occupational Behavior, 2,* 99–113.

Maslash, C., Schaufeli, W., & Leiter, M. (2001). Job burnout. *Annual Review of Psychology, 52,* 397–422.

Meyersburg, C., Bogdan, R., Gallo, D., & McNally, R. (2009). False memory propensity in people reporting recovered memories of past lives. *Journal of Abnormal Psychology, 118*(2), 399–404.

Neimeyer, G., Taylor, J., & Wear, D. (2010). Continuing education in psychology: Patterns of participation and aspects of selection. *Professional Psychology: Research and Practice, 41*(4), 281–287.

Osborn, C. (2004). Seven salutary suggestions for counselor stamina. *Journal of Counseling & Development, 82,* 319–328.

Roberts, M., Borden, K., Christiansen, M., & Lopez, S. (2005). Fostering a culture shift: Assessment of competence in the education and careers of professional psychologists. *Professional Psychology: Research and Practice, 36*(4), 355–361.

Rodolfa, E., Bent, R., Eisman, E., Nelson, P., Rehm, L., & Ritchie, P. (2005). A cube model for competency development: Implications for psychology educators and regulators. *Professional Psychology: Research and Practice, 36*(4), 347–354.

Smith, S., Gleaves, D., Pierce, B., Williams, T., Gilliland, T., & Gerkens, D. (2003). Eliciting and comparing false and recovered memories: An experimental approach. *Applied Cognitive Psychology, 17,* 251–279.

Spruill, J., Rozensky, R., Stigall, T., Vasquez, M., Bingham, R., & Olvey, C. (2004). Becoming a competent clinician: Basic competencies in intervention. *Journal of Clinical Psychology, 60*(7), 741–754.

Stebnicki, M. (2008). *Empathy fatigue: Healing the mind, body, and spirit of professional counselors.* New York, NY: Springer.

Wilcoxon, A., & Hawk, R. (1990). Continuing education services: A survey of state associations of AACD. *Journal of Counseling & Development, 69,* 93–94.

Chapter 8

DIVERSITY AND MULTICULTURAL COMPETENCE

CHAPTER OBJECTIVES

- Understand the definition of *diversity* and various categories of diverse groups
- Develop an understanding of specific diverse groups based on race/ethnicity, gender, disability, sexual orientation, religion, and socioeconomic status and the possible unique characteristics of each group
- Develop an understanding of how diversity affects counseling

---

Case

Jim is a school counselor at a high school in a suburb of a large city. He has worked at this school for 5 years, but since the economy has been slow, the school is laying off several support staff including Jim. He is devastated by the loss of this position; he enjoys working with the students, who are of middle- and upper-class socioeconomic status (SES). They typically have high career expectations, and Jim likes seeing these students with such promise for success. He starts a job search, and a position is open in an inner-city school with students of low SES. The majority of the students are African American and Latino. Jim has never worked with inner-city students, and he grew up in the suburbs. He has had little interaction with those from minority groups. Jim likes being a school counselor, and he wants to continue his career. He goes for the interview, and he likes the other school counselors, the principal, and other school personnel. They seem to like him, and he thinks it would be okay to spend a few years working in this environment until another position in the suburbs opens up. Jim is offered the job, and he is trying to decide whether to accept it. He consults his advisor at the university from which he received his counseling degree. The advisor asks Jim a few questions such as the following: "What counseling competencies will you need to be successful in this position?" "Have you acquired any of these competencies from previous coursework or work experience?" Jim has difficulty answering these questions. He does not know what he should do—accept the job or keep looking.

INTRODUCTION

Recall from Chapter 7 that competence can be understood based on foundational competencies that include ethical/legal understanding, cultural diversity, and reflective practice. We have discussed reflective practice, and this book addresses the ethical and legal issues of counseling. Diversity and multicultural competence are important issues in the training of counselors (J. Hansen, 2010). J. Hansen (2010) suggested that diversity and multicultural orientations are significant components of the professional counselor's identity. He also noted that the primary value of multiculturalism is an appreciation of diversity. Pederson (1998) suggested that multiculturalism is potentially viewed as the "fourth force" in psychology and counseling. (The other three forces are psychoanalytic, behaviorist, and humanistic approaches.) Various definitions of *diversity* have been offered (Banks, 2009; S. Silverman, 2010). Rubel and Ratts (2011) noted there are differences between the definitions of *multiculturalism* and *diversity.* Diversity encompasses the term *multiculturalism,* which is focused on differences based on race and ethnicity. Diversity includes group and individual differences in race and ethnicity and other characteristics such as gender, SES, disability, sexual orientation, and religion (Rubel & Ratts, 2011). The Association of American Colleges and Universities (www.aacu.org/compass/inclusive-excellence.cfm) offers the following broad definition of *diversity:* "individual differences (e.g., personality, learning styles, and life experiences) and group/social differences (e.g., race/ethnicity, class, gender, sexual orientation, country of origin, and ability as well as cultural political, religious, or other affiliations)" (p. 3).

A significant question, given the currently diverse and multicultural population, is, What role should diversity and multicultural competence play in the training and ethics of professional counselors? According to the U.S. Census Bureau (www.census.gov/popest/national/asrh/NC-EST2006/NC-EST2006-03.xls), the population estimates of major minority groups in the United States, such as Asian, Black, and Latino groups, are approximately 104 million (33% of the total U.S. population). The projected population of Asians, Blacks, and Latinos residing in the United States is more than 223 million by the year 2050, constituting more than 50% of the total U.S. population (http://www.census.gov/population/www/projections/summarytables.html).

Conversely, those providing counseling services are primarily European American (S. Wang & Kim, 2010). Developing multicultural competence is essential to provide counseling to minority populations based simply on the number of minorities currently living in and projected to reside in the United States in the near future. S. Wang and Kim (2010) cited the number of missed appointments by those who are minorities. One might hypothesize that part of the reason minority individuals sometimes do not follow through on counseling is a misunderstanding of multicultural issues by counseling and counseling professionals.

In addition to minority groups that fit traditional definitions, there are those groups against whom people discriminate: those who choose an alternative sexual orientation such as gay or lesbian and those who have disabilities. Rutter, Estrada, Ferguson, and Diggs (2008) noted that those who choose lesbian, gay, or bisexual as a sexual orientation have difficulty finding counseling services primarily due to lack of understanding by those who provide counseling services. They noted that many counselors have homophobic attitudes and lack understanding of alternative sexual preferences.

The use of the term *diversity* is broad as has been noted to include individual and group affiliation based on such categories as gender, SES, disability, sexual orientation, and religion as well as race and ethnicity (multiculturalism). Given that diversity is quite broad and includes a number of categories that are relevant for counselors developing competence, we want to address multiculturalism (race and ethnicity), disability, sexual orientation, gender, SES, and religion.

Balcazar, Suarez-Balcazar, and Taylor-Ritzler (2009) suggested there are four elements of diversity and multicultural competence:

1. self-awareness;

2. cultural knowledge;

3. the ability to communicate understanding through empathy, particularly advanced empathy; and

4. the ability to apply the previous three in the appropriate context.

Balcazar et al. (2009) described the importance of having self-awareness particularly of one's own biases and prejudices. One may conclude, maybe even somewhat defensively, that he or she holds no such prejudices. However, reflection on attitudes and behaviors may result in an awareness that in fact one does hold certain biases and prejudices toward members of other groups and specifically toward those from minority groups or groups that are different from one's own.

MULTICULTURAL COMPETENCE

Sue, Arredondo, and McDavis (1992) provided an introduction to multicultural competencies. General categories of multicultural competencies include counselor awareness of his or her own values and biases, understanding of the worldview of the culturally different client, and development of appropriate intervention strategies and techniques for working with those who are culturally different. These authors further outlined these competencies based on beliefs and attitudes, knowledge, and skills. Counselor awareness is based on attitudes and beliefs: "Culturally skilled counselors are aware of their own cultural background and experiences, attitudes, and values" (Sue et al., 1992, p. 81). A knowledge example is Sue et al.'s statement that "culturally skilled counselors possess knowledge and understanding about how oppression, racism, discrimination, and stereotyping affect them personally and in their work. This allows them to acknowledge their own racist attitudes, beliefs, and feelings" (p. 81). Sue et al. provided examples of skills in regard to counselor awareness:

> Culturally skilled counselors seek out educational, consultative, and training experiences to enrich their understanding and effectiveness in working with culturally different populations. Being able to recognize the limits of their competencies, they (a) seek consultation, (b) seek further training or education, (c) refer to more qualified individuals or resources, or (d) engage in a combination of these. (p. 82)

Sue et al. (1992) provided concrete examples of competencies for counselors based on understanding the worldview of clients, those who are culturally different in particular. Sue et al. described counselors' beliefs or attitudes:

> Culturally skilled counselors are aware of their negative emotional reactions toward other racial and ethnic groups that may prove detrimental to their clients in counseling. Counselors are willing to contrast their own beliefs and attitudes with those of their culturally different clients in a nonjudgmental fashion. (p. 82)

In regard to knowledge and understanding of worldviews, Sue et al. suggested that a competency is demonstrated by culturally skilled counselors' showing knowledge of the impact of race, culture, and so forth. Counselors understand how worldview affects the development of mental health problems, and the counselor should select interventions based on an understanding of the worldviews of culturally different clients. Also, understanding worldviews may involve attending and participating in cultural experiences such as particular community celebrations.

The Association of Multicultural Counseling and Development has identified three competencies: (a) an awareness of a counselor's own worldviews and biases, (b) an awareness of the worldviews of clients, and (c) the skills necessary to provide culturally appropriate interventions to those who are culturally different (Arredondo et al., 1996). They proposed that such competencies include attitudes and beliefs as well as knowledge and skills for each of the three competencies (http://www.amcdaca.org/amcd/competencies.pdf).

Pedersen (2007) suggested that multicultural competency and awareness is a three-stage developmental process. The first stage in developing cultural competency is "awareness of culturally learned assumptions" (p. 8). The second stage is an understanding of culturally relevant facts (p. 8). The third stage is development of culturally appropriate interventions (p. 8). Essentially, cultural competence requires the development of awareness, knowledge, and skill. Pedersen concluded that if counselors do not have a balance in the development of these three stages, they will not be successful in acquiring cultural competence.

COMPETENCE AND RACE/ETHNICITY

Early efforts to address culture and counseling focused on race as a primary difference. Weinrach and Thomas (2002) stated,

No analysis of the Competencies would be complete without addressing the underlying assumptions and beliefs about race that appear to have influenced the content of Competencies and their apparent purpose to advocate primarily for African-Americans, Asian Americans, Native Americans, and Latinos. (p. 24)

The U.S. Surgeon General's (2001) *Report on Mental Health* provides a brief history of how racism and discrimination in America have developed. The report noted,

Since its inception, America has struggled with its handling of matters of race, ethnicity, and immigration. The histories of each racial and ethnic minority group attest to long periods of legalized discrimination. . . . Ancestors of many of today's African Americans were forcibly brought to the United States as slaves. The Indian Removal Act of 1830 forced American Indians off their land and onto reservations in remote areas of the country that lacked natural resources and economic opportunities. The Chinese Exclusion Act of 1882 barred immigration from China to the U.S. and denied citizenship until it was repealed in 1952. (p. 37)

Many perceive the term *race* as a way to categorize humans based on biological characteristics (Satcher, 2001). People seem to associate certain biological characteristics, such as skin color and the shape of the eyes or face, with race. However, there is no clear biological basis for differentiating or categorizing humans in such a way. Racial differences may be understood through the definition of *phenotype,* which refers to physical characteristics interacting with social influences on an organism/human. *Genotype* refers to the genetic makeup of the organism/human. Most important, only genotype—not phenotype—differentiates humans. Smedley (1999) noted that prior to the 18th century, connotations of and references to race were minimal. Western perspectives focused on differentiating humans based on class and status. In essence *race* was a socially constructed term used primarily to differentiate humans based on physical features and denoting status and class (Smedley, 1999).

The U.S. Surgeon General's (2001) *Report on Mental Health* noted important issues to consider, such as family factors, coping styles, attitudes of mistrust, and issues of stigma, when working with consumers of mental health services. Research on counselor competencies has shown mixed results (Chao, Chu-Lien, Good, & Flores, 2011). Some research has demonstrated differences in multicultural competencies based on race, for example, racial minorities were found to have higher levels of multicultural competence than Whites (Constantine, 2001; Neville, Spanierman, & Doan, 2006). Alternatively, other researchers have found no differences based on racial background and counselor multicultural competence (Manese, Wu, & Nepomuceno, 2001). Researchers have concluded that individual characteristics of the counselor play an important role in levels of multicultural competence (Sue & Sue, 2008). One characteristic of the counselor identified as relevant is his or her color-blind racial attitudes (Chao et al., 2011). Color-blind racial attitudes are marked by a denial that race matters and a belief that race no longer has a social impact (Chao et al., 2011). Those counselors who hold higher levels of color-blind attitudes have demonstrated bias in counseling activities such as diagnosing those from minority groups (Gushue, 2004). Counselors achieving multicultural and diversity competence are characterized by a level of self-reflection and specifically reflection about personal attitudes of color blindness.

An understanding of the concerns of different racial groups also is relevant to developing multicultural counseling competence. Considerations in working with/ counseling African Americans include an understanding of family structure, income, and education (Satcher, 2001). Moore-Thomas and Day-Vines (2010) described the African American family: Having "roots in indentured servitude and slavery, the African American family has survived the African holocaust" (p. 53).

They further noted that these early experiences in African American history have resulted in certain values and behavioral patterns that still continue. Characteristics of African American families include valuing the extended family, providing support among family members, and taking shared responsibility for child rearing within the family, including the extended family (Moore-Thomas & Day-Vines, 2010).

Satcher (2001) noted that the family structure for African Americans is unique and may affect the counseling process. For example, 38% of African American children grow up in two-parent families compared to 69% of all children in the United States. In addition, most children in single-parent families live with the mother. Satcher noted that any negative impact of growing up in such single-parent families is offset by the extensive support of extended family members. In regard to economics and income, African Americans are comparatively poor, with approximately 22% of such families living below the poverty line (U.S. Census Bureau, 2001). It is important to note that African Americans have experienced a significant increase in educational achievement during the past several decades. Rates of completion of high school and college are comparable to the rates of the rest of Americans (U.S. Census Bureau, 2001). An example of how counselor knowledge and awareness is relevant in working with African Americans is the impact of the extended family. Ignoring the impact of the extended family, for example, promoting autonomous, independent decision making, may interfere with family functioning. Many African Americans are significantly involved in religion and church activities (Kanel, 2003). The role of religion can be an important issue in counseling African American clients. Kanel (2003) suggested that intervention skills that may be helpful with African American clients are identification of specific problems and concrete goal setting. Insight-oriented approaches also have been found to be helpful (Kanel, 2003).

Multicultural counseling competencies in working with Asian Americans are unique, although all such competencies share some commonalities. Satcher (2001) described Asian American family structure as composed of family households, with only 14% being female-headed families. Parenting styles among Asian Americans are based on more of an authoritarian approach (Park, Kim, Chiang, & Ju, 2010). Asian Americans in general marry later in life, and they have fewer children. Education distinguishes Asian Americans from other groups in that Asian Americans have high rates of higher education; 44% have college degrees (compared to 28% of Whites; U.S. Census Bureau, 2001). The income of Asian American families is high, but it is based on total household income, which does not reflect individual family members' income. However, the data provide information about the amount of income that is available to the family for daily living. In Asian families, the family's needs are many times placed ahead of an individual's needs, and a counselor needs to be aware of such family perspectives. Another important issue in working with Asian American clients is the worldview concerning fulfilling obligations and bringing shame to the family (Kanel, 2003). Asian American families may deny or not disclose important information that is necessary for treatment of clients (Kanel, 2003). An Asian American client's communication with the counselor may be different due to accepted interactional patterns such as avoiding eye contact. This may be perceived by the counselor as not attending or indicating indifference in the counseling relationship versus having attitudes and behaving consistently with the culture.

Latinos are the fastest growing minority in the United States (Satcher, 2001). It is estimated that by the year 2050 approximately one fourth of the U.S. population will be Latino (Satcher, 2001). The Latino worldview includes a focus that is strongly family oriented. Latinos remain in the family home typically until they marry. Latino families have the largest number of children younger than 18 compared to other racial/ethnic groups (Satcher, 2001). Latinos' educational achievement is typically lower compared to other racial/ ethnic groups (Lewis, 2008); 56% graduate from high school compared to 83% of all groups nationally (U.S. Census Bureau, 2000). There is a difference in the Latino community in regard to economic success and income. Those from Cuban backgrounds typically have higher incomes compared to other Latino groups such as those from Puerto Rican or Mexican backgrounds (Satcher, 2001). In addition, Latino families commonly send money back to relatives in their home countries (Lewis, 2008). Kanel (2003) discussed research into Latino client preferences for type of treatment and specified a theoretical approach. Most Latinos reported that a more direct approach that included specific advice giving was preferred. Other interesting findings were that Latinos did not find it particularly helpful to discuss childhood experiences but did find it helpful to focus on current problems and issues.

Native Americans compose about 1.5% of the U.S. population (U.S. Census Bureau, 2001). The number of Native American families headed by single women has increased during the past several decades. Currently, the number of single-parent, female-headed, Native American households is higher than the national average (Satcher, 2001). In addition, Native American families are generally larger than the national average. In regard to education, Native Americans have increased graduation rates; however, these rates still lag behind the national average (Satcher, 2001). Limb and Hodge (2009) noted that Native American families use and value spirituality, which may be understood differently than the spirituality of other groups that value more traditional religion.

Satcher (2001) noted that Native American children perform similarly to other groups in early elementary grades but gradually fall behind. It has been speculated that such losses occur as a consequence of differences in how information is processed (Satcher, 2001). Incomes of Native Americans are typically lower than other groups'. This is due in part to the restricted economic opportunities found in many Native American communities (Satcher, 2001).

Gone (2010) noted the importance of counselors' having competence in and understanding of traditional healing methods within Native American culture. He noted that a professional may not necessarily be able to conduct traditional healing methods but that he or she should be knowledgeable about them and determine how they may be integrated with more traditional therapy approaches that are consistent with Native American views. Gone also noted that because of the complexity of integrating traditional counseling with traditional healing methods, competence in working with Native Americans may require significant training and experience.

COMPETENCE AND DISABILITIES

The U.S. Census Bureau reports that approximately 54 million Americans, or approximately 19% of the population, have disabilities (http://www.census.gov/hhes/www/disability/sipp/disable05.html). Houser and Domokos-Cheng Ham (2004) suggested that one type of evidence demonstrating that those with disabilities fit within a minority or diverse group is found in their significantly lower employment rate. Those with disabilities are 4 times more likely to be out of the workforce than are those without disabilities, despite having the desire to work (Cook et al., 2006). In addition, there are numerous historical examples of discrimination against those with disabilities, including the ancient Greek perspective that they should be eliminated because they are "weak and damaged" (Rubin & Roessler, 2008, p. 3). Also, there is considerable historical evidence that those with disabilities may be considered an oppressed minority (Batavia, 2001).

People with disabilities have faced discrimination and bias similar to those faced by (multicultural) minority group members (Cornish, Gorgens, Olkin, Palombi, & Abels, 2008; Williams & Abeles, 2004). A key issue underlying the multiculturalism and minority status perspective is that minority groups experience significant oppression, and many with disabilities have similar experiences (Cornish et al., 2008; Strike, Skovholt, & Hummel, 2004). Strike et al. (2004) concluded that the dominant model of minority groups includes seeing a difference versus a deficit. The view that those with disabilities have a difference versus a deficit fits with many current views of disabilities (Dell Orto & Power, 2007).

Suggestions for professional competence in working with those with disabilities have been proposed (Cornish et al., 2008; Strike et al., 2004). Common competencies for professionals to have include the following (Aubry, Flynn, Gerber, & Dostaler, 2005; Cornish et al., 2008; Strike et al., 2004):

- awareness of one's attitudes toward disabilities,
- awareness of societal attitudes toward those with disabilities,
- knowledge of laws and regulations for those with disabilities,
- awareness of barriers and obstacles for those with disabilities,
- knowledge of disability models, and
- knowledge and skills for treating those with disabilities.

Counselors need to be knowledgeable about laws protecting those with disabilities such as the Americans With Disabilities Act. The Americans With Disabilities Act essentially prohibits discrimination based on a disability in terms of employment, access to accommodations, access to public transportation, and the use of telecommunications (http://www.ada.gov/). Awareness of one's own biases toward those with disabilities is necessary to act ethically and act competently when working with those with disabilities. People with disabilities frequently encounter barriers, many of which are physical barriers such as access to public facilities. An example of such barriers that one can easily identify occurs when department stores and grocery stores clog the aisles with specials, blocking access for those who use wheelchairs or need space to maneuver. Reflecting on and identifying such barriers may help a counselor begin to develop competence in this area. Disability models vary significantly, and early models utilized the medical model, which is founded on the belief that a disability is a deficiency that needs to be remediated or corrected (Dell Orto & Power, 2007). There are numerous other models such as the social constructionist and biopsychosocial models. Recently there have been attempts to identify the best treatments for those with disabilities based on evidence-based practice (Kaiser & McIntyre, 2010). Key in many treatments for those with disabilities is the inclusion of individualized treatment, similar to treatment for those without disabilities. Counselors who work with those with disabilities should be aware of research-supported, evidence-based practice to ensure competence. Kaiser and McIntyre (2010) provided an example of how knowledge of evidence-based practice can be used when working with those with intellectual and developmental disabilities. They stated, "The integration of functional analyses of behavior with communication interventions has shown consistently positive outcomes for individuals with significant disabilities" (p. 357).

COMPETENCE AND SEXUAL ORIENTATION

Development of competencies in working with those whose sexual orientation is lesbian, gay, bisexual, or transgender (LGBT) may be understood from a multicultural and diversity perspective (Grove, 2009; Rutter et al., 2008). Those who hold LGBT sexual orientations have had a long history of significant negative reactions including violence and discrimination (Whitley, 2001). One can easily conclude that individuals who are LGBT have experienced discrimination and oppression. They also have been considered deviant and different and as a result have been rejected (Franklin, 2000; Sullivan, 1999).

Carroll and Gilroy (2001) noted the limitations in training beginning counselors to work with clients who are LGBT and stated,

> Educating trainees about GLBT [gay, lesbian, bisexual, or transgender] issues is deemed a priority, yet ambivalence exists concerning the manner in which this is to be accomplished. Evidence indicates that most training programs do not offer specialized coursework or formal training in working with sexual minority clients. (p. 49)

Rutter et al. (2008) described the lack of experience of counselors in providing services to clients who are LGBT. Clients who are LGBT seek out counselor services 5 times more frequently than do clients who are heterosexual (Rutter et al., 2008). Rutter et al. cited the lack of satisfaction of clients who are LGBT with the counseling services they do receive. Clearly there is a need for competent counselors to provide treatment to those who are LGBT.

A place to start in developing competence in working with people who are LGBT is understanding related theory and research. Jagose (2009) discussed the development of theories of sexual orientation such as queer theory. De Lauretis (1991) introduced queer theory in an effort to include sexual orientation in context with other minority categories such as gender and race. Halperin (2003) noted that queer theory initially was intended to bring about changes in perceptions of and research into the LGBT field. Also, De Lauretis did not have a comprehensive theory to offer but wanted to begin a discussion that went beyond traditional attempts at interpreting and understanding LGBT concerns within conventional interpretations from a heterosexual perspective. Others have offered further explanations of what queer theory of LGBT perspectives includes (Morland & Willox, 2005; Seidman, 1996). Seidman (1996) described the underpinnings of queer theory, which include (a) a view of sexuality wherein sexual power is understood in terms of social life and defined by social boundaries and expectations, for example, in regard to traditional sexual relationships; (b) the identification of nonheterosexual acts as problems by others and an attempt to understand how LGBT identity may develop differently from traditional heterosexual identity; (c) the use of strategies that are alternatives to accepted civil rights efforts; and (d) an exploration of areas of LGBT life beyond sexuality.

There has been discussion about whether LGBT as a category may be understood in combination with feminism theory (Jagose, 2009). Within the LGBT literature, there are differences in perceptions and beliefs about the acceptance of those who are bisexual or transgender (Erickson-Schroth & Mitchell, 2009). There has been debate about whether bisexual identity is truly one that exists (B. Carey, 2005) or whether it is an attempt by those who are gay, lesbian, or heterosexual who want to present themselves as being more open.

As with other diverse groups, an understanding of and sensitivity to LGBT perspectives is important for counselor competence. Also, awareness of oneself and the implications of one's views of LGBT is critical to provide competent counseling. An understanding of the status of reparative therapy is an important issue for counselor competence in work with clients who are LGBT. Reparative therapy is defined as conversion from an LGBT sexual orientation to a heterosexual orientation. Hein and Mathews (2010) stated, "Reparative therapy, also known as conversion therapy, is a general term for approaches aimed at changing lesbian, gay, and bisexual people to a heterosexual orientation" (p. 29). The outcomes of reparative therapy have been mixed in terms of success (Hein & Mathews, 2010; Nicolosi, Byrd, & Potts, 2000: Shidlo & Schroeder, 2002). The American Psychological Association ([APA] 1997) has concluded that reparative therapy is harmful and should not be used. Hein and Mathews described the ethical issue in providing the treatment of reparative therapy:

> Proponents of reparative therapy cite a patient's right to self-determination (or a parent's right to govern their child) as the basis for their efforts, stating that it is unethical to deny treatment to those who would seek it. . . . However, to refuse to provide a potentially harmful treatment to someone requesting it would hardly be deemed as prohibiting self-determination. (p. 32)

COMPETENCE AND GENDER

Counselor competence with gender is one of the variables that has been shown to influence counseling outcomes (Owen, Wong, & Rodolfa, 2009). Owen et al. (2009) investigated gender, competence, and counseling outcomes. They noted that a therapist's competence may be associated with his or her ability to comprehend clients' values, beliefs, and attitudes. There have been considerable writings about the specific characteristics and effects of gender (APA, 2007; Hartung & Widiger, 1998; Houser & Domokos-Cheng Ham, 2004). APA (2007) has suggested 11 guidelines for promoting the practice of gender- and culture-sensitive treatment for women and girls. The guidelines are organized under three major categories: professional responsibility, diversity and power, and practice applications (APA, 2007). One guideline under diversity and power concerns the development of an awareness of how socialization and stereotyping affect girls and women. For example, research on the socialization of girls and women has found that they may develop attitudes about being devalued and seen in specific ways. This socialization may result in a focus on physical appearance as well as subservience to and caretaking of others. Most important, such socialization may result in girls' and women's seeing restrictions in roles and opportunities in areas such as employment.

Another guideline proposed by APA (2007) focused on practice applications; it encouraged the use of appropriate interventions that have been found to be effective for working with girls and women. Particularly important is the use of evidence-based research to match interventions to the population or clients served. An example of careful application of evidence-based research concerns modification of negative internalized self-attitudes related to eating disorders (Thompson-Brenner, Glass, & Western, 2003). Therapy approaches that treat distorted thinking are examples of matching the intervention to the client, in this case girls and women.

A third general category, professional responsibility, may involve a counselor's awareness of his or her own personal development and socialization affecting his or her practice. APA (2007) suggested that lack of personal self-awareness may hinder the appropriate use of interventions and thus affect competence. Most important, the counselor's lack of self-awareness may reinforce societal attitudes that affect girls and women negatively. Such lack of personal self-awareness may be held by both male and female counselors; female and male counselors may hold a particular view of potential jobs that women may pursue.

Competence in gender and counseling involves an understanding of social impact, for example, socialization. Clients enter into treatment already socialized in ways that may hinder their development. Counselors have a responsibility to understand how socialization may interfere with growth and development, particularly because a counselor may seek to facilitate goals in contradiction to societal expectations.

COMPETENCE AND SOCIOECONOMIC STATUS

SES is an interesting concept in the United States because many would suggest no formal structure exists (Russell, 1996). There are different theories of SES, but one main theory concerns differentiating status through occupational position (Berberoglu, 1994). Essentially the occupational position one holds produces a certain income, which is based on the complexity and skill required for the position (Berberoglu, 1994). Parsons (1961) proposed that social class stratification provides society with information about rules and behaviors for interaction.

The significance of SES is important in understanding diversity (J. Pope & Arthur, 2009; L. Smith, 2008). The impact of SES, particularly on those of lower SES, is significant. J. Pope and Arthur (2009) described how lower SES is associated with many mental health and health problems relative to higher SES. They noted that lower SES is not a consequence of health problems, but lower SES can be a contributor to health problems. If one does not have the funds to pay for health insurance or a job that pays for health insurance, then he or she has a higher rate of health problems. Major detractors from well-being originating from lower SES are stressors that one experiences. These stressors include concerns about funding basic needs such as housing, health insurance, and food. In addition, those of lower SES have less family and community support than those of higher SES (J. Pope & Arthur, 2009). Many families of lower SES are not intact, and lower SES families frequently include single-parent families. Pope and Arthur suggested that a professional may hold negative attitudes toward those of lower SES; this is called classism. Professionals, it has been found, prefer not to work with those of lower SES (Leeder, 1996).

J. Pope and Arthur (2009) cited important skills and competencies needed to work with particularly low-SES clients. As with other diverse groups, an awareness of the group's issues and characteristics is important. Counselors need to be up to date on current information concerning the effects of SES. For example, continuously living in a lower SES across generations may result in lower self-esteem and feelings of helplessness. Pope and Arthur proposed that counselors use a strength-based approach to treatment, one that focuses on client positive attributes/assets, when working with those of lower SES. Such an approach highlights the client's assets and does not point out deficits. Those of lower SES have been found to have lower levels of self-esteem, and focusing on assets reduces the emphasis on the negative (Lorant et al., 2003).

COMPETENCE AND RELIGION/SPIRITUALITY

The relevance of religion and spirituality in the lives of humans has a long history and is well established. Recent surveys of Americans have found that 95% report belief in God (Gallup & Lindsay, 1999). In addition, 75% of Americans have noted the importance of religion and spirituality in their lives (University of

Pennsylvania, 2003). Religion and spirituality are associated with beliefs in God or a higher power (Morrison, Clutter, Pritchett, & Demmitt, 2009). Standard, Sandhu, and Painter (2000) noted the differences between and definitions of *religion* and *spirituality*. They stated, "Spirituality is a more subjective experience, whereas religion is a set of beliefs or doctrines that are institutionalized" (p. 205). Both involve beliefs in the sacred. There is a wide variety of approaches to the practice of religion and spirituality. Major world religions include Christianity, Judaism, Islam, Hinduism, Buddhism, Confucianism/Taoism (Chinese religions), and Primal or Indigenous. Religion has resulted in considerable disagreements and at times even violence; for example, the Christian Crusades with their focus on removing Muslims from their holy city (Jerusalem) offer an example of how religion can result in violence between groups. More recently there has been considerable disagreement between Christians and Muslims about locations of mosques, for example, a New York City mosque near Ground Zero (http://www.nytimes.com/2010/08/04/nyregion/04mosque.html?_r=1).

J. Young, Wiggins-Frame, and Cashwell (2007) discussed spirituality and counselor competence. They identified nine competencies for counselors:

1. an ability to explain the difference between spirituality and religion,

2. an ability to explain religious and spiritual beliefs from various perspectives,

3. an awareness of the counselor's own religious and spiritual beliefs,

4. an ability to clarify various religious models and beliefs,

5. an ability to accept others' views of religious and spiritual beliefs,

6. an ability to identify one's limitations in understanding religious and spiritual beliefs,

7. an ability to assess the client's spiritual and religious beliefs,

8. an ability to link religious and spiritual beliefs to the counseling process, and

9. an ability to use the client's religious and spiritual beliefs as is appropriate in counseling goals.

SUMMARY

Diversity in the United States continues to grow and increasingly becomes a challenge for counselors and their competence. The term *diversity* is broad as has included individual and group affiliations based on categories such as gender,

SES, disability, sexual orientation, and religion as well as race and ethnicity (multiculturalism). Counselor competence with diversity requires considerable education and experience because of the broad definition. A counselor achieving competence with diversity starts with an awareness of his or her own limitations, beliefs, and attitudes. Knowledge of specific background information about diverse groups is another important step in gaining competence. In addition, counselor competence with diversity involves knowledge and skills in providing interventions appropriate to those needed by a member of a diverse group.

Case Analysis and Reflection

Reread the case at the beginning of the chapter. Based on what you have subsequently read in this chapter, what advice do you have for Jim? Should he take this job or not? Are there any other options that would ensure Jim is competent to successfully do the job in the urban school?

Questions for Further Reflection

1. For which diverse groups do you feel you have the competence to provide counseling services?

2. What additional training or experience will help you become competent with diverse groups other than those listed in your response to Question 1?

3. Does one's ethical developmental level affect diversity competence? Explain.

Additional Recommended Readings

Aubry, T., Flynn, R., Gerber, G., & Dostaler, T. (2005). Identifying the core competencies of community support providers working with people with psychiatric disabilities. *Psychiatric Rehabilitation Journal, 28,* 346–353.

Batavia, A. (2001). The new paternalism. *Journal of Disability Policy Studies, 12,* 107–117.

Berberoglu, B. (1994). *Class structure and social transformation.* Westport, CT: Praeger.

Cook, J., Mulkern, V., Grey, D., Burke-Miller, J., Blyer, C., Razzano, L., . . . Steigman, P. (2006). Effects of local unemployment rate on vocational outcomes in a randomized trial of supported employment for individuals with psychiatric disabilities. *Journal of Vocational Rehabilitation, 25,* 71–84.

Cornish, J., Gorgens, K., Olkin, R., Palombi, B., & Abels, A. (2008). Perspectives on ethical practice with people who have disabilities. *Professional Psychology: Research and Practice, 39*(5), 488–497.

Erickson-Schroth, L., & Mitchell, J. (2009). Queering queer theory, or why bisexuality matters. *Journal of Bisexuality, 9,* 297–315.

Franklin, K. (2000). Antigay behaviors among young adults: Prevalence, patterns and motivators in a non-criminal population. *Journal of Interpersonal Violence, 15*(4), 339–362.

Gone, J. (2010). Psychotherapy and traditional healing for American Indians: Exploring the prospects for therapeutic integration. *The Counseling Psychologist, 38*(2), 166–235.

Gushue, G. (2004). Race, color-blind racial attitudes, and judgments about mental health: A shifting standards perspective. *Journal of Counseling Psychology, 51,* 398–407.

Harlperin, D. (2003). The normalization of queer theory. *Journal of Homosexuality, 45,* 339–343.

Hartung, C., & Widiger, T. (1998). Gender differences in the diagnosis of mental disorders: Conclusions and controversies of the DSM-IV. *Psychological Bulletin, 123,* 260–278.

Hein, L., & Matthews, A. (2010). Reparative therapy: The adolescent, the psych nurse, and the issues. *Journal of Child and Adolescent Psychiatric Nursing, 23*(1), 29–35.

Houser, R., & Domokos-Cheng Ham, M. (2004). *Gaining power and control through diversity and group affiliation.* Westport, CT: Praeger.

Jagose, A. (2009). Feminism's queer theory. *Feminism & Psychology, 19*(2), 157–174.

Kaiser, A., & McIntyre, L. (2010). Editorial: Introduction to special section on evidence-based practices for persons with intellectual and developmental disabilities. *American Journal on Intellectual and Developmental Disabilities, 115*(5), 357–363.

Leeder, E. (1996). Speaking rich people's words: Implications of a feminist class analysis and psychotherapy. In M. Hill & E. Rothblum (Eds.), *Classism and feminist therapy: Counting costs* (pp. 45–58). New York, NY: Haworth.

Lewis, M. (2008). Familias in the heartland: Exploration of the social, economic, and cultural realities of Latino immigrants. *Families in Society, 89*(2), 193–201.

Limb, G., & Hodge, D. (2009). Utilizing spiritual ecograms with Native Americans families and children to promote cultural competence in family therapy. *Journal of Marital and Family Therapy, 37*(1), 81–94.

Lorant, V., Deliege, D., Eaton, W., Robert, A., Philipott, P., & Ansseau, M. (2003). Socioeconomic inequalities in depression: A meta-analysis. *American Journal of Epidemiology, 157,* 98–112.

Moore-Thomas, C., & Day-Vines, N. (2010). Culturally competent collaboration: School counselor collaboration with African-American families and communities. *Professional School Counseling, 14*(1), 53–62.

Morland, I., & Willox, A. (2005). *Queer theory.* New York: NY: Palgrave Macmillan.

Morrison, J., Clutter, S., Pritchett, E., & Demmitt, A. (2009). Perceptions of clients and counseling professionals regarding spirituality in counseling. *Counseling and Values, 53,* 183–194.

Park, Y., Kim, B., Chiang, J., & Ju, C. (2010). Acculturation, enculturation, parental adherence to Asian cultural values, parenting styles, and family conflicts among Asian American college students. *Asian American Journal of Psychology, 1*(1), 67–79.

Pedersen, P. (2007). Ethics, competence, and professional issues in cross-cultural counseling. In P. Pedersen, W. Lonner, J. Draguns, & J. Trimble (Eds.), *Counseling across cultures* (pp. 5–20). Thousand Oaks, CA: Sage.

Pope, J., & Arthur, N. (2009). Socioeconomic status and class: A challenge for the practice of psychology in Canada. *Counseling Psychology, 50*(2), 55–65.

Rubel, D., & Ratts, M. (2011). Diversity and social justice issues in counseling and psychotherapy. In D. Capuzzi & D. Gross (Eds.), *Counseling and psychotherapy* (5th ed., pp. 29–58). Alexandria, VA: American Counseling Association.

Russell, G. (1996). Internalized classim: The role of class in the development of self. In M. Hill & E. Rothblum (Eds.), *Classism and feminist therapy: Counting costs* (pp. 59–72). New York, NY: Haworth.

Rutter, P., Estrada, D., Ferguson, L., & Diggs, G. (2008). Sexual orientation and counselor competency: The impact of training on enhancing awareness, knowledge and skills. *Journal of LGBT Issues in Counseling, 2*(2), 109–125.

Seidman, S. (1996). *Queer theory/sociology.* Cambridge, MA: Blackwell.

Shen, Y., Lowinger, R., & Jay, R. (2007). School counselor's self-perceived Asian American counseling competence. *Professional School Counseling, 11*(1), 69–71.

Smedley, A. (1999). "Race" and the construction of human identity. *American Anthropologist, 100*(3), 690–701.

Smith, L. (2008). Positioning classism within counseling psychology's social justice agenda. *The Counseling Psychologist, 36,* 895–924.

Standard, R., Sandhu, D., & Painter, L. (2000). Assessment of spirituality in counseling. *Journal of Counseling & Development, 78,* 204–210.

Strike, D., Skovholt, T., & Hummel, T. (2004). Mental health professionals' disability competence: Measuring self-awareness, perceived knowledge, and perceived skills. *Rehabilitation Psychology, 49*(4), 321–327.

Sue, D., & Sue, D. (2008). *Counseling the culturally different: Theory and practice* (2nd ed.). New York, NY: John Wiley.

Wang, S., & Kim, B. (2010). Therapist multicultural competence, Asian American participants' cultural values, and counseling process. *Journal of Counseling Psychology, 10,* 1–8.

Wilcoxon, A., Remley, T., & Gladding, S. (2012). *Ethical, legal, and professional issues in the practice of marriage and family therapy.* Boston, MA: Pearson.

Young, J., Wiggins-Frame, M., & Cashwell, C. (2007). Spirituality and counselor competence: A national survey of American Counseling Association members. *Journal of Counseling & Development, 85,* 47–52.

Chapter 9

USE OF TECHNOLOGY AND ETHICS

Case

Susan is a marriage and family counselor who is employed in a mental health agency/ clinic serving a rural population in the Southeast. She has a master's degree in marriage and family counseling, and she graduated 10 years ago. She has not had much exposure to the use of technology in providing counseling. The director of the clinic recently articulated a need to begin using technology in recording client information and completing intake assessments online. The clinic is considering contracting with a software company that provides online client intake assessment and client record keeping. The clinic director has formed a committee of three staff members to make a final recommendation, and Susan is a member of this committee. Susan is concerned about maintaining confidentiality and the privacy of her families. She has heard about some issues with confidentiality when using cloud drives. Also, Susan has requested that her supervisor review the validity and reliability of the instrument to be used for intake. She is concerned that the intake assessment instrument be inclusive in assessing family issues. The ethical issues for Susan are maintaining confidentiality and privacy in using the computer intake assessment and, second, determining whether the online intake assessment is inclusive of family issues. She does not want to be an obstructionist in moving the clinic forward but wants to ensure that any decision considers all of the ethical issues.

INTRODUCTION

The percentage of Americans who use technology has increased to almost 60% of the adult population (K. Young, 2005). There are a number of uses of technology in the practice of counseling (Beutler & Harwood, 2004; Casper, 2004; Mallen & Vogel, 2005; O'Dell & Dickson, 1984). Online counseling has grown during the past 10 years, and there are professional codes specifically designed to address its ethical concerns (Casper, 2004). In 1995 it was difficult to find an online counselor; however, 5 years later there were more than 250 online clinics and more than 700 therapists listed as providing online counseling (Alleman, 2002). Electronic record keeping is a second ethical issue arising from the use of technologies. Federal laws have been enacted (e.g., the Health Insurance Portability and Accountability Act [HIPAA]). Privacy is an ethical concern because so many client records are entered into online databases. Computer-based assessment is another potential area for ethical concern with the use of technology. Issues of accuracy and privacy arise when using online assessment. Last, the use of virtual reality in counseling potentially creates new and possibly significant ethical concerns about how counselors may actively affect client thinking and even memories.

ONLINE COUNSELING

Online counseling is relatively new to the counseling profession and has been identified as starting around 1972 (G. Jones & Stokes, 2009). Rochlen, Zack, and Speyer (2004) defined Internet therapy as "any type of professional therapeutic interaction that makes use of the Internet to connect qualified mental health professionals and their clients" (p. 270). G. Jones and Stokes (2009) have identified some reasons counselors may decide to use online counseling. These include a curiosity about a new approach to counseling, an attempt to increase the number of clients one treats, and the desire to provide counseling to those who need such services but may not have access (e.g., in more rural areas). They also identified reasons counselors may choose not to engage in online counseling: a belief that one cannot establish a therapeutic relationship, a belief that online counseling does not work, a questioning of the safety of online counseling, and concerns about the maintenance of confidentiality.

Researchers have found that online counseling is rated favorably by many clients (Haberstroh, Duff, Evans, Gee, & Trepal, 2007; K. Young, 2005). However, ratings comparing online to in-person counseling find there is a slight difference in satisfaction; those attending in-person counseling have higher ratings of satisfaction (Leibert, Archer, Munson, & York, 2006). One of the key issues for online clients appears to be the lack of nonverbal communication (Haberstroh et al., 2007). Sanchez-Page (2005) has suggested that online counseling may be most appropriate for a restricted client population. She concluded that those who are young, affluent, well educated, and highly functioning appear likely to benefit the most from online counseling. Also, she proposed that racial differences may influence the use of and access to online counseling, with Whites having the easiest access to the technology needed for participation in online counseling.

There are several methods used with online counseling: asynchronous e-mail, synchronous chat, and videoconferencing (see Table 9.1). Asynchronous methods involve mostly e-mail formats, and this was one of the earlier approaches to online counseling. Some have defined the use of e-mail counseling as "online letter writing" (Mallen & Vogel, 2005). Haberstroh et al. (2007) mentioned that as the use of online counseling and e-mail are "an interactive form of therapeutic writing, interventions delivered in this environment may combine the power of the written word with therapeutic conversations" (p. 270). Murphy and Mitchell (1998) coined the term "therap-e-mail" to describe the use of e-mail as part of counseling practice. The use of e-mail in counseling provides the client an opportunity to have saved transcripts of communication with a counselor. This can provide both the client and the counselor an opportunity for ongoing reflection and opportunities to concretely evaluate progress (Mallen & Vogel, 2005). Other benefits of using asynchronous e-mail are that the counselor may carefully decide how to respond in a thoughtful and reflective way, which may not be as possible with in-person counseling. Also, the counselor may consult with a supervisor or peers to gather further information about an appropriate response.

Websites have been set up to facilitate online counseling, for example, Therapy Online (www.therapyonline.ca). Therapy Online states that its intention is to provide a level of care similar to what one would receive in person. It also states that online counseling with its service is completed by highly qualified and experienced counselors. All counseling is done through e-mail, an asynchronous approach. Another website that offers professional counseling is Ask the Internet

Table 9.1	Methods of Online Counseling

Method	Description
Asynchronous e-mail	Counselor-client exchanges via e-mail or message board, not in real time
Synchronous chat	Real-time chats through instant messaging using Internet Relay Chat (IRC): Comments are typed that can be seen by the recipient and sender
Videoconferencing	Use of videoconferencing such as Skype, using images (via a camera typically built into a laptop computer) and voice in real time

Source: Jones and Stokes (2009).

Therapist (www.asktheinternettherapist.com). The site lists qualified therapists who reportedly hold various state licenses and provide specific types of counseling, for example, addiction or marriage and family counseling. Clients can choose to participate in both asynchronous (e-mail) and live synchronous chats.

Professional codes of ethics, such as the *ACA Code of Ethics* (American Counseling Association [ACA], 2005), have been designed to address ethical concerns with online counseling. There are several professional codes from the *ACA Code of Ethics* that potentially apply to online counseling. Standard A.12.b, Technology-Assisted Services, states, "When providing technology-assisted distance counseling services, counselors determine that clients are intellectually, emotionally, and physically capable of using the application and that the application is appropriate for the needs of the client." A second standard, A.12.c, Inappropriate Services, states, "When technology-assisted distance counseling services are deemed inappropriate by the counselor consider delivering services face to face." A third standard, A.12.d, Access, states, "Counselors provide reasonable access to computer applications when providing technology-assisted distance counseling services." Another standard is A.12.g, Technology and Informed Consent, which states, "As part of the process of establishing informed consent, counselors do the following: address issues related to the difficulty of maintaining the confidentiality of electronically transmitted communications." All of these standards provide counselors with direction for ethical actions when providing online counseling services.

Several concerns and ethical issues have been raised about online counseling (Bloom, 1998; Mallen & Vogel, 2005). One ethical issue is the maintenance of confidentiality. An online environment may not be secure because of the activities of hackers. Hackers attempt to access secure information on the Internet, which poses particularly important issues about confidentiality. Counselors can use virus protection and security software to protect against hacking and exposure to breaches of confidentiality. Also, clients should be encouraged to purchase such software to protect their side of the interaction on their computers. Confidentiality of records and counseling sessions is always an issue whether counseling is conducted in an office setting or online; ACA Standard A.12.g (ACA, 2005) addresses electronically transmitted communications. Recently cloud drives have been introduced; these are online storage systems that allow the user to access information and files from any computer because data are stored on company computers accessible online. There are still questions about the security of cloud drives. Counselors need to maintain up-to-date security measures, and this seems particularly important in an online environment. Bloom identified another ethical issue pertinent to online counseling: the lack of counselor understanding of specific geographical and/or local contexts. Counselors need to be aware of specific attitudes, laws, and local influences on the client. A counselor providing services at a distance may not be aware of such specifics due to the client's location. This can be important for those living, for example, in rural areas, which may include unique worldviews that can affect the counseling process. The counselor can address this issue through systematically gathering information, which can be accomplished by reading local newspapers and asking the client to describe his or her perceptions of the community. Consultation with another counselor who is aware of community values and the context of the community can be helpful. Another issue or ethical concern is a question of justice or fair access to services (Bloom, 1998). It has been noted that most who use and benefit from online counseling are more affluent, highly functioning Whites who have access to the Internet (Sanchez-Page, 2005). Lack of fair access to online counseling services is difficult to remedy. Those who do not have the financial resources to purchase computers and Internet services clearly miss out on online counseling services. *ACA Code of Ethics* Standard A.12.d, Access, states, "Counselors provide reasonable access to computer applications when providing technology-assisted distance counseling services." Counselors need to consider alternative ways of helping such underserved clients, particularly in more rural areas where counselors are not readily available. One option is for counselors to collaborate in the development of funding for the purchase of laptops and Internet services for those who cannot afford them. These laptops may be loaned to clients during the online counseling process and returned for other users once counseling is complete.

Another major concern and ethical issue is how the relationship develops in an online environment (Casper, 2004). The relationship in counseling is considered an essential ingredient for success. How does such a relationship develop in an online environment, particularly when one only uses e-mail or asynchronous communication? An ethical issue arises when one attempts to assess the success of treatment and there are questions about the efficacy of such an approach; see *ACA Code of Ethics* Code A.12.a, Benefits and Limitations (ACA, 2005). Casper (2004) stated,

> Maybe we should not accept traditional therapeutic relationships as a standard, but look at what is missing. Maybe new forms of relationship will develop which are not generally (but maybe for some patients and situations) better or worse than a traditional therapeutic relationship. (p. 225)

There has been research into what is termed "telepresence" in an online environment (Rochlen, Zack, et al., 2004). Rochlen, Zack, et al. (2004) defined *telepresence* as "the feeling (or illusion) of being in someone's presence without sharing any immediate physical space" (p. 272). Further research into telepresence in counseling and how it affects the counseling relationship is necessary. A counselor using an online format and particularly asynchronous methods needs to assess and determine whether such a presence exists and evaluate the quality of the therapeutic relationship.

A final ethical issue that can arise in online counseling is the problem of licensure and state approval to practice. Online counseling can go across state and approved licensure boundaries. A counselor licensed in one state, for example, Virginia, may provide online counseling to someone in another state, for example, Alabama. Which laws and professional codes does the counselor follow? Ohio State Licensure Law 4757-5-13, Standards of Practice and Professional Conduct: Electronic Service Delivery (Internet, Email, Teleconference, etc.), states that anyone practicing online counseling with a resident of Ohio must be licensed by the state. In addition, the law states that an Ohio licensed counselor offering online counseling outside of Ohio must comply with the jurisdiction in which the counseling is provided. Not all states currently address online counseling and regulate online counseling. Online counseling creates professional issues for counselors and what transpires across state boundaries. An important question is whether it is feasible for those providing online counseling to address each state's laws and requirements.

ELECTRONIC RECORD KEEPING

The use of electronic records or electronic medical records (EMRs) has increased significantly during the past several years because of the benefits associated with this approach (DeLettre & Sobell, 2010; Richards, 2009). One of the major benefits is that professionals from within an organization may have access to patient/client records, and they can best coordinate services. Richards (2009) noted that employing a multidisciplinary team is many times desired to enhance treatment and sharing among professionals; use of EMRs allows this to happen.

One of the major changes in record keeping recently is federal legislation, for example, HIPAA. For a summary of HIPAA legislation, see http://www.hhs.gov/ocr/privacy/hipaa/understanding/summary/privacysummary.pdf.   The   U.S. Department of Health and Human Services states that the

> HIPAA Privacy Rule provides federal protections for personal health information held by covered entities and gives patients an array of rights with respect to that information. At the same time, the Privacy Rule is balanced so that it permits the disclosure of personal health information needed for patient care and other important purposes. The Security Rule specifies a series of administrative, physical, and technical safeguards for covered entities to use to assure the confidentiality, integrity, and availability of electronic protected health information. (http://www.hhs.gov/ocr/privacy/hipaa/understanding/index.html)

In addition, it is stated that one of the major goals of the act is to ensure the protection of health information of individuals while at the same time promoting the free flow of information necessary for the health care of the individual. *ACA Code of Ethics* (ACA, 2005) Section A.12.g, Technology and Informed Consent, addresses issues of privacy in an online/electronic environment. An extension of HIPAA is the Health Information Technology for Economic and Clinical Health Act of 2009. The purpose of the act is to set up the Office of National Coordinator for Health Information Technology with the intent of coordinating the electronic use of patient health information. The focus is on improving the quality of health and reducing medical errors. Economic incentives are used to promote the use of electronic secure resources in patient care.

Richards (2009) identified the benefits and limitations of EMRs. One benefit is that coordination among professionals reduces the risk of errors in treatment. A second benefit is that treatment among professional becomes more efficient and duplication of services does not occur as often. EMRs also may be used to remind professionals about annual screenings and required immunizations (Richards, 2009). Last, EMRs allow for patient/client participation. Patients/clients can enter data directly into the system (medical, social information, etc.), and they can access treatment information including lab results.

Richards (2009) identified the potentially high cost of participating in EMR systems. This can be particularly problematic for private practitioners with small practices. Another problem that exists with EMRs is that a computer system can crash and information can be lost. Last, and this is probably one of the more important issues of concern for the professional, is that there is a potential for breach of security. Hacking is a common practice, and an EMR system containing confidential patient/client records may be an attractive secured system to conquer.

M. Wells, Mitchell, Finkelhor, and Becker-Blease (2007) has suggested that professionals seek to understand HIPAA guidelines, professional codes of ethics, and other federal guidelines on record keeping, for example, the Federal Education, Records and Privacy Act. In addition, counselors need to be aware of agency or school policies on record maintenance and protection. School or agency policies may be different than professional codes. An example is when a school has a policy about contacting parents if a child engages in high-risk behavior, for example, the use of drugs. Contacting the parents violates most professional codes of ethics regarding confidentiality.

COMPUTER-BASED ASSESSMENT

The use of technology and assessment in counseling has a relatively long history, with career-based assessment developed in the 1950s (Butcher, Perry, & Hahn, 2004). Early efforts, which involved the use of assessment and computers, concerned simply scoring in an effort to improve the accuracy of scoring. In the 1960s, Eliza, a computer program designed to assess client feelings, was introduced (J. Epstein & Klinkenberg, 2001). Eliza was set up as a Rogerian counselor and elicited responses from clients, who were to explain their feelings. Eliza served as the first approach to computer-assisted interviewing (CAI). There have been a number of CAI programs developed since the 1960s that are designed to assess clinical areas such as depression, suicide risk, and psychological functioning (Davis, Hoffman, Morse, & Luehr, 1992; Greist et al., 1973; McCullough, 1983). J. Epstein and Klinkenberg (2001) described the benefits of CAI, which include consistency in the interview, client control over the interview and the pace of questions, and a detailed report summarizing the findings. Counselors might let personal mood and affect impact the interview and the questions asked. There is little opportunity for the client to have as much control over the pace of a face-to-face interview. Last, entering results directly into a computer allows for ease of storage with minimal need for space.

Alternatively, Esptein and Klinkenberg (2001) described limitations of and concerns with CAI. One concern is that CAI does not have the flexibility to conceptualize the case as a whole, and therefore there may be a tendency to focus on specific elements of the responses. There is a belief that CAI is a cold and distant approach to gathering information from the client. Counselors believe that they can be more flexible in crafting the questions and pursuing questions that may not be typically programmed into computer software.

Computers have been used in counseling in ways other than CAI, such as personality assessment, neurological assessment, adaptive testing, and career assessment (Butcher et al., 2004; J. Epstein & Klinkenberg, 2001). Personality assessment has been one of the common uses of computers and assessment. An example of tests administered through computers is the Minnesota Multiphasic Personality Inventory (MMPI/MMPI-2; Butcher et al., 2001). Researchers have found a high correlation between computer-administered and paper-and-pencil-administered MMPI/MMPI-2 results (Pinsoneault, 1996). Butcher et al. (2004) concluded that computer-administered personality tests such as the MMPI/MMPI-2 had several benefits: Their interpretation is more reliable, and their administration is cost effective compared to paper-and-pencil administration. Costs are reduced when a test administrator is not required and a respondent can complete the test on a computer.

A potential ethical issue in the use of technology and assessment is maintaining privacy and confidentiality with assessment findings. *ACA Code of Ethics* (ACA, 2005) Code A.12.g, Technology and Informed Consent, provides information about maintaining ethical behavior with respect to using technology. Another possible ethical issue concerns the appropriateness of using an electronic/technology-assisted assessment. There may be some clients who have difficulty using the technology for assessment, who would need additional assistance, or who would not benefit from this type of delivery of psychological services; refer to *ACA Code of Ethics* Section A.12.b, Technology-Assisted Services.

VIRTUAL REALITY IN COUNSELING

In Norcross, Hedges, and Prochaska's (2002) survey of psychologists that asked about their predictions of future counseling interventions, psychologists predicted that the use of virtual reality was the third most likely to increase and change counseling activities/interventions. The use of virtual reality has grown; increasingly researchers have noted that it is an exciting opportunity to use in counseling (Riva & Vincelli, 2001). Glantz, Durlach, Barnett, and Aviles (1996) described the potential of virtual reality: "Perhaps the key feature of VR [virtual reality] is its ability to create environments that simulate real experiences so vividly as to evoke many of the same emotions that a comparable real-world experience would produce" (p. 464).

Virtual reality has been used with a number of mental health issues such as a range of anxiety disorders:

- fears and phobias, for example, fear of flying, acrophobia, social phobias, panic disorder, fear of public speaking, and
- posttraumatic stress disorder (Meyerbroker & Emmelkamp, 2010).

Other non-anxiety-involved conditions that have been treated with the use of virtual reality are

- pain management, eating disorders, and obesity, and
- sexual disorders (Riva, 2009).

Fear of flying can be treated through virtual reality with simulation of flying without the actual experience of taking off and landing. Virtual images of the experience of flying can be introduced to the client while he or she is coached through self-control methods such as the use of relaxation techniques.

S. Harris, Kemmerling, and North (2002) have described the use of virtual reality in the treatment of mental health problems through immersion in computer-generated virtual environments. There are various technological devices associated with virtual reality. These include head-mounted displays and data gloves that are equipped with position trackers (Riva & Vincelli, 2001). The use of virtual reality typically involves both software and hardware components. Changes in technology, both software and hardware, are rapid and require frequent updates in knowledge and skills.

There are several ethical codes that apply to the use of virtual reality in counseling (e.g., ACA, 2005). The potential for using new virtual reality technology is exciting and provides counseling with a new creative modality for treating a range of mental health issues. However, there are a number of ethical issues and concerns that need to be considered. One possible ethical issue is the competence needed to use the technology; according to *ACA Code of Ethics* (ACA, 2005) Standard C.2.a, "Boundaries of Competence—Counselors practice only within the boundaries of their competence based on their education, training, supervised experience, state and national professional credentials, and appropriate professional experience." Because this is a relatively new technology, there are not many who can provide supervision in implementation through this modality. As with other areas in counseling, competence is an important ethical concern.

A second possible ethical issue concerns how virtual reality technology is used. Many researchers have used virtual reality with stress-management techniques. However, a counselor could use virtual reality to create memories. An important question is, How does the brain process a virtual experience? If the brain processes virtual reality information similar to how it processes real-life experiences, is it possible to create new memories from virtual events? Certainly this can be an ethical issue if the counselor can create new memories and experiences for clients. This could be used either positively or negatively. Creating a new memory could be used positively, to remediate unpleasant difficult memories and replace them with a more positive memory, although one must question the ethical nature of implanting such a memory. Alternatively, the counselor could use virtual reality to create a memory that is negative or adds to the client's problems. For example, a counselor could implant a memory that creates an ongoing problem and therefore a need for the client to see the counselor, creating a long-term dependence.

SUMMARY

The use of technology among Americans has increased significantly during the past 10 years. There are a number of uses of technology in the practice of counseling including direct provision of counseling through the Internet, that is, online counseling. Electronic record keeping is another ethical issue stemming from the use of technology. A third potential ethical issue involving technology is the use of computer-based assessment. The potential use of virtual reality in counseling also creates new and significant ethical concerns about how counselors may actively affect client thinking and even implant memories.

Case Analysis and Reflection

Reread the case at the beginning of the chapter. Do you have a new understanding of Susan's concerns about the use of computer-based assessment? What further questions do you believe are relevant in helping Susan resolve her ethical concerns?

Questions for Further Reflection

1. What is your level of knowledge and expertise in using technology? What are your limitations? How would these affect your ethical behavior?

2. Given that technology is constantly changing and potentially will affect the future of counseling, what do you see as areas for growth and opportunities? How will you develop new technology skills and maintain current knowledge necessary to practice ethically?

Additional Recommended Readings

Alleman, J. (2002). Online counseling: The Internet and mental health treatment. *Psychotherapy: Theory/Research/Practice/Training, 39*(2), 199–209.

Beutler, L., & Harwood, T. (2004). Virtual reality in psychotherapy training. *Journal of Clinical Psychology, 60*(3), 317–330.

Davis, L., Hoffman, N., Morse, R., & Luehr, J. (1992). Substance use disorder diagnostic schedule (SUDDS): The equivalence and validity of a computer-administered and interviewer-administered format. *Alcoholism: Clinical & Experimental Research, 16*(2), 250–254.

Glantz, K., Durlach, N., Barnett, R., & Aviles, W. (1996). Virtual reality (VR) for psychotherapy: From the physical to the social environment. *Psychotherapy, 33*(3), 464–473.

Greist, J., Gustafson, D., Strauss, F., Rowse, G., Laughren, T., & Chiles, J. (1973). A computer interview for suicide risk prediction. *American Journal of Psychiatry, 130*, 1327–1332.

Haberstroh, S., Duff, T., Evans, M., Gee, R., & Trepal, H. (2007). The experience of online counseling. *Journal of Mental Health Counseling, 29*, 269–282.

Harris, S., Kemmerling, R., & North, M. (2002). Brief virtual reality therapy for public speaking anxiety. *Cyberpsychology & Behavior, 5*(6), 543–550.

Jones, G., & Stokes, A. (2009). *Online counseling: A handbook for practitioners.* New York, NY: Macmillan.

Leibert, T., Archer, A., Munson, M., & York, Y. (2006). An exploratory study of client perceptions of Internet counseling and the therapeutic alliance. *Journal of Mental Health Counseling, 28*, 69–83.

Mallen, M., & Vogel, D. (2005). Introduction to the major contribution: Counseling psychology and online counseling. *The Counseling Psychologist, 33*, 761–774.

McCullough, L. (1983). The development of a microcomputer based information system for psychotherapy research. *Problem Oriented Systems & Treatment Post, 6*(1), 3–4.

Meyerbroker, K., & Emmelkamp, P. (2010). Virtual reality exposure therapy in anxiety disorders: A systematic review of process-and-outcome studies. *Depression and Anxiety, 27*, 933–944.

Norcross, J., Hedges, M., & Prochaska, J. (2002). The face of 2010: A Delphi poll on the future of psychotherapy. *Professional Psychology: Research and Practice, 33*(3), 316–322.

Riva, G. (2009). Virtual reality: An experiential tool for clinical psychology. *British Journal of Guidance & Counselling, 37*(3), 337–345.

Young, K. (2005). An empirical examination of client attitudes towards online counseling. *Cyberpsychology & Behavior, 8*, 172–177.

Chapter 10

SUPERVISION AND ETHICS

CHAPTER OBJECTIVES

- Acquire an understanding of the definition of *supervision* in counseling
- Develop an understanding of the different roles of a supervisor in the counselor-supervisor relationship
- Develop an understanding of the phases or stages of counselor development and how they may be employed in counseling and supervision
- Acquire an understanding of the characteristics of the competent supervisor
- Develop an understanding of multicultural issues in the supervisor-supervisee relationship
- Acquire an understanding of the legal responsibilities associated with supervision in counseling

Case

Jim is a mental health counselor working in a community mental health center in the western United States. He has just received his state licensure, and he feels good about his counseling skills and his knowledge. He is self-assured and confident in his abilities. He asks his supervisor if he can have an intern from a local university to supervise. He hopes to eventually enter more formal supervisory and administrative roles in the future, so he thinks it would be good to get experience in supervision. Jim's supervisor agrees to give him an intern, and he is assigned one. Jim meets with the intern and goes over how he plans to provide the supervision. The intern listens and appears to be interested in what Jim has to say. Jim begins meeting with the intern and provides what he considers good advice and clear direction. After a few months Jim begins to notice that the intern does not share as much information as she did when they first started supervision.

He begins to question the intern's abilities, and when he asks the intern about what is happening in her sessions, she questions his knowledge and experience in providing supervision. The student's challenging Jim and his ability to supervise irritates him, so he becomes much more assertive, almost aggressive, in the supervisory sessions. This conflict extends for several months, until the end of the first part of the internship for the student. Jim meets with the university supervisor and expresses concern about the student's openness to supervision and the competency of the student. When asked by the university instructor what grade he would give the student, Jim states, "An F"; he does not feel the student should pass the internship. The university supervisor acknowledges Jim's comments. The university supervisor later suggests to Jim that he enroll in a course at the university focused on supervision because this is an interest of his. The question is, What will he discover in the supervision class that may shed light on any ethical issues in his supervision of the student intern whom he wanted to fail?

INTRODUCTION

Ladany and Bradley (2010) described the importance of counselor supervision and stated, "Counselor supervision is arguably the primary way in which educators facilitate or inhibit counselor competence" (p. 3). Casile, Gruber, and Rosenblatt (2007) suggested that supervision is a major factor in promoting ethical, legal, and professional practice by counselors. Supervision is an integral part of the counseling process, and we note that it is an important element in ethical decision making based on a hermeneutic model (see Figure 4.1 in Chapter 4). Supervisors' values, beliefs, professional identity, and so forth influence the horizon of the ethical decision-making process. Ladany and Bradley defined supervision as

> dyadic activity whereby the supervisor facilitates the provision of feedback to the supervisee, which is based on the interpersonal communication between both members of the dyad and can pertain to the work in supervision, the supervisee, the supervisee's clients or the supervisor.

I. Bernard and Goodyear (1998) noted that supervision concerns "overseeing" others. They provided a formal, detailed definition of *supervision* as the following:

> an intervention provided by a more senior member of a profession to a more junior member or members of that same profession. This relationship is evaluative, extends over time, and has the simultaneous purposes of enhancing the professional functioning of the more junior person(s), monitoring the quality of professional services offered to the client. (p. 6)

It is important to note that supervision includes an effort to monitor and improve the quality of services provided, and this may be accomplished through evaluative methods. In addition, this intervention—supervision—facilitates the growth of the junior professional into the profession. There are many ethical issues that arise when one considers efforts to improve the quality of services to clients through supervision or overseeing of a junior professional.

The Association for Counselor Education and Supervision ([ACES] 1993) identified four major supervisory roles. These roles include monitoring client welfare; encouraging compliance with relevant legal, ethical, and professional standards for professional practice; monitoring clinical performance and professional development of supervisees; and evaluating and certifying current performance and potential of supervisees for academic, screening, placement, employment, and credentialing purposes. In addition to these supervisory roles, the role of the supervisor may be understood based on the counselor job functions that are being supervised, for example, administrative or clinical (Tromski-Klinghirm, 2007). Tromski-Klingshirm (2007) noted that a clinical supervisor may be understood as "a senior member of the profession who helps the supervisee or 'junior member' develop therapeutic competence" (p. 54). The key here is the development of therapeutic competence. A supervisor who acts in the role of clinical supervisor needs to have advanced therapeutic or counseling skills to successfully provide clinical supervision.

A second job function for a supervisor is administrator (Tromski-Klingshirm, 2007). The administrative role is focused on the management of services. Tromski-Klingshirm (2007) identified the following tasks of the administrative function: supervising agency records; ensuring agency policies and procedures are followed; performing the activities of hiring, firing, and remediating employees; and evaluating employee performance.

There are a number of models of counselor supervision (I. Bernard & Goodyear, 1998; Casile et al., 2007; Ladany & Bradley, 2010). These include stage models (I. Bernard & Goodyear, 1998; Casile et al., 2007; Ladany & Bradley, 2010), counseling- and therapy-based models (I. Bernard & Goodyear, 1998; Casile et al., 2007; Ladany & Bradley, 2010), and social role models (I. Bernard & Goodyear, 1998; Casile et al., 2007). In addition, there has been a considerable amount of writing about counseling supervision during the past 30 years (J. Bernard, Clingerman, & Gilbride, 2011; Borders & Brown, 2005; Casile et al., 2007; Ladany & Bradley, 2010; Ronnestad & Skovholt, 1993; Wheeler, 2007). It is not the intention of this text to address counselor supervision in detail beyond identifying the major elements of supervision and the impact of supervision on ethical practice.

One relevant ethical issue in counselor supervision is promoting the development of the counselor (Dye & Borders, 1990). A second ethical issue is general competence and training in becoming a supervisor. Many supervisors are promoted to the position without any training because they are good at counseling. Another important ethical issue in regard to supervision is culturally competent supervision. We live in a diverse society, and as with counselor multicultural competence, it is important for a supervisor to be culturally competent to provide ethical supervision. The ethical issue that arises with the two primary functions of supervision, clinical and administrative, concerns the dual roles that can develop. One function, clinical supervision, may delve more into personal counselor issues affecting counseling, whereas the administrative function includes evaluation. The two functions can potentially create an ethical dilemma, a dual relationship. A supervisor hearing personal information may use the information in evaluating the supervisee. Finally, a supervisor has responsibility for the ethical and legal issues of his or her supervisee in working with clients. A supervisor may be held responsible/ accountable for his or her counselor supervisee's actions.

SUPERVISION AND COUNSELOR DEVELOPMENT

One of the major competencies of a supervisor is an understanding of the counselor developmental process and an ability to apply it in supervision (Dye & Borders, 1990). A helpful approach to understanding ethical issues in supervision and counseling is through comprehensive understanding of the developmental process of a counselor's career (Ronnestad & Skovholt, 2003). Ronnestad and Skovholt (2003) concluded that counselor development of a career has certain characteristics. They stated that "(a) development always implies change of some sort, (b) the change is organized systematically, and (c) the change involves succession over time" (p. 7). Based on extensive interviewing of counselors, Ronnestad and Skovholt identified six phases of counselor development. The six phases are the lay helper, beginning student, advanced student, novice professional, experienced professional, and senior professional phases (see Table 10.1). The first phase is identified through experiences of and approaches to helping that are based on no professional training; however, the individual may receive reinforcement for helping others informally. This may include helping friends, family, and colleagues. It may involve more lay helping such as working in summer camps or even working as a residence hall assistant in a college dormitory. The process the individual uses is characterized by the individual's experiencing strong emotions in response to the situation followed by giving advice based on one's own personal experiences. Ronnestad and Skovholt described the lay helper's approach as the use of "one's own solutions for the problems encountered" (p. 10). In addition, the lay helper frequently has issues with boundaries, including overidentification with the helpee and inserting one's own values and beliefs into the solution of the

| Table 10.1 | Phases of Professional Development |

Phase	*Characteristics of Development*
Lay helper	This stage involves experiences of informally helping others such as friends and family. There are overidentification with the helpee, strong emotional experiences, and sympathy.
Beginning student	In this stage, the counselor develops an understanding of the difference between a lay helper and a professional helper. There is a heightened sensitivity to criticism. The focus is on receiving external feedback in directing counseling efforts. Ideally the counselor is open to learning.
Advanced student	This phase is most associated with a student engaged in an internship. The task for the student is to develop a professional identity and develop skills necessary to function as a professional. The counselor is fairly rigid in applying techniques—almost mechanical—versus using a more flexible approach. An external frame of reference is maintained, and the student looks for others to provide feedback on success and evaluation of skills.
Novice professional	The first few years of professional practice are associated with this phase. The counselor in this phase of development experiences some conflict about what was learned in professional training and what happens in actual practice; much of the knowledge and many of the skills are found not always to work the way they were presented. The counselor still has difficulty with personal versus professional boundaries, and he or she may become overly invested in the client's life.
Experienced professional	The counselor has practiced for a number of years, and there is increased congruence between professional life (professional and ethical identity) and personal/individual identity. The counselor notes the importance of the counselor-client relationship in bringing about positive results. There is increased flexibility in choosing techniques and interventions. Boundaries between counseling sessions and other activities, such as personal life, are clear.
Senior professional	This phase is exemplified by a professional who has worked in the field for more than 20 years and is viewed by colleagues as a leader, someone who is knowledgeable. There is a continued commitment to learning and growing professionally. Typically there is a sense of accomplishment and feelings of self-acceptance.

Source: Adapted from Ronnestad and Skovholt (2003).

problem. The layperson is likely to use more sympathy than empathy in understanding the situation. The lay helper also frequently has difficulty managing personal emotions and reactions to hearing the problem and the situation. Personal reactions may be strong, and the lay helper may not separate his or her feelings from those experienced by the person seeking help.

The second phase is the beginning student phase, which coincides with the individual's beginning his or her professional academic training (Ronnestad & Skovholt, 2003). Generally upon entrance into a professional graduate program, the beginning student understands there is a difference between helping as a lay helper and helping as a professional counselor, or it is hoped the student will acquire this understanding soon after entering the program. An early experience, for many but not all, is an attempt to judge whether one has the ability and potential to become a successful counselor (Ronnestad & Skovholt, 2003). Ronnestad and Skovholt (2003) suggested that students in this phase are particularly sensitive to criticism from faculty or supervisors. A major task for the beginning student is meeting clients for the first time and managing the stress and anxiety associated with the ambiguity of this new situation. Students entering practicum settings frequently wonder what they will say in such sessions and how they will manage a conversation for a 50-minute period of time. Researchers have linked cognitive development to early graduate training (Granello, 2002; Lyons & Hazler, 2002). In addition, beginning counseling students have been found to have a somewhat rigid view, which results in their seeking to find absolute truths in counseling (Granello, 2002). Many beginning students seek to find structure in the counseling session where none may exist. In addition, there are opportunities for feedback from faculty, peers, and clients. How the feedback is presented is important to beginning students, and harsh criticism may significantly affect them in a negative way. It can be helpful for a student to have understanding of and skill in easily applied counseling theories and models (Ronnestad & Skovholt, 2003). There are many things for the beginning student to focus on in counseling, and a simple approach during this early clinical experience is important. It is similar to learning to ride a 10-speed versus a single-speed bike. One does not need to learn on a 10-speed bike, and generally he or she will not use the multiple speeds early in the learning process because it is too distracting (and likely to result in spills and accidents). The same may be true in counseling; a single, simple approach may be best and may reduce confusion and anxiety for the beginning counselor. Another important characteristic of a beginning counselor is openness to learning. A beginning counselor who "knows it all" can be a problem, and a know-it-all attitude can hurt one's learning of the necessary knowledge and skills. Ronnestad and Skolholt noted that a closed attitude to learning may result in "professional stagnation."

Phase 3, the advanced student phase, is associated with the internship and the later stage of counselor training (Ronnestad & Skolholt, 2003). The primary task in this phase is learning the basic knowledge and skills of a professional counselor. There may be continued anxiety and doubt for the first few weeks of the internship, but typically intern students begin to feel comfortable and competent after this initial early experience. Many students even express that after 4 or 5 months in an internship, they are ready to accept a full-time professional position even though they have another semester of internship. Students in this phase of development recognize the benefits of their academic training and see that what they have learned does apply in actual practice (Ronnestad & Skolholt, 2003). Counselors in this phase remain focused on external feedback as a point of reference for determining professional competence. Researchers have found that there is not a significant change in this phase in cognitive development and in openness to a flexible approach to understanding the counseling process (Granello, 2002). Granello (2002) stated, "The differences in cognitive development between individuals at the beginning of their counseling graduate programs and those at the end were rather small" (p. 290). Ronnestad and Skovholt (2003) have found that students in this phase express concern that they have not had many opportunities to observe more advanced professional counselors. Students frequently continue to use primarily one theory or model but seem to be open to exploration of others.

Phase 4, the novice professional phase, encompasses the first few years after graduation from the counseling program (Ronnestad & Skovholt, 2003). One may think about these early professional years as flying solo. Ronnestad and Skovholt (2003) suggested that there is an attempt to verify that what was learned in the graduate training applies in actual practice. At times there is conflict between what was learned and how well it applies in practice, so the professional in this phase may experience some disillusionment and need to adjust through self-reflection and additional training. A good part of this process is that when the novice counselor experiences this lack of congruency between training and needed skills and knowledge in the actual work setting, it may influence the counselor to seek additional information, for example, learn new theories and modalities of counseling. Also, the novice counselor is still attempting to define professional versus personal boundaries. A concrete example of this boundary problem is an understanding that one needs to leave professional concerns at work and freely enter one's personal life after work is done. The novice counselor begins to develop a more complex view of counseling including a better understanding of the significance of the counseling relationship, which potentially is greater than the theory or modality used (Ronnestad & Skovholt, 2003). A significant change in this phase is the development of more of an inner-focused approach to evaluating and seeking effectiveness (Ronnestad & Skovholt, 2003). So there is a change from an external frame of reference to an internal frame in seeking to be an effective counselor.

The fifth phase of development is the experienced professional counselor phase (Ronnestad & Skovholt, 2003). This phase involves the counselor engaged in practice for a number of years in which he or she has worked with a range of clients in a variety of settings. Ronnestad and Skovholt (2003) proposed that the primary task of this phase is the development of an integrated and congruent perspective between a counseling role and self-perceptions (professional identity and professional ethical identity) and personal values. Development of a professional identity that is congruent with self-perceptions and individual or personal identity is likely essential for the counselor to continue in the profession. The counselor in this phase continues to develop a deeper understanding of the role of the client-counselor relationship and how important it is in success in counseling. Another characteristic of this phase is the development of a more flexible and adaptive approach to the application of counseling techniques and interventions. Counselors trust their professional judgment, which allows them to be more flexible. In addition, the counselor in this phase may realize that at times there are not clear solutions to problems encountered, which is curious given the counselor's level of experience. This may be interpreted as the counselor's developing a more pragmatic understanding of the limitations of his or her efforts. Ronnestad and Skovholt further proposed that the counselor deepens the distinction in his or her boundaries; he or she focuses on being present and working with clients while in session but, once the session is complete, moves on to other clients or home and personal life, as is appropriate. Another interesting point in this phase is that the counselor is able to connect information and experience from other sources of knowledge and disciplines as it applies to practice. An example is a counselor who sees a connection with a movie or book as it applies in the counseling process or with a particular client. Counselors learn from clients during this phase and express openness to examining differences in outcomes to inform the use of interventions and techniques.

The last phase of counselor development is the senior professional phase. Ronnestad and Skovholt (2003) described this phase's being exemplified by a professional counselor who has more than 20 years of experience. This phase is associated with the counselor's being seen by colleagues as a seasoned professional. He or she is sought out for advice and guidance by other counselors. The counselor in this phase has a sense of accomplishment and is self-accepting. It is interesting that even in this late phase of development, the professional counselor continues to learn and grow. This probably contributes to a sense of excitement and commitment to the profession.

Both counselors and supervisors can use this phases of professional development model to facilitate understanding and interpretation of ethical issues. For example, in early career developmental phases (beginning student and advanced student), the supervisor and student are focused on competence and building the skills necessary to be successful as a counselor. The supervisor needs to monitor carefully complex ethical decision making during these early phases of career development. The counselor himself or herself needs to be cognizant that there will be situations and circumstances, which he or she needs to identify, that involve ethical issues and consultation with the supervisor. There are times when the beginning counselor may feel he or she does not need to consult a supervisor about ethical issues (a need for autonomy by the counselor), but generally most counselors in these early phases should consult regularly with supervisors and even be overly cautious in seeking assistance with potential ethical issues. The novice counselor in Phase 4 may benefit from feedback and supervision about integration of what was learned during his or her graduate education and the practical applications of being a novice counselor. The potential for a novice counselor to quickly engage and burn out can be a concern, and experienced supervisors can address the development of professional boundaries and how to manage them so the novice counselor does not become overwhelmed.

SUPERVISOR COMPETENCE

Supervision is a significant element in the ethical decision-making process based on the hermeneutic model (see Figure 4.1; Houser, Wilczenski, & Ham, 2006). A competent supervisor is critical to ensure effective and quality contributions from this element in the ethical decision-making model. An important question is, What constitutes a competent supervisor? Can one become a supervisor simply through acquiring a certain number of years of experience? A way to think about the development of a competent supervisor is a review of what it takes to become a supervisor (Casile et al., 2007). Casile et al. (2007) described the process of becoming a supervisor: "In the counseling profession, many practitioners are promoted to the supervisory position as a result of their seniority, exceptional work as a counselor, or desire to be a supervisor" (p. 6). The American Counseling Association's ([ACA] 2005) *ACA Code of Ethics* Section F.2.a, Supervisor Preparation, states, "Prior to offering clinical supervision services, counselors are trained in supervision methods and techniques. Counselors who offer clinical supervision services regularly pursue continuing education activities including both counseling and supervision topics and skills." Saccuzzo (2005) discussed the ethics of supervisor competence and noted that first the supervisor must be competent to supervise others. Succuzzo stated that "the supervisor is qualified to supervise by education, training, supervised experience, consultation, study or professional experience" (p. 11). ACES identified 11 standards for counseling supervisors; these standards are identified in terms of personal traits, knowledge, and competencies (Dye & Borders, 1990). The 11 standards are further differentiated through specific subparts (see Table 10.2).

Table 10.2 Standards for Counseling Supervisors

Standard	Subpart Example
Professional counseling supervisors are effective counselors whose knowledge and competencies have been acquired through training, education, and supervised employment experience.	1.1 The counseling supervisor demonstrates knowledge of various counseling theories and systems and their related methods.
Professional counseling supervisors demonstrate personal traits and characteristics that are consistent with the role.	2.2 The counseling supervisor is sensitive to individual differences.
Professional counseling supervisors are knowledgeable regarding ethical, legal, and regulatory aspects of the profession and are skilled in applying the knowledge.	3.2 The counselor supervisor demonstrates and enforces ethical and professional standards.
Professional counseling supervisors demonstrate conceptual knowledge of the personal and professional nature of the supervisory relationship and are skilled in applying this knowledge.	4.4 The counselor supervisor is sensitive to the evaluative nature of supervision and effectively responds to the counselor's anxiety relative to performance evaluation.
Professional counseling supervisors demonstrate conceptual knowledge of supervision methods and techniques and are skilled in using this knowledge to promote counselor development.	5.4 The counselor supervisor can perform the supervisor's functions in the role of teacher, counselor, or consultant as appropriate.
Professional counseling supervisors demonstrate conceptual knowledge of the counselor developmental process and are skilled in applying this knowledge.	6.1 The counselor supervisor understands the developmental nature of supervision.
Professional counseling supervisors demonstrate knowledge and competency in case conceptualization and management.	7.1 The counselor supervisor recognizes that a primary goal of supervision is helping the client of the counselor.
Professional counselor supervisors demonstrate knowledge and competency in client assessment and evaluation.	8.1 The counselor supervisor monitors the use of tests and test interpretation.
Professional counseling supervisors demonstrate knowledge and competency in oral and written reporting and recording.	9.3 The counselor supervisor assists the counselor in establishing and following policies and procedures to protect the confidentiality of client and supervisory records.
Professional counseling supervisors demonstrate knowledge and competency in the evaluation of counseling performance.	10.2 The counselor supervisor can identify the counselor's professional and personal strengths as well as weaknesses.
Professional counseling supervisors are knowledgeable regarding research in counseling and counselor supervision and consistently incorporate this knowledge into the supervision process.	11.2 The counseling supervisor reads, interprets, and applies counseling and supervisory research.

Source: Adapted from Dye and Borders (1990).

Based on the standards identified, the complexity of the counselor supervisor competencies is significant, and not fulfilling these standards potentially can result in ethical issues. One example is a counselor supervisor who does not keep up to date on the current research literature and is not able to discuss and apply such research results effectively. It would be similar to a head surgeon's not being current on the most innovative surgical techniques when supervising other surgeons. A second example is a supervisor's not monitoring and assisting in the interpretation of assessments or tests. Those who supervise novice counselors who do not monitor test interpretation or results may facilitate incorrect use and interpretation of results, which could injure a client. Not having a competent supervisor places more pressure on the counselor to make ethical decisions. The importance of competent supervision cannot be underestimated in promoting counselor development and ethical practice in counseling.

SUPERVISOR-COUNSELOR ETHICAL AND LEGAL RESPONSIBILITIES

Many beginning/new supervisors are likely excited about their new position. They may not realize that as a consequence of their position, they are suddenly legally responsible for the actions of their supervisees (Guest & Dooley, 1999; Saccuzzo, 2002). What this also means is that a counselor himself or herself may place the supervisor in jeopardy legally through his or her actions and ethical decisions. Tannenbaum and Berman (1990) noted that "today's psychotherapy supervisor is ultimately responsible for every act or omission of his or her supervisee" (p. 76). This is a rather sobering interpretation of the ultimate responsibility of the supervisor. The parameters of legal responsibility of supervisors remain to be fully developed (Guest & Dooley, 1999). However, there has been speculation about whether supervisees themselves could initiate successful lawsuits for inadequate supervision (Robiner, Fuhrman, & Bobbitt, 1990).

There are several ethical and legal concerns that may place both the counselor and the supervisor at risk, for example, lawsuits or criminal charges. These include allegations of malpractice, violations of confidentiality, acts of omission (not reporting child abuse), and violation of boundaries such as sexual contact between the counselor and client. Counselors may become involved in either civil or criminal charges; see Chapter 12 for more detail about legal issues, counselors, and supervisors. Criminal charges result from violations of criminal laws, and these might include acts such as not reporting abuse. For example, Wisconsin's statute Wisconsin 940.22, Sexual Exploitation by a Therapist: Duty to Report, is an example of a criminal law that could affect a counselor. All 50 states have laws requiring professionals such as counselors to report suspected child abuse. An example is Massachusetts's mandating reporter requirements and consequences of violation of this statute, for example, a possible fine if suspected child abuse is not reported. A recent update (July 1, 2010) to the Massachusetts child abuse law states,

> Any mandated reporter who willfully fails to report child abuse or neglect that resulted in serious bodily injury or death can be punished by a fine of up to $5,000 and up to 2½ years in jail, and be reported to the person's professional licensing authority. (Massachusetts Department of Children and Families, 2009)

Certainly, this is a significant consequence for the counselor and potentially the supervisor. Civil law is focused on noncriminal suits, which are designed to resolve differences about such things as violations of contracts or acts resulting in harm. A civil law resulted in the court ruling in *Tarasoff v. Regents of the University of California* (1976). Counselors/therapists have a duty to warn an intended victim of a violent crime, for example, when someone makes a threat toward another person in a counseling session and the intent is plausible (see Chapter 12 for further explanation of duty to warn).

The important ethical issue for supervisors and counselors is to understand which laws apply to ethical problems and their practice. There are several complexities that arise in understanding laws affecting counseling practice. One concern is where the counselor and supervisor practice, for example, in a specific geographic location or online. Another complexity is knowing which laws potentially apply; counselors are not trained in the law. In cases wherein the counselor and supervisor are not sure about the legal implications of an ethical dilemma, the supervisor or counselor should consult with a lawyer. Many agencies and schools have access to legal services, and counselors and supervisors should not hesitate to consult as necessary.

DUAL RELATIONSHIPS BETWEEN SUPERVISOR AND SUPERVISEE

Similar to the possible ethical problems associated with dual relationships between client and counselor, there can be ethical problems with dual relationships between supervisee and supervisor. There are several dual relationships that present ethical issues in the counseling supervisee–supervisor relationship. One possible ethical dilemma centers on the possible conflict between the roles and job tasks of a supervisor (Tromski-Klingshirm, 2007). It is common for a supervisor to perform the roles of both clinical supervisor and administrative supervisor. A dual role of administrative and clinical supervisor possibly creates an ethical dilemma because of the different tasks that are required by each. Clinical supervision involves promoting therapeutic/counseling competence. The task may involve exploring personal counselor issues that could interfere with the client-counselor relationship. The supervisee in this relationship may disclose personal information that is sensitive and exposes the supervisee to perceptions of fallibility. One of the major tasks of the administrative function for the supervisor is evaluating a supervisee. If the supervisor is responsible for both clinical supervision and administrative supervision, the dual relationship may make it difficult to separate the information obtained in clinical supervision (which may be personal and show fallibilities of the supervisee) and evaluation data on counselor performance. The ACA's (2005) *ACA Code of Ethics* addresses this potential ethical issue and a dual role with clinical and administrative supervision in Section F.3.a, Relationship Boundaries With Supervisees:

> Counseling supervisors clearly define and maintain ethical, professional, personal, and social relationships with their supervisees. Counseling supervisors avoid nonprofessional relationships with current supervisees. If supervisors must assume other professional roles (e.g., clinical and administrative supervisor, instructor) with supervisees, they work to minimize potential conflicts and explain to supervisees the expectations and responsibilities associated with each role. They do not engage in any form of nonprofessional interaction that may compromise the supervisory relationship.

In actual practice it is more common to have a supervisor who performs both administrative and clinical supervision (Tromski-Klingshirm, 2007). Consequently, both the supervisor and the supervisee should be cognizant of the possible impact in the relationship when both roles are combined in a supervisory role. One possible solution that provides some clarity and is consistent with the *ACA Code of Ethics* (ACA, 2005) is to develop a written contract outlining the various activities and tasks that will be addressed in supervision. Also, separating the roles in terms of supervisory session times can be helpful. This means discussing clinical supervisory issues separately from administrative issues, particularly any evaluative feedback. Clearly noting the change in roles can be helpful in separating the possible dual relationship.

A second type of dual relationship that may occur in supervision is sexual relations between the supervisor and supervisee. Researchers have found that from 1% to 6% of supervisors had sexual relations with supervisees (K. Pope,

Tabachmick, & Kieth-Spiegel, 1987). The ACA's (2005) *ACA Code of Ethics* is explicit about sexual relationships between supervisor and supervisee. Code F.3.b states, "Sexual or romantic interactions or relationships with current supervisees is prohibited." The issue here concerns the differential amount of power in the relationship, or the question of coercion; the supervisor has power over the supervisee in evaluating him or her. This type of dual relationship is rather simple to understand, but clearly it still occurs. The question is, Why do sexual relations between supervisor and supervisee occur given the clarity of the problems with such a dual relationship? There are many organizations that have employee guidelines forbidding supervisors from having personal relationships with supervisees.

A third issue or dual relationship involves nonprofessional relationships. Nonprofessional relationships may involve friendships between supervisors and supervisees, and this type of dual relationship is more likely/common than many others. ACES's (1993) Ethical Guideline 2.10 states, "Supervisors should not participate in any form of social contact or interaction that would compromise the supervisor-supervisee relationship. Dual relationships with supervisees that might impair the supervisor's objectivity and professional judgment should be avoided and/or the supervisory relationship terminated." This is a difficult ethical problem. In many schools and mental health agencies, staff become friends and socialize outside of the workplace. If a supervisor does engage in such personal relationships outside the work setting, others in the organization may question the objectivity of the supervisor. Also, the supervisor may have difficulty completing either a positive or a negative evaluation of the supervisee given the dual relationship.

MULTICULTURAL ISSUES AND SUPERVISION

It has been noted that competence in multicultural/diversity supervision is an important factor in counselor development (Ancis & Marshall, 2010). Ancis and Marshall (2010) cited research that found when cultural issues are discussed in supervision, supervisees report greater satisfaction with the supervisor-supervisee relationship. Gloria, Hird, and Tao (2008) described the importance of multicultural supervision competence and stated, "Competence in multicultural supervision is imperative given the findings that receiving multicultural supervision significantly predicted trainees' self-reported multicultural counseling competence" (p. 129). Not addressing multicultural issues in supervision, it has been noted, is associated with problems and barriers to effective and competent supervision (Constantine, 1997; Gloria et al., 2008; Helms & Cook, 1999). It is interesting to note that researchers have found that only 30% of supervisors received multicultural counseling training compared to 70% of supervisees (Constantine, 1997). This may be changing as more recent graduates who likely had multicultural training receive promotions to supervisors. Certainly if supervisors did not receive training in multiculturalism, it may be hard for them to address diversity in supervision sessions. Burkhard et al. (2006) proposed that supervisors may intentionally choose to ignore or not address cultural issues in supervision; the authors referred to this as culturally unresponsive supervision. Furthermore, supervisors who are culturally unresponsive tend to dismiss the relevance of cultural issues in counseling (Burkhard et al., 2006).

There are different ways in which counselors may develop their own multicultural/diversity awareness. One way is through classes specifically focused on diversity and multicultural awareness. A second method is through supervision during field experiences such as the internship. We are concerned with how culturally competent supervision is a necessity for those acting ethically. In addition, counselors' awareness of the responsibilities of culturally competent supervisors can provide them with the necessary understanding and background to advocate for effective supervision. Casile et al. (2007) identified ways to ensure cultural sensitivity in the supervisory relationship. They identified the following four methods:

1. Identify and discuss multicultural issues that may exist in counseling sessions and in supervisory sessions.

2. Utilize the working alliance that develops between the supervisor and supervisee in an effort to promote collaboration in determining the effect of culture on the supervisory relationship.

3. Foster the development of trusting and open communication in the supervisory relationship that facilitates discussions addressing cultural issues in both the supervisory and the client-counselor sessions.

4. Maintain respectful responses to cultural differences, and utilize culturally appropriate interventions.

An effective ethical approach to supervision involves first the supervisor's developing his or her own competence in cultural/diversity competence. As has been noted, many supervisors may not have gone through training programs and may not have had extensive exposure to cultural/diversity training (Burkard et al., 2006). The *ACA Code of Ethics* (ACA, 2005) emphasizes the importance of supervisor cultural competence. *ACA Code of Ethics* Code F.2.b, Multicultural Issues/Diversity in Supervision, states, "Counseling supervisors are aware of and address the role of multiculturalism/diversity in the supervisory relationship." The ACA codes also cite the importance of supervisors' being trained in providing supervision (see Code F.2.a, Supervisor Preparation). Continued training beyond initial training as a supervisor is important, as is the counselor's continued development. Those who are providing supervision may benefit from ongoing training or continued education (ACA, 2005). One method of continued training is peer groups' engaging in discussions about cultural/diversity competence among supervisors. Regular participation in group discussions between supervisors, both beginning and more mature supervisors, can be beneficial to promote and enhance culturally competent supervision. Counselors would benefit from multicultural/diversity discussion in supervision sessions. As has been noted, both supervisees and supervisors benefit from such an open discussion of multiculturalism/diversity in supervision. These types of discussions increase the chances that competent counseling services are provided to clients. In addition, both counselors and supervisors with cultural/diversity competence are part of ethical practice.

SUMMARY

Supervision is a major contributor to ethical, legal, and professional practice by counselors. Supervision is an important element in ethical decision making based on a hermeneutic model; for example, supervisors' values, beliefs, and professional identity influence the horizon of the ethical decision-making process. There are a number of ethical issues that potentially arise from a supervisor-supervisee relationship. One ethical issue in counselor supervision is promoting the development of the counselor, the responsibility of fostering the growth of the counselor based on his or her developmental level and needs. Another potential ethical issue in regard to supervision is general competence and training in becoming a supervisor. Few supervisors receive training in being a supervisor before receiving a promotion to the position. These counselors often receive the promotion because they have demonstrated skill at counseling, which is important. Another important ethical issue is culturally competent supervision. Culturally competent supervision is separated from general competence because of the importance it plays in providing sensitive, effective services. An ethical issue that arises with the two primary functions of supervision—clinical and administrative—concerns the dual roles that can develop. Finally, supervisors have responsibility for the ethical and legal issues of their supervisees in working with clients. Supervisors need to make judgments about how much monitoring to do with each counselor to ensure clients are not harmed or injured.

Case Analysis and Reflection

Reread the case at the beginning of the chapter. Jim has not received training in being a supervisor, and his own supervisor did not provide any direction. Jim certainly is creating an ethical dilemma through his lack of competence in supervision. What might be the appropriate course of action for Jim to address this ethical issue? Should Jim even have volunteered to provide the supervision without first receiving training? What responsibility does Jim's supervisor have in contributing to and resolving this ethical dilemma?

Questions for Further Reflection

1. Consider the developmental phases and how counselors think about working with clients. Which phase represents your development?

2. How do you feel about a supervisor's having responsibility for your actions, for example, if you by chance harm a client? He or she may be just as liable as you under a lawsuit. Is this fair?

3. How would you feel about assuming the role of a supervisor in the future? What would make it attractive? Unattractive?

4. What role may your own ethical/moral developmental level have on your use of supervision or your providing supervision in the future?

Additional Recommended Readings

Ancis, J., & Marshall, D. (2010). Using a multicultural framework to assess supervisees' perceptions of culturally competent supervision. *Journal of Counseling & Development, 88,* 277–285.

Borders, L., & Brown, L. (2005). *New handbook of counseling supervision* (2nd ed.). Mahwah, NJ: Lawrence Erlbaum.

Burkard, A. W., Johnson, A. J., Madson, M., Pruitt, N., Contreras-Tadych, D., Kozlowski, J. M., . . . Knox, S. (2006). Supervisor responsiveness and unresponsiveness in cross-cultural supervision. *Journal of Counseling, 53,* 288–301.

Campbell, J. (2000). *Becoming an effective supervisor: A workbook for counselors and psychotherapists.* London, UK: Routledge.

Gloria, A., Hird, J., & Tao, K. (2008). Self-reported multicultural supervision competence of White predoctoral intern supervisors. *Training in Education in Professional Psychology, 2*(3), 129–136.

Granello, D. (2002). Assessing the cognitive development of counseling students: Changes in epistemological assumptions. *Counselor Education & Supervision, 41,* 279–292.

Ladany, N., & Bradley, L. (2010). *Counselor supervision* (4th ed). New York, NY: Routledge.

Ladany, N., & Inman, A. (in press). Training and supervision. In E. A. Almaier & J. Hansen (Eds.), *Oxford handbook of counseling psychology.* New York, NY: Oxford University Press.

Lyons, C., & Hazler, R. (2002). The influence of student development level on improving counselor student empathy. *Counselor Education & Supervision, 42,* 119–130.

Massachusetts Department of Children and Families. (2009). *Child abuse & neglect reporting: A guide for mandated reporters.* Boston: Author.

Pope, K., Tabachmick, B., & Keith-Spiegel, P. (1987). Ethics of practice: The beliefs and behaviors of psychologists as therapists. *American Psychologist, 42,* 993–1006.

Ronnestad, M., & Skovholt, T. (2003). The journey of the counselor and therapist: Research findings and perspectives on professional development. *Journal of Career Development, 30*(1), 5–42.

Chapter 11

ETHICAL USE OF RESEARCH IN COUNSELING PRACTICE

CHAPTER OBJECTIVES

- Acquire an understanding of the definition of *evidence-based* specific to counseling
- Develop strategies to promote and utilize evidence-based practice, for example, establishing evidence-based practice work groups
- Develop an understanding of the benefits of evidence-based practice in counseling
- Acquire an understanding of the limitations of evidence-based practice in counseling
- Identify possible specific counseling issues or problems and gold-standard treatments/interventions
- Understand the possible future impact of evidence-based practice on counseling

Case

Michelle is a rehabilitation counselor in a state vocational rehabilitation agency in the Southwest. She has worked in the state agency for 20 years, and she feels she is competent at her job. She comes to work and completes the necessary job tasks to help her clients/consumers obtain jobs and maximize their potential. She graduated with a master's degree in rehabilitation counseling more than 20 years ago, and she has periodically read journal articles when colleagues have brought them to work and recommended them to her. She maintained her membership in the American Rehabilitation Counseling Association for a few years after graduation but did not want to pay the ongoing dues, so she ceased being a member. She recalls that her least favorite course while she was a student was the research course. She maintains today that reading research is not that helpful to her in doing her job. She believes her 20 years' experience provides her with the necessary skills to do her job. Michelle has developed an expertise in her caseload, working primarily with those with severe mental illness. In addition, she has developed knowledge of substance abuse treatment because many of her consumers with major mental illness have substance abuse problems. Michelle has several clients who have been diagnosed with schizophrenia who also have had heroin addictions. Two of her consumers are participating in a methadone medical maintenance program in a local community agency.

Michelle is assigned an intern, Stephanie, who is enthusiastic and wants to learn as much as she can. Initially Michelle appreciates her enthusiasm for learning, but one day Stephanie brings up a study she read about how the research evidence on the effectiveness of methadone medical maintenance programs is inconclusive. Stephanie wonders how Michelle could support continuing methadone medical maintenance given the lack of evidence-based research. Michelle is offended that this student intern would challenge her knowledge. Michelle believes, based on her experience, that she can readily conclude whether the program works. The student offers to bring in the article for Michelle to read, but Michelle declines, saying she is too busy to read articles that contradict her experiences. Days later, Michelle begins to wonder if she should get the article and read it; she does want to be an ethical rehabilitation counselor. Work becomes very busy during the next few weeks, and Michelle forgets about the issue.

INTRODUCTION

Professions are defined in part by a foundation of practice based on research (Cruess, Johnston, & Cruess, 2004). Professions develop over time, and professional journals are introduced and provide practitioners with information sources for professional training and practice. Evidence-based practice (EBP) was first introduced in medicine (Sackett, Rosenberg, Gray, Haynes, & Richardson, 1996), then introduced later in other professions such as psychology (APA Presidential Task Force on Evidence-Based Practice, 2006) and counseling (Sue & Sue, 2008). There has been considerable discussion in the professional literature supporting (or not) the use of EBP (J. Carey & Dimmitt, 2008; Chan, Tarvydas, Blalock, Strauser, & Atkins, 2009; S. Cooper, Benton, Benton, & Phillips, 2008). The APA Presidential Task Force on Evidence-Based Practice (2006) offered a definition of *EBP* and concluded that EBP "is the integration of the best available research with clinical expertise in the context of patient characteristics, culture, and preferences" (p. 273). Several other definitions of EBP have been proposed (Hunsley, 2007; Whaley & David, 2007). Mayer (2004) provided one of the earliest definitions from medicine, stating that EBP is "the conscientious, explicit, and judicious use of the best evidence in making decisions about the care of individual patients" (p. 9). Common concepts of these definitions are statements about, first, identifying the best available research and, second, using reflection and evaluation in choosing the practices to be used. It has been suggested frequently that key in the preparation of the counseling professional is training in the use and application of research (Houser, 2009; Kettlewell, 2004). It is easy to recognize that we want to receive services from professionals who are highly competent and who are up to date on the most recent treatment approaches. No one wants to see a physician who has not maintained his or her knowledge and skills based on current methods or the most effective treatment methods. The ethical use of EBP in medicine may appear to be comparable to applying it in counseling, but there may be additional ethical issues for counseling (Berke, Rozell, Hogan, Norcross, & Karpiak, 2011). Intuitively, it may appear that accepting EBP does not raise any ethical issues, but there have been questions about its use (Berke et al., 2011). A review of the pros and cons of using EBP in counseling may help identify the ethical issues.

Kettlewell (2004) identified several benefits of using EBP. One benefit is that EBP can offer guidance for providing treatment and is consistent with expectations that professionals are current and competent. A second potential benefit is that the use of scientific approaches allows the professional to evaluate implementation of treatment, which then can inform future treatment. The professional can make adjustments to the intervention based on the evaluation results obtained. Kettlewell noted that over time the professional can develop a fund of information about best practices in his or her field, in this case counseling. A third rationale for using EBP is that one needs to be efficient and choose interventions and treatments that do not waste resources. This includes choosing interventions that are effective and do not waste health care resources, for example, the number of available counseling sessions covered by health insurance. A final argument for using EBP is that the use of science in making treatment decisions likely will advance the profession. Again, in a profession there is a body of knowledge, and developing a strong research base can promote the advancement of counseling.

Our society values science and the benefits that have developed, and this view provides credibility to evidence-based treatment (EBT)/evidence-based practice. The alternative is shifting the focus, making counseling an art or a practice based on one's personal experience. This may be compared to training in the trades, where one learns a trade through observing and working with a master practitioner. Such an approach has its benefits, but one of its limitations is that counseling is much more complex than learning a trade and requires more objectivity.

Berke et al. (2011) observed the following about EBP:

Evidence-based practice (EBP) is, arguably, the most consequential and controversial development in mental health during the past decade. On the face of it, every practitioner acknowledges the value of identifying, disseminating, and practicing treatments that entail the thoughtful synthesis of research evidence, clinical expertise, and patient values. But deciding what qualifies as veracious research and weightings . . . are complicated matters with deep philosophical traditions and huge practical consequences. (p. 329)

Key in this statement is the point that the research evidence from counseling may not be so clear (as it might be in medicine). Consequently, what are the ethical implications of making treatment or EBP decisions based on fuzzy results?

There has not been total acceptance of EBP, and there has been some criticism of the approach (Wampold, Goodheart, & Levant, 2007). Wampold et al. (2007) suggested caution in using and interpreting EBP information. The caution centers on the view that not enough is known to suggest that there is evidence that can be used to guide practice. The authors point out that one may miss the importance of the subjective experience of counseling or therapy. Counseling has been called an art, and losing subjectivity of the experience may interfere with this aspect of the process (Nystul, 1999). Wampold et al. (2007) pointed out that the evidence in psychology and counseling is not unambiguous and that "evidence is not data, nor is it truth" (p. 616). Several important questions arise with these criticisms. One question is, How much of the subjective aspect of counseling should be part of the practice? Professions have been identified and defined in terms of having a basis of knowledge (Weikel & Palmo, 1996). Despite the practice of counseling having a subjective component, counselors need to substantiate their practices on a basis of knowledge, specifically a research basis. Another question is, What level or amount of evidence is needed to use evidence-based research in practice? What has been suggested is to select the best available evidence and use it but, most important, evaluate the impact or effect.

There is an assumption in counseling that counselors' efforts are always positive and, because they are for the most part well intentioned, do not result in harm. However, there is evidence that counseling can cause harm (Lilienfeld, 2007). Lilienfeld (2007) noted studies showing that anywhere between 3% and 10% of clients in counseling actually deteriorate after counseling. In addition, he noted that harm may occur with family and friends as a consequence of counseling with a client; for example, clients may learn to behave differently, which affects those close to them in a negative way. Lilienfeld concluded that because there is no formal monitoring of treatments, for example, by a federal agency such as the Federal Drug Administration, counseling/psychology professionals need to monitor potentially harmful therapies. The use of EBP may help reduce the frequency and impact of potentially harmful therapies, but only if certain criteria are used to make good decisions about the interventions used in counseling. Ensuring counselor competence and selection of appropriate therapies/techniques is an ethical issue because not doing so may increase the likelihood of employing potentially harmful therapies or techniques. One example of how counselors sometimes jump to provide new approaches that turn out to be potentially harmful therapies is the recovered memories technique, which was not based on research or adequate evidence (Lilienfeld, 2007). Geraerts et al. (2007) found that recovered memories that were inconsistent and originated within therapy were less reliable and were questionable. Essentially the question posed was whether counselors/ therapists contributed to recovering memories that were constructed and not corroborated from other sources. Colangelo (2007) noted that recovered memories and False Memory Syndrome resulted in many individuals' being falsely accused of sexual abuse as a consequence of counselors' engaging in recovered memory work/counseling. Lilienfeld identified a number of other potentially harmful therapies such as boot camp interventions. Counselors acting ethically need to be alert to feedback and information that suggest the potential for harm. Including EBP information (professional knowledge) is an element in the hermeneutic ethical decision-making model and needs to be considered when one is confronted with an ethical dilemma (see Figure 4.1).

APPROACHES TO EVIDENCE-BASED PRACTICE

There have been several suggestions about how to effectively and ethically use EBP and the selection and evaluation of evidence (Mayer, 2004). Mayer (2004) proposed six steps in the EBP approach that are important to using it effectively in practice. The first step is the identification of a question; for example, What needs to be answered? Important in constructing this question is the identification of the outcome desired. The second step is a careful review of the professional literature that is relevant to the question to be answered. The goal is to discover the best information available on the topic. The third step is the identification of a study that most closely resembles the issue to be addressed and the evaluation of the outcomes achieved in the study; for example, Are the outcomes those desired by the practitioner? The fourth step is an evaluation of the study to determine its quality and use. Step 5 is an assessment of how the study outcomes may be applied to the current issue. The last step, Step 6, is an evaluation of how successful the efforts are in practice once implemented by the practitioner/counselor. A limitation of this approach is that much of the evaluation is accomplished by the practitioner. However, it does provide a systematic approach the individual counselor can use to evaluate and use EBP effectively and ethically.

Other approaches to effectively and ethically employ EBP have been proposed (Rousseau & McCarthy, 2007). Rousseau and McCarthy (2007) offered several principles in using EBP. The first principle, according to Rousseau and McCarthy, is, "Focus on principles where the science is clear" (p. 85). What are the basic principles of the discipline? Some basic principles in counseling are findings about human development, counseling techniques, and multiculturalism. A counselor then focuses on research findings addressing human development. A second principle proposed by Rousseau and McCarthy is, "Develop decision awareness in professional practice" (p. 87). The process involves sharing among colleagues in evaluating and critiquing practices (Rousseau & McCarthy, 2007). A third principle is a focus on the identification of underlying factors that involve practice decisions (Rousseau & McCarthy, 2007). The basic idea is for the practitioner to identify questions that are designed to diagnose the problem to be addressed with EBP. A counselor needs to have an understanding that there is an issue with how clients are functioning and to determine whether something can be done to improve their lives through counseling. Rousseau and McCarthy suggested the next principle concerns an understanding of the context of the situation, the issue to be addressed, and how the counselor adapts the information/research to the setting. There is a level of judgment that is required of the counselor in adapting the research evidence to the clinical situation. Some counselors are likely better at connecting the research evidence to the practical situation. The next principle, according to Rousseau and McCarthy, is the use of colleagues in applying research evidence in practice. Unfortunately, most practitioners do not engage in discussions with colleagues about research evidence and how it might be used in practice. J. Carey and Dimmitt (2008) proposed that counselors should develop "evidence-based" practice teams. The focus of the teams is to link evidence-based research to practice and discuss how this may be accomplished. This is an interesting and thoughtful approach to implementing evidence-based practice and promoting ethical practice through group discussion and feedback. The last principle concerns counselors' reading current research literature and attending conferences where they may be exposed to new ideas and EBP knowledge (Rousseau & McCarthy, 2007).

As was mentioned earlier, we as consumers of services such as medical services want professionals who are knowledgeable and who have up-to-date knowledge and skills in providing our treatment. Certainly, our clients have the same expectations of counselors. In addition, the American Counseling Association concludes that counselors have a responsibility to the public to provide research-based practice; *ACA Code of Ethics* Section C, Professional Responsibility, states, "Counselors have a responsibility to the public to engage in counseling practices that are based on rigorous research methodologies" (American Counseling Association, 2005).

COUNSELING RESEARCH EVIDENCE: EXAMPLES OF EVIDENCE-BASED PRACTICE INFORMATION

There have been a number of writings about and summaries of EBP focusing on specific issues in counseling (Gowers, 2006; Kaiser, 2007; Stenhoff & Lignugaris-Kraft, 2007). The Substance Abuse and Mental Health Services Administration lists a registry of evidence-based programs and practices addressing alcohol and substance abuse (www.nrepp.samhsa.gov/ViewAll.aspx). *Mental Health: A Report of the Surgeon General* provides a review of current mental health practices and focuses on specific mental health treatment such as mood disorders (www.surgeongeneral.gov/library/mentalhealth/home.html). Another source of EBP reviews is the Cochran Collaboration website (www.cochrane.org/about-us). It is not the purpose of this text to review all of the evidence-based counseling publications, but a review of several will provide examples of what is available to the practitioner. Keel and Haedt (2008) provided a comprehensive review of EBTs for eating disorders. Results of their review of more than 20 studies identified specific treatment effectiveness for anorexia nervosa, for example, family therapy for treating anorexia nervosa. The Cochrane Collaboration cited 13 studies that support the use of family therapy with clients who are diagnosed with anorexia nervosa (www2.cochrane.org/reviews/en/ab004780.html). Gowers (2006) provided EBP information for counseling adolescents with eating disorders using cognitive-behavioral therapy. Gowers concluded that the research evidence for the treatment of bulimia nervosa using cognitive-behavioral therapy is comparatively good and is considered the "gold standard treatment" for bulimia. However, he further concluded that the research evidence for using cognitive-behavioral therapy with anorexia nervosa is not quite as clear and that there needs to be further research before one can conclude that it fits as a gold standard of treatment for anorexia nervosa. One can see that the evidence that family therapy is effective with anorexia nervosa is complex (Keel & Haedt, 2008), but cognitive-behavioral therapy is not effective with anorexia nervosa (Gowers, 2006). The implication for practitioners using EBP is that there needs to be careful research into which methods work in which particular situations. This does not mean that one cannot use a certain intervention, and this may be particularly true if there is no other gold standard available. Counselors should choose the best available documented intervention when the information is available.

W. Silverman, Pina, and Viswesvaran (2008) analyzed more than 30 studies focusing on treatments for phobia and anxiety disorders in children and adolescents. Based on the review, they concluded that certain interventions such as cognitive-behavioral therapy and group cognitive-behavioral therapy do show probable effectiveness in treating phobias. No consistent research supports a particular treatment focused on anxiety disorders. Again, there were specific findings related to the treatment of certain conditions.

There has been extensive research on changing health-risk behavior (Baban & Craciun, 2007). Baban and Craciun (2007) focused on health-risk behaviors including smoking, sexual behavior, alcohol abuse, eating habits, screening behaviors, and medication adherence. They discussed different approaches to changing health-risk behavior such as the Health Action Process Approach and the Transtheoretical Model of Change approach (Prochaska & Norcross, 2010). Baban and Craciun provided information about approaches that may be used with various health-risk behaviors, and they cited the effectiveness of each based on research outcomes. For example, the Transtheoretical Model of Change approach was noted to be effective with smoking, alcohol abuse, and screening behaviors. The Transtheoretical Model of Change is not found to be as effective with sexual behavior or medication adherence. There may be several explanations for why it was not found to be effective; one may be that there is not enough research to support such a conclusion.

SUMMARY

Counselor competence is based in part on the use of an EBP approach and maintaining current knowledge. Acting ethically using EBP is not simple, and a counselor needs to develop systematic strategies for implementing EBP. It may be too complex for an individual counselor to evaluate the research literature alone, but meeting with colleagues and discussing current research is a way to begin evaluating research. Members of such a professional work group could share their own literature review findings and evaluate the level and quality of the evidence focused on a particular treatment strategy or mental health problem. If one cannot find or develop such a group, developing a simple strategy such as that proposed by J. Carey and Dimitt (2008) may be a solution in practicing ethically. The strategy J. Carey and Dimitt proposed requires carefully identifying the problem, reviewing evidence-based research, and finally evaluating the outcomes. Key in evaluating the evidence is noting whether a number of studies have been conducted on the topic and they have used rigorous research methods. Simply the publication of a study or a description of a new approach does not raise the evidence high enough. Consistent outcome results showing the effectiveness of a treatment approach are necessary to qualify for the strong evidence that is necessary to practice ethically. Full disclosure to clients is important in acting ethically. This means that sharing with clients the evidence available about the outcomes of using a particular treatment is part of ethical practice. We as consumers of health care want to know the possible outcomes of particular treatments, and similarly consumers of counseling want information about possible outcomes and strategies. In cases wherein the evidence is not strong, clients should be informed of the status of the treatments or inventions. We recognize that not all mental health problems have well-established evidence for practice, and in such cases informing clients of that status or level of evidence maintains ethical practice.

Thomason (2010) made several predictions about the use and status of EBP. One prediction is that at some point liability insurance covering counselor practice will cover only treatments supported by EBP. In essence, if a counselor is sued after using a treatment not based on EBP, he or she may not be covered/protected. This seems extreme given that not all mental health problems have enough evidence to demonstrate effectiveness. Certainly if there is evidence available and it is not used, the insurance industry may choose not to cover any lawsuit charges. A second prediction by Thomason is that only EBTs will be reimbursed by health insurance and that those client problems that do not have adequate evidence must be treated without health coverage. This too seems drastic, but health insurers may require the use of EBT when it is available to reimburse for treatment. These predictions, if they become reality, add to the ethical issues in counseling practice. Health insurers limiting payment or liability coverage to only EBTs place counselors in difficult positions about what to treat. We propose that fully informed disclosure is ethical and reasonable in using EBP. As has been noted, there are conditions and treatments that currently do not have the evidence necessary to claim acceptable levels for treatment outcomes. This does not mean that treatments and approaches not reaching levels of quality evidence should not be used. The key is giving the client full information about the level of evidence or lack of evidence and engaging him or her in a discussion about the course of counseling to follow.

Case Analysis and Reflection

Reread the case at the beginning of the chapter. You are the intern, and you see a supervisor who has years of experience not using the research literature and EBP strategies. What do you do? What will you do in your practice to avoid being this supervisor after 20 years of practicing counseling?

Questions for Further Reflection

1. How comfortable are you in using professional research and reading research? Is your competence in reading research adequate to understand EBP, or do you need to develop these skills more? How can you increase these skills?

2. Discuss with colleagues how you might establish an EBP work group once you enter the profession. How can such a work group be maintained over time?

3. What are your thoughts about full disclosure and informing a client that in some cases there is little research support for a particular treatment?

4. Is there any connection to your ethical/moral development and how you implement EBP?

Additional Recommended Readings

APA Presidential Task Force on Evidence-Based Practice. (2006). Evidence-based practice in psychology. *American Psychologist, 61*(4), 271–285.

Carey, J., & Dimmitt, C. (2008). A model for evidence-based elementary school counseling: Using school data, research, and evaluation to enhance practice. *Elementary School Journal, 108*(5), 422–430.

Colangelo, J. (2007). Recovered memory debate revised: Practice implications for mental health counselors. *Journal of Mental Health Counseling, 29*(2), 93–120.

Cruess, S., Johnston, S., & Cruess, R. (2004). Profession: A working definition for medical educators. *Teaching and Learning in Medicine, 16*(1), 74–76.

Gowers, S. (2006). Evidence-based research in CBT with adolescent eating disorders. *Child and Adolescent Mental Health, 11*(1), 9–12.

Kaiser, A. (2007). Addressing challenging behavior: Systematic problems, systematic solutions. *Journal of Early Intervention, 29,* 114–118.

Kamps, D., Abbott, M., Greenwood, C., Arrega-Mayer, C., Wills, H., Longstaff, J., . . . Walton, C. (2007). Use of evidence-based, small-group reading instruction for English language learners in elementary grades: Secondary-tier interventions. *Learning Disability Quarterly, 30,* 153–168.

Keel, P., & Haedt, A. (2008). Evidence-based psychosocial treatments for eating problems and eating disorders. *Journal of Clinical Child & Adolescent Psychology, 37*(1), 39–61.

Kettlewell, P. (2004). Development, dissemination, and implementation of evidence-based treatments: Commentary. *Clinical Psychology: Science and Practice, 11*(2), 190–194.

Lilienfeld, S. (2007). Psychological treatments that cause harm. *Perspectives on Psychological Science, 2,* 53–68.

Mayer, D. (2004). *Essential evidence-based medicine.* Cambridge, UK: Cambridge University Press.

Nystul, M. (1999). *Integrative approach to teaching counseling psychology.* Boston, MA: Allyn & Bacon.

Odom, S., Brantlinger, E., Gersten, R., Horner, R., Thompson, B., & Harris, K. (2005). Research in special education: Scientific methods and evidence-based practices. *Exceptional Children, 71*(2), 137–149.

Rousseau, D., & McCarthy, S. (2007). Educating managers from an evidence-based perspective. *Academy of Management Learning & Education, 6*(1), 84–101.

Sackett, D., Straus, S., Richardson, W., Rosenberg, W., & Haynes, R. (2000). *Evidence-based medicine: How to practice and teach EBM.* New York, NY: Churchill Livingston.

Silverman, W., Pina, A., & Viswesvaran, C. (2008). Evidence-based psychosocial treatments for phobic and anxiety disorders in children and adolescents. *Journal of Clinical Child & Adolescent Psychology, 37*(1), 105–130.

Stenhoff, D., & Lignugaris-Kraft, B. (2007). A review of the effects of peer tutoring on students with mild disabilities in secondary settings. *Exceptional Children, 74,* 8–30.

Sue, D., & Sue, D. (2008). *Foundations of counseling and psychotherapy: Evidence-based practices for a diverse society.* Hoboken, NJ: John Wiley.

Thomas, G., & Pring, R. (2004). *Evidence-based practice in education.* Maidenhead, UK: Open University Press.

Wampold, B., Goodheart, C., & Levant, R. (2007). Clarification and elaboration on evidence-based practice in psychology. *American Psychologist, 62,* 616–618.

Weikel, W., & Palmo, A. (1996). *Foundations of mental health counseling* (2nd ed.). Springfield, IL: Charles C Thomas.

Chapter 12

PROFESSIONAL CODES OF ETHICS AND THE LAW

CHAPTER OBJECTIVES

- Acquire an understanding of how laws affect counseling practice
- Develop an understanding of factors to consider in duty to warn and duty to protect ethical issues
- Develop an understanding of the factors to consider in duty to warn when a client has sexually transmitted diseases and is not informing partners of his or her condition
- Acquire an understanding of elements of the horizon in hermeneutic ethical decision making that affect a decision to make a child abuse and neglect report
- Be able to recognize and apply professional codes in ethical decision making

Case

Jane is a rape counselor working in a nonprofit agency in the Midwest. She received her graduate degree in mental health counseling more than 10 years ago. She is licensed as a professional counselor in her state, and she is one of the more seasoned counselors in her agency.

She has been providing counseling for the past 2 months to an 18-year-old woman, Janice, who was raped by a man at a party within the first month of her beginning college. Janice had been drinking, and she admits she probably drank too much and was not careful enough in being aware of her environment and those around her. She reported the rape, which took place in a fraternity house; she was lured into a room on the premise that she was to be shown a new computer game. She recalls clearly telling the man "no," but he overpowered her and raped her. She reported the rape to campus police, who arrested a suspect and charged him with forcible rape, a criminal offense. The suspect was charged and released on bail. Janice had difficulty sleeping and eating and decided to seek counseling at local counseling center.

The defense attorney discovers that Janice is in counseling and obtains a subpoena for the counseling records. Jane consults with her supervisor and decides not to comply with the court-ordered subpoena. Jane feels strongly that the counseling records should be confidential and that the records particularly should not be used to help the defense build a case. She feels this would be a second effort to harm her client, not giving her justice if the defendant is not found guilty. The judge in the case cites Jane with contempt of court and orders her to release the counseling records. He gives Jane 2 days to release the records or she will be arrested and placed in jail until she releases the records. After consulting with the agency attorney, Jane decides to appeal the subpoena to a higher court. Jane was arrested at work after 2 days and is now locked up in jail awaiting the higher court's decision on her appeal. She is wondering whether she is doing the right thing in withholding the records. What should she do now?

INTRODUCTION

An introduction to the legal system is an important place to start in understanding the impact of laws on counselor practice and ethical practice. There are two major types of laws that potentially affect counselors: civil and criminal laws. Criminal laws start with an understanding that an offense is against the state, and the consequences may be fines, imprisonment, or death (Carp & Stidham, 1998). *Black's Law Dictionary* (Garner, 2004) describes *criminal law* as "the body of law defining offenses against the community at large, regulating how suspects are investigated, charged, and tried, and establishing punishments for offenders" (p. 431). A crime may also be understood as an obligation to society and generally involves an overt act or behavior causing harm to person, property, and so forth. Carp and Stidham (1998) noted that most crimes are those that everyone in society agrees are not acceptable forms of human behavior. Laws that are defined as crimes need to be clear and clearly determined. Legally one cannot charge someone with a crime if no law exists even if the act is one that harms others and may appear to require punishment (Carp & Stidham, 1998).

Geldhart and Yardley (1995) differentiated civil law and criminal law and stated,

> The difference between civil law . . . and criminal law turns on the difference between objects which the law seeks to pursue—redress or punishment. The

object of civil law is the redress of wrongs by compelling compensation or restitution, the wrongdoer is not punished, he only suffers so much harm as is necessary to make good the wrong he has done. The person who has suffered gets a definite benefit from the law, or at least he avoids a loss. On the other hand, in the case of crimes, the main object of law is to punish the wrongdoer; to give him and others a strong inducement not to commit the same or similar crimes, to reform him if possible, and perhaps to satisfy the public sense that wrongdoing ought to meet with retribution. (p. 174)

Both criminal and civil laws affect counseling practice. One criminal behavior that counselors have engaged in is fraudulent billing for client services (www .psychcrime.org/database/). It is estimated that mental health professionals submit billions of dollars in fraudulent billing each year. Fraudulent billing is a criminal offense and can involve significant fines and imprisonment. Another criminal act with which mental health professionals have been charged is sex with minors (www.psychcrime.org/database/). Some states have criminal laws against having sex with patients, regardless of age (www.bbs.ca.gov/pdf/publications/lawsregs .pdf). Another criminal activity that counselors have engaged in is taking bribes for service referrals and failing to file income taxes. It is clear that counselors may be convicted of crimes related to their professional activities that go outside normal/professional actions, resulting in criminal behavior and convictions.

A counselor may be sued for malpractice in a civil lawsuit (A. Roberts, Monferrari, & Yeager, 2008). This type of lawsuit is focused on the plaintiff's alleging harm (this typically is not covered under criminal law, but it can be covered under criminal law) with the intention of receiving monetary compensation from the defendant. One of the more frequent reasons for such lawsuits against counselors is the client's committing suicide. A. Roberts et al. (2008) noted that some of the largest monetary judgments against counselors for malpractice were the consequence of clients' committing suicide; the families brought the lawsuits. There has been a range of lawsuits against counselors for various malpractice reasons. Appelbaum (2001) noted the number of lawsuits brought based on counselors'/therapists' generating false memories in clients; many of these lawsuits were brought by third parties to counseling (those not in counseling) who were accused of sex abuse through recovered memories. Appelbaum reviewed such cases in various states and concluded that there is no uniform view on whether counselors/therapists may be sued by third parties for generating false recovered memories. Third-party lawsuits have been successful in some courts and not others.

Good advice for counselors in regard to criminal law issues is to be knowledgeable about state and federal laws that apply. Also, being knowledgeable about trends in court decisions on lawsuits for malpractice is important. The reality is that counselors, or anyone, can be sued for any actions or behaviors. One can act ethically and still be sued. This is one reason it is important to thoughtfully reason through ethical dilemmas. Including a review of state and federal laws and court decisions in the hermeneutic ethical decision-making process is important (review Figure 4.1).

PROFESSIONAL CODES OF ETHICS

It has been suggested that a characteristic of a profession is the establishment of professional codes of ethics (Walden, Herlihy, & Ashton, 2003). Lunt (1999) suggested that "codes may provide bottom-line rules or prescriptions for behavior or aspirational guidelines" (p. 245). Freeman (2000) also attempted to clarify the role of professional codes and concluded that "ethical standards are self-imposed regulations that provide rough guidelines for professional behavior and attempt to specify the nature of the ethical responsibilities of members, at least minimally" (p. 19). Counseling programs, particularly accredited programs, require students to accept professional codes (the American Counseling Association [ACA] ethical codes, the American Mental Health Counseling Association ethical codes, etc.) and adhere to their standards. Information about expectations of students adhering to professional codes often is stated in student handbooks. The important ethical question is, What role do the professional codes play in the counseling practice? It is important to note that each student/graduate in counseling should be very familiar with the professional codes of ethics of his or her discipline. Professional codes of ethics have been developed for a number of counseling specialties (see Table 12.1).

Table 12.1   Codes of Ethics for Various Counseling Specialties

Counseling Specialty	Professional Code	Web Link
American Counseling Association	ACA Code of Ethics	www.counseling.org/Resources/CodeOfEthics/TP/Home/CT2.aspx
American Mental Health Counseling Association	Principles for AMHCA Code of Ethics	www.amhca.org/assets/news/AMHCA_Code_of_Ethics_2010_w_pagination_cxd_51110.pdf
American Association of School Counseling	Ethical Standards for School Counselors	asca2.timberlakepublishing.com//files/EthicalStandards2010.pdf

Commission on Rehabilitation Certification	CRC/CRCC Code of Ethics	www.crccertification.com/pages/crc_ccrc_code_of_ethics/10.php
American Association for Marriage and Family Therapy	AAMFT Code of Ethics	www.aamft.org/imis15/content/legal_ethics/code_of_ethics.aspx
National Career Development Association	NCDA Code of Ethics	associationdatabase.com/aws/NCDA/asset_manager/get_file/3395/code_of_ethicsmay-2007.pdf

How does a counselor use professional codes? Codes are considered guidelines for practice. In reviewing the codes, you may see where standards that address confidentiality are in conflict with codes that focus on protecting others (and result in a breach of confidentiality). There are other possible standards that conflict, and the counselor must try to determine a course of action. A hermeneutic model of ethical decision making (see Figure 4.1) provides a format for working through complex ethical issues; one sees the total horizon and does not have tunnel vision (considering only one element of the horizon). Focusing on only one source of information such as a code of ethics hinders a full understanding of an ethical dilemma. Also, professional codes of ethics may be in conflict with state and/or federal laws. Finally, codes of ethics may be in conflict with personal ethical values and ethical theories.

DUTY TO WARN/DUTY TO PROTECT/DUTY TO CONTROL

One particularly important court decision concerning duty to warn is *Tarasoff v. Regents of the University of California.* Duty to warn is much more complex than what has been taught and presented in many counseling programs. Frequently duty to warn is associated with the California case that was the result of events occurring in 1969 (www.stanford.edu/group/psylawseminar/Tarsoff%20I.htm). The case involved a lawsuit brought by the parents of Tatiana Tarasoff, who was murdered by Prosenjit Poddar, against a psychologist employed at the University of California, Berkeley; the university police; and the director of the counseling center. Mr. Poddar had become friends with Ms. Tarasoff, and he interpreted their relationship as more than friendship. Once he expressed his interest in more than a friendship, Ms. Tarasoff rejected his efforts. She left for Brazil for several months. Mr. Poddar was depressed and upset that he had been rebuked by

Ms. Tarasoff. Prosenjit Poddar sought counseling from the university counseling center. Dr. Lawrence Moore saw Mr. Poddar for several months. In one session, Mr. Poddar stated he wanted to murder a woman who was easily identified as Ms. Tarasoff. The psychologist contacted campus police and requested that Mr. Poddar be detained and evaluated for dangerousness. The campus police briefly detained Mr. Poddar and released him, concluding that he was not dangerous. The counseling center supervisor concluded that no further action was needed, and he had records of the counseling sessions destroyed (Buckner & Firestone, 2000). No university personnel warned Ms. Tarasoff, who was out of the country at the time, about the threat made by Mr. Poddar. When she returned to California, Mr. Poddar murdered Ms. Tarasoff. The complaints by Ms. Tarasoff's parents against the counseling center and university involved four assertions: the therapist's failure to have Mr. Poddar detained; a failure to warn Ms. Tarasoff or her family; the choice of the center director, Dr. Powelson, not to pursue detention; and finally, breach of primary duty. The court found in favor of the parents/plaintiffs. The conclusion was that counselors, psychologists, and so forth do have a responsibility, a duty to warn an intended victim of a violent act. The fact that Mr. Poddar was free and not confined required that the mental health professionals and those with knowledge of the situation had a duty to warn Tatiana Tarasoff and/or her family members of the potential danger. *Tarasoff* is based on the perspective that counselors, psychologists, social workers, and so forth have a duty to use reasonable care to protect identified others from harm from their clients/patients. *Tarasoff* did include an interpretation that such a standard of care is based on the client's/patient's identification of an intended victim. Vague reference to a victim who is not easily identified does not fall under *Tarasoff* (Buckner & Firestone, 2000). Duty to warn and the laws and court decisions associated with it fit into the hermeneutic model under review of local, state, and federal laws (see Figure 4.1).

The ethical decision based on the hermeneutic model is further complicated by states' having different perspectives on duty to warn and duty to protect (see Appendix A). In addition, the ACA suggests that a universal ethical approach is to warn those who can potentially be harmed by a client. *ACA Code of Ethics* (ACA, 2005) Section B.2.a, Danger and Legal Requirements, states,

> The general requirement that counselors keep information confidential does not apply when disclosure is required to protect clients or identified others from serious and foreseeable harm or when legal requirements demand that confidential information must be revealed. Counselors consult with other professionals when in doubt as to the validity of an exception.

Despite the ACA code, state laws and court interpretations of duty to warn vary from state to state (Barbee, Combs, Ekleberry, & Villalobos, 2007). For example, Texas law does not support duty to warn. The Texas court decision *Thapar v. Zezulka* found that state law does not support disclosure to a third party in a case of identified threat from a client. In fact, it is contrary to Texas state law, which encourages maintaining confidentiality (Barbee et al., 2007). Barbee et al. (2007) noted that "Licensed Professional Counselors and other licensed mental health professionals in Texas should be aware that their allegiance must be to state law or significant penalties may result" (p. 22). There have been numerous subsequent court cases and state laws that affect counselor actions about duty to warn and duty to protect. Counselors need to consider this element in the hermeneutic model (review local, state, and federal laws and court decisions; see Figure 4.1) when making decisions about an ethical dilemma (see Appendix A for a list of state laws and court decisions affecting counseling practice and duty to warn).

TYPES OF CONFIDENTIALITY: BROAD CONFIDENTIALITY AND PRIVILEGED COMMUNICATION

A basic foundation of the counselor-client relationship is confidentiality. Professional codes of ethics espouse the importance of maintaining confidentiality. Confidentiality is seen as an element in establishing trust between a counselor and a client. Clients enter counseling with an expectation that the counseling sessions are confidential (Glosoff, Herlihy, & Spence, 2000). Most beginning counselors also believe that counseling sessions are confidential and may believe that confidentiality in counseling has legal status. Beginning practicum students have been heard to tell clients that everything said in the sessions is totally confidential. The broad term *confidentiality* does not have any legal status and is not protected from legal proceedings. Glosoff, Herlihy, Herlihy, and Spence (1997) described the relationship between counseling and the legal system: "The ethic of confidentiality is not a legally recognized excuse for failing to obey a court order to disclose information relevant to a case" (p. 573). Broadly, confidentiality is established through professional organizations such as the ACA, the American Mental Health Counseling Association, the American School Counseling Association, the Commission on Rehabilitation Counselor Certification, the American Association for Marriage and Family Therapy, and so forth. These professional codes provide broad guidelines outlining the special circumstances under which confidentiality may be breached. These circumstances include such incidences as the client's intention to harm himself or herself or others, child abuse, and compliance with legal proceedings. Increasingly, the courts and legal system have utilized counseling services, and as a consequence they seek information about what transpires in counseling. The legal system may be interested in client progress and compliance with counseling services. As a consequence, it is not easy for the counselor to offer or maintain a guarantee of confidentiality. Counseling with children and adolescents is another source of possible conflict surrounding breach of confidentiality. Parents are legally responsible for their children, and consequently they may request information about their children's progress. In addition, schools frequently have policies about parental notification when there is a risk or danger to the child, for example, concerning use of drugs or threats of suicide. Bodenhorn (2006) surveyed school counselors and found that more than 90% concluded the most difficult ethical issue concerns maintaining student confidentiality. Confidentiality is complex in schools because counselors have relationships with teachers who may seek out counselors for advice about working with a child. Parents may seek out information from counselors about counseling with their child. School administrators may seek information to make determinations about discipline decisions.

Family therapists have ethical dilemmas with confidentiality because they potentially have a whole family in counseling. For example, if family therapists see children in the family separately, they may be encouraged by parents to share what transpires in sessions. In addition, if there is any information about possible child abuse, confidentiality may be breached (confidentiality and reporting child abuse are addressed in subsequent sections of this chapter). Clearly there are numerous possible ethical dilemmas facing counselors in maintaining confidentiality and deciding whether to break confidentiality.

A more narrow type of confidentiality is privileged communication. Privileged communication is commonly associated with the relationship between lawyers and clients, clergy and parishioners, and doctors and patients. Glosoff et al. (2000) described privileged communication in regard to legal proceedings: "Only privileged communication, which is established by statute, can protect clients from disclosure in legal proceedings" (p. 78). Herlihy and Sheeley (1987) attempted to identify the extent of privileged communication according to state statutes for various professionals such as psychologists, family therapists, counselors, and social workers. They noted that counselors more than two decades ago did not have the legal protection of privileged communication. However, a more recent study of state statutes and privileged communication finds that this has changed significantly. State statutes recognizing privileged communication for counselors have expanded to include more than 45 states' offering some degree of privileged communication protection for counseling clients (Glosoff et al., 2000). Glosoff et al. noted that privileged communication historically, in all professions, includes four criteria: confidentiality is critical to the professional relationship; the disclosure is communicated predicated on the belief that it would not be disclosed outside the professional relationship; the community/public respects the maintenance of protected communication between the professional and client; and any damage as a consequence of the disclosure would likely result in greater harm than the benefits of court proceedings or legal proceedings. Despite privileged communication's having a legal basis, there are limitations to the extent to which it is implemented. States that have statutes for privileged communication for counselors vary as to what the exceptions are. Glosoff et al. surveyed states and identified many of the exceptions to maintaining privileged communication. One of the most common exceptions is when there is a conflict between the counselor and client. A client's initiating a complaint is an exception to the privilege (the counselor needs to be able to defend himself or herself from any allegations). A second common exception to privileged communication written into state laws concerns the issue of mental illness and the possible question of an insanity defense in a court hearing. A second circumstance involving mental illness is when a client wants to pursue a complaint that an injury caused him or her to seek out mental health services. Counselors should be aware of whether privileged communication is extended to counselors in the jurisdictions in which they operate. A review of the hermeneutic model (see Figure 4.1) and the elements of the horizon addressing state, local, and federal laws and professional codes of ethics provides additional insight about the importance of systematically thinking about ethical dilemmas.

CONFIDENTIALITY AND TRANSMITTED DISEASES

Another important ethical issue involving confidentiality is working with clients who have sexually transmitted diseases. DiMarco and Zoline (2004) asked the question, "What are the ethical and legal duties of mental health professionals who learn that an HIV-infected client is endangering others by knowingly exposing them to the virus?" (p. 68; see Appendix A). Many writers have attempted to interpret and answer this question through state laws and court decisions founded on *Tarasoff* and duty to warn (Alhazo, Upton, & Cioe, 2011; Burkemper, 2002; DiMarco & Zoline, 2004; Huprich, Fuller, & Schneider, 2003). Alhazo et al. (2011) discussed how counselors may consider applying duty to warn to a situation involving an identified partner of a client who is infected with HIV/AIDS and who has not informed his or her partner of the disease. The three essential elements of duty to warn are a special counseling relationship, a reasonable prediction of immediate harm communicated by the client, and the ability to identify the potential victim (Alhazo et al., 2011). The ethical question arises in the interpretation of the second element with HIV/AIDS. Is there an immediate danger of harm, and is it possible for the counselor to identify the intention to harm directly?

A review of both professional codes of ethics and state laws shows a potential conflict for counselors (see Appendix A). *ACA Code of Ethics* (ACA, 2005) Section B.2.b, Contagious, Life Threatening Diseases, states,

> When clients disclose that they have a disease commonly known to be both communicable and life threatening, counselors may be justified in disclosing information to identified third parties if they are known to be at demonstrable and high risk of contracting the disease. Prior to making a disclosure, counselors [must] confirm that there is such a diagnosis and assess the intent of clients to inform the third parties about their disease or engage in any behaviors that may be harmful to an identified third party.

The ACA code provides guidelines to counselors outlining that they should implement duty to warn when working with clients who have HIV/AIDS and whose situation fulfills the three criteria, that is, a special counseling relationship, a reasonable ability to predict harm, and identification of the potential victim. In essence, if a counselor becomes aware that his or her client has a sexually transmitted disease such as HIV/AIDS and has not disclosed the information to his or her sexual partner (and is engaging in unprotected sex), then the counselor contacts the third party, the partner of the client, to inform him or her of the client's sexually transmitted disease status.

A conflict arises for counselors using the ACA code with many states' having laws that prohibit breaking confidentiality to disclose HIV/AIDS status. A report to the U.S. Centers for Disease Control and Prevention (epic.org/privacy/medical/cdc_survey.html) summarizes a survey of state statutes on rules for maintaining privacy/confidentiality for those with HIV. The state statutes address issues such as who can release such information and to whom. Gostin, Lazzarini, and Flaherty (1995) reported in a survey of state statutes outlining protection of those with HIV/AIDS from inappropriate disclosure and breach of confidentiality that some state laws allowed for release of information about HIV/AIDS status under specific circumstances. The most frequent reason for disclosing HIV/AIDS status is to share information about health care professionals. The second most common reason for releasing information about HIV/ADS status concerns sharing of needles or sexual partners (37 states have such statutes).

Also, state laws may spell out who is able to share HIV/AIDS status with sexual partners. In many cases the identified professional who is able to disclose HIV/AIDS status to sexual partners is a physician or medical professional. For example, the Illinois state law on disclosing information about HIV/AIDS status to sexual partners allows only a physician to disclose such information (www .health.state.ny.us/diseases/aids/facts/helpful_resources/confidentiality_law .htm). Consequently, counselors in Illinois have a conflict about whether to follow professional codes, such as the ACA code, or state laws for guidance regarding breaking confidentiality and informing a sexual partner if a client has HIV/AIDS and is engaging in unprotected sex. In addition, Illinois state law includes a statement that unauthorized disclosure may result in a criminal offense, possible jail time, or a fine. According to Pennsylvania state law, HIV/AIDS status may be disclosed to a sexual partner only by a physician. Case law addressing inappropriate disclosure of HIV/AIDS status varies from state to state (Webber, 2004). Not all states or jurisdictions have case law outlining whether any violations will result from disclosure.

REPORTING ABUSE: CHILD, ELDER, OR DISABILITY ABUSE

There are almost 2 million reports of child abuse made in the United States each year (McDaniel, 2006). All states have child abuse laws, and they have identified mandated reporters including counselors (see Appendix B). Counselors are confronted with ethical decisions about reporting suspected child abuse and neglect; it rarely is a simple decision. Researchers have discovered that ethical decisions about whether to report child abuse and neglect are complex and not easily determined (Carleton, 2006; McDaniel, 2006; Zellman, 1990). One of the biggest issues facing counselors in reporting child abuse and neglect is the way that state laws are written and the lack of clear description of what constitutes abuse and neglect. Zellman (1990) concluded that definitions in state laws regarding child abuse are "vague and nonbehavioral" (p. 325). This places mandated reporters in a dilemma as they try to interpret what constitutes abuse and neglect. Child abuse may be reported to state departments of child protection (designations vary from state to state, and they may be called departments of social services) by both professionals/mandated reporters and nonprofessionals (the general public). Researchers have found that slightly more than 50% of child abuse reports are completed by mandated reporters and the remainder are completed by neighbors and family members. In addition, it has been found that approximately 40% of child abuse cases reported nationally are substantiated, which means that 60% are not substantiated (McDaniel, 2006). It could be concluded that the significantly low rate of substantiated child abuse cases is the result in part of vague definitions of abuse stated in public laws. Others have discovered that many counselors/professionals do not have confidence in state departments of protective services and consequently will not make child abuse reports but work with their clients to reduce the abuse.

A counselor's familiarity with his or her state's laws is essential to making ethical decisions and reporting suspected child abuse (see Appendix B). An ethical decision to submit a report should cause the counselor considerable deliberation. A report of suspected child abuse or neglect may significantly affect a family and a child. A counselor's submitting a report may break the trust between a client and counselor if the client thinks everything said in counseling is confidential. Conversely, not reporting child abuse and neglect may place a child in significant danger and may result in a juvenile client's sense of distrust ("You are not protecting me"). An easy answer to the question of whether to report child abuse or neglect is not possible given the complexity of each circumstance. Reviewing the elements of the horizon that are present in the hermeneutic model should help one make an ethical decision (see state laws, professional codes, and relevant ethical theories in Figure 4.1).

FEDERAL LAWS AND CONFIDENTIALITY AND PRIVILEGED COMMUNICATION

There are several federal laws and court decisions that address confidentiality for counselors. The Health Insurance Portability and Accountability Act (HIPAA) and the Family Education Right Privacy Act (FERPA) address confidentiality in regard to health and psychological records and educational records, respectively. Another federal law that protects a specific population is the Code of Federal Regulations, Title 42–Part 2, Confidentiality of Alcohol and Drug Abuse Patient Records. HIPAA was passed by Congress in 1996 with the initial intention of reducing health care costs. Bragg (2009) cited the specific goals of HIPAA, which are to promote access to health insurance (allow workers to maintain health insurance when changing jobs); cut fraud, abuse, and waste; and increase the efficiency of health care. HIPAA applies to health care providers, including those providing mental health services. There are rules for protecting the privacy of health care records, including counseling records, called Protected Health Information. Protected Health Information is defined in terms of Individually Identified Health Information (Bragg, 2009). Individually Identified Health

Information includes (www.hhs.gov/ocr/privacy/hipaa/understanding/summary/ privacysummary.pdf):

- a person's past, present, and future physical or mental health condition;
- the actual provision of health care and mental health care to the client; and
- past, present, and future payment for health care and mental health care.

Individually Identified Health Information also includes such specific information as a client's name, address, social security number, and so forth. Disclosure of information requires patient/client consent; however, there are exceptions. The exceptions include emergencies, subpoenas, and audits by state agencies. In addition, HIPAA includes exceptions for psychotherapy notes. The Office of Civil Rights described an exception for psychotherapy notes:

> A covered entity may use or disclose, without an individual's authorization, the psychotherapy notes, for its own training and to defend itself—in legal proceedings brought by the individual . . . to avert a serious and imminent threat to public health or safety. (www.hhs.gov/ocr/privacy/hipaa/understanding/ summary/privacysummary.pdf)

Disclosure to avert serious threat and imminent danger to public health or safety may involve ethical issues discussed earlier such as duty to warn for physical threats and/or sexually transmitted diseases.

A second federal law that is important in ethical decision making for counselors is FERPA (Wise, King, Miller, & Pearce, 2011). FERPA is primarily focused on protecting the privacy of student records. First, FERPA gives a parent the right to access his or her child's student records in school. Second, once a student is 18 years or older, he or she may access his or her school records. Parents and students have the right to review school records; however, schools are not required to provide copies of the records (unless the parent or student lives at a distance from the school and cannot come to the school to review the records). Also, parents and students have the right to ask schools to correct any inaccurate records. Parents and students must grant permission to release any information from school records. There are exceptions to releasing records without appropriate permission (see Table 12.2).

Release of educational information may be completed without release of records from parents and/or students in emergency situations that involve threat to the health or safety of students or others. An example is a student who has been disciplined for aggressive behavior and threats made to others. Disclosure of information such as documented aggressive behavior to appropriate officials, that is, police or paramedics, when safety or health is threatened, may fall under this exception.

Table 12.2	Exceptions to the Prohibition of Releasing Student Records (Family Education Right Privacy Act Guidelines)

Records may be released to

- school officials with legitimate educational reasons,
- another school where the student is transferring,
- officials conducting an audit or evaluation,
- accreditation organizations,
- other parties in adherence to legal requirements and in cases of court subpoena, and
- appropriate officials in cases of health and safety emergencies.

Source: www2.ed.gov/policy/gen/guid/fpco/ferpa/index.html.

A third federal law that is relevant in considering ethical actions particularly focused on the release of information and confidentiality is the Confidentiality of Alcohol and Drug Abuse Patient Records codes (Code of Federal Regulations, Title 42–Part 2, Public Health). This legislation provides protection for those in substance abuse and alcohol treatment. The legislation prohibits disclosure of the following records of those in such treatment: identity (not even acknowledging that the person is receiving treatment), diagnosis, prognosis, and/or treatment. In addition, no information about those in substance abuse or alcohol treatment may be used in any criminal charges against the client, although there are exceptions. One exception is if there is a court order to release the information. Also, information may be disclosed in the following circumstances: a crime on the premises of a treatment program, communication to emergency personnel to address a medical emergency, and reports of suspected child abuse and neglect.

SUMMARY

Applying the hermeneutic model in counseling ethics includes a number of elements of the horizon, for example, state and federal laws, professional codes of ethics, ethical theories, and client personal values. Counselors should become familiar with state and federal laws that affect their counseling practice. This means acquiring copies of state and federal laws that apply and being aware of the applications to counseling. Also, counselors should be aware of and be current on court decisions that affect practice. Breaking confidentiality and consideration of duty to warn varies from state to state, and counselors should be aware what the laws are in the jurisdictions in which they practice. Another ethical concern involving maintaining confidentiality arises when a client has HIV/AIDS and has not informed his or her sexual partner. What responsibility does the counselor have under duty to warn and duty to protect in such cases? Again, state and federal laws should be reviewed in determining the best ethical decision.

A specific type of confidentiality that holds more protection is privileged communication. The amount of legal protection counseling sessions are granted varies from state to state, and counselors should be aware of the limits of confidentiality in the regions of their practice. Three federal laws potentially apply to counseling: HIPAA, FERPA, and the Confidentiality of Alcohol and Drug Abuse Patient Records codes. Child abuse and neglect create significant and complex ethical dilemmas. All states have child abuse and neglect laws that identify mandated reporters, and counselors are considered mandated reporters of child abuse and neglect. A problem is that all states have laws that are vague in defining what child abuse and neglect are, and therefore making a report is difficult. Once a counselor breaks confidentiality and makes a suspected child abuse and neglect report, he or she may negatively affect the counseling relationship and potentially even fracture it to the point where the client will not continue. Professional codes of ethics provide guidelines for counseling practice. There are specific codes for various counseling specialties, and a review of relevant codes in making an ethical decision is necessary to make the best decision possible. We suggest a careful review of state and federal laws, court decisions, and professional codes when making an ethical decision based on the hermeneutic model. Remember that the hermeneutic model is a dynamic process, and elements of the ethical horizon are interpreted simultaneously once the information is identified; it is not considered in a linear fashion.

Case Analysis and Reflection

Reread the case at the beginning of the chapter. What would you decide to do if a court ordered you to release counseling records and break confidentiality in such a case? Would you be willing to go to jail to protect a client's counseling records and defy a court order? Which state laws might apply to this case in the area in which you live? Review the ACA codes of ethics that apply, and identify the standards that possibly apply.

Questions for Further Reflection

1. It is important to develop a statement to share with clients about the extent of confidentiality. Write a statement about the limits of confidentiality that you might use in counseling.

2. Discuss with a colleague how you would go about sharing with clients examples of situations in which you would be required to break confidentiality.

3. Remaining current on changes in state and federal laws and court decisions is challenging. Which strategies could you use to remain current?

Additional Recommended Readings

Appelbaum, P. (2001). Law and psychiatry: Third party suits against therapist in recovered memories cases. *Psychiatric Services, 52,* 27–28.

Bodenhorn, N. (2006). Exploratory study of common and challenging dilemmas experienced by professional school counselors. *Professional School Counseling, 10*(2), 195–202.

Bragg, M. (2009). *HIPAA for the general public.* Chicago, IL: American Bar Association.

Buckner, F., & Firestone, M. (2000). Where the public peril begins: 25 years after Tarasoff. *Journal of Legal Medicine, 21*(2), 187–222.

Wilcoxon, A., Remley, T., & Gladding, S. (2012). *Ethical, legal and professional issues in the practice of marriage and family therapy.* Boston, MA: Pearson.

Section III

Ethical Theories and Cases

Chapter 13

WESTERN THEORIES OF ETHICS

CHAPTER OBJECTIVES

- Acquire an understanding of virtue ethics and relevant concepts
- Acquire an understanding of natural law ethics and relevant concepts
- Acquire an understanding of utilitarian ethics and relevant concepts
- Acquire an understanding of respect for persons ethics and relevant concepts
- Acquire an understanding of feminine/feminist ethics and relevant concepts

We suggest that including ethical theories in ethical decision making is an essential element of the process. We want to introduce Western ethical theories first and discuss how they may be applied to a counseling ethical dilemma. The five Western theories that are addressed include virtue, natural law, utilitarian, respect for persons, and feminism/feminist ethics. Each perspective provides methods for interpreting ethical dilemmas and provides insight into what counselors may consider in choosing ethical actions. Professional codes of ethics are typically founded on several of these theories, for example, virtue ethics and utilitarian ethics.

VIRTUE ETHICS

In Western philosophical thought it is common to view the field as primarily defined by three main approaches for determining what is right and wrong. The oldest of these three is virtue ethics, which focuses on moral character and attends to the characteristics of the individual that lead to moral actions. This view can be contrasted to theories that emphasize moral duties or rules (e.g., deontological approaches, respect for persons) or the moral consequences of an action (e.g., utilitarian approaches).

The history of virtue ethics begins with the ancient Greek philosophers including Plato, Socrates, and especially Aristotle, who is most associated with current models of virtue ethics. Taken together, these theorists helped to define what the good life entails and how one ought to live, what are the standards for a characteristic to be good, and how one should act to attain happiness. It is interesting to note that some have identified a Chinese influence on Greek thinking, and it may be more than a coincidence that Chinese and Greek models have a similar focus on moral character and an interest in finding a compromise between extreme positions (e.g., Buddhism; see Chapter 14). For most of Western history, virtue ethics was the dominant perspective; this lasted until the Enlightenment when interest in other moral systems took hold (Shanahan & Wang, 2003). However, since the 1950s there has been a renewed interest in virtue ethics, and more recently many of those in the character education movement rely on virtue ethics to define the character elements that they hope to foster (Carr & Steutel, 1999).

Major Concepts

Professionals are trained to develop the skills associated with best practice in their fields and a clear sense of their responsibility to society at large (Beauchamp & Childress, 2001; Jordan & Meara, 1990). The claim is that through direct instruction and socialization, professionals come to understand this responsibility to society through the development of an identity that includes an ethical component. To illuminate this ethical component, the profession typically lists the principles or virtues that define a professional ethical identity (see Table 13.1). In the helping professions, these core virtues include the following:

1. nonmalevolence, the duty to do no harm;

2. benevolence, the duty to do good for clients and the larger society;

3. justice, the duty to treat all fairly;

4. fidelity, keeping a promise—maintaining confidentiality; and

5. respect for autonomy, the duty to ensure that the individual's right to make decisions is maintained.

More specifically, *nonmalevolence* refers to the central duty to do no harm either through intention or by entering into any action that may indirectly cause harm in others. Professionals must be vigilant to ensure that their actions maximize the good across their interactions with clients. In counseling, concerns about entering into or terminating treatment, the use of confidential information, and whether to inform interested parties about information learned during treatment are central to concerns about the possibility of doing harm.

At first blush, benevolence appears to be simply the flipside of nonmalevolence. However, whereas nonmalevolence suggests that one must refrain from actions that do harm, benevolence directs one to take active steps to promote the welfare of others. The professional should help members of society who could benefit from his or her expertise and should actively seek these people out. Similarly, the professional should make every effort to be current in his or her knowledge to maximize the good that can be achieved in professional interactions. Similarly, decisions about clients should be constructed to maximize the clients' well-being and potential development.

Justice refers to treating all persons in a fair and equitable way. All professionals must ensure that their professional help is available to all persons in need without undue consideration of noncentral characteristics of the individual such as group affiliation, beliefs, and life situation. In particular, professionals ought not to practice in a way that discriminates against others. Furthermore, justice requires professionals to address inequities in access to their care and services.

Respect for autonomy refers to a professional's duty to respect the client's right to self-determination. A professional addresses respect for autonomy by telling the truth about his or her plans, actively consulting the client throughout the process, and ensuring that the client understands the ramifications of any treatment options. Furthermore, respect for autonomy requires that the professional gain informed consent for any treatment plans and that all matters of privacy are respected.

In addition to these core virtues, it is expected that the professional be truthful, be faithful, maintain confidentiality, and respect the privacy of others: fidelity. As we noted above, these values fall from the core virtues but are typically explicitly stated. By attending to these virtues and values, it is hoped that over time and through the growth of professional wisdom, these virtues will become part of the professional's identity and as such, his or her character. Furthermore, it is assumed that these virtues as character elements will be used to inform ethical decision making. Or put another way, the professional will develop virtuous habits of mind that will be applied wisely to specific situations (Beauchamp & Childress, 2001).

| Table 13.1 | Summary of Ethical Concepts for Virtue Ethics |

Ethical Concept	Definition/Description
Nonmalevolence	Obligation to do no harm
Benevolence	Obligation to promote the welfare of others, for example, clients
Justice	Obligation to treat others fairly, for example, avoid special treatment in distribution of services
Autonomy	Right to make free informed choices, one's own free will
Fidelity	Keeping a promise such as a promise of confidentiality

NATURAL LAW ETHICS

Aristotelian philosophy and virtue ethics influenced the development of natural law. Humans follow natural law in what they do by nature; this is a law based on conscience. Natural law decisions or actions are right because they fulfill human nature, which is communicated by God. The intent is to discover that nature or natural law. Natural law is interpreted as universal and unchangeable, as moral absolutism (C. E. Harris, 2007). C. E. Harris (2007) described natural law and stated that the theory is based on the view that humans have free will and they must decide whether to act ethically. Because natural law derives from nature, it is believed to be binding on human behavior even beyond the laws established by humans (eternal law).

There were several early contributors to natural law. St. Augustine in the 4th century CE and St. Thomas Aquinas in the 13th century CE offered a Christian version of Aristotle's ethics (Shanahan & Wang, 2003). Shanahan and Wang (2003) described Augustine and Thomas Aquinas as the Plato and Aristotle of the middle ages. Thomas Aquinas was the primary proponent of natural law theory (C. E. Harris, 2007). Shanahan and Wang described Thomas Aquinas's life as "devoted to studying, writing, teaching and traveling. It was by general agreement, one of the most philosophically productive lives anyone has ever lived" (p. 57). Natural law is associated closely with the Catholic Church.

Natural law theory is a morally absolute theory; it is not relativistic. What this means in practice is that the principles of natural law are applied uniformly across situations, across cultures, and do not vary as a consequence of a particular situation. Natural law theorists believe that there are objective standards of morality independent of the individual. Ethical laws are natural, and they apply to all human beings regardless of the customs, beliefs, and values of a particular society. Natural law is based on a nonconsequential perspective. The outcomes of an act are not necessarily relevant, but the intentions of the individual are. Determining whether an act is ethical includes determining the intentions of the individual: Did he or she have good intentions? An absolute value, according to natural law, is that of human life; consequently, a single life should not be sacrificed to save several lives. For example, a person can choose to visit a sick relative and help him or her out in an effort to ensure getting into the will, or the person can perform the same behaviors to ensure the relative is safe and feels someone cares. The intentions are different even though the behaviors may be the same, and an evaluation of intentions provides insight into the morality of the act.

Major Concepts

We want to present the primary concepts in natural law theory and the basic information necessary to understand and apply the theory (see Table 13.2). Natural law is based on the idea that humans operate from free will, which suggests that humans can decide how they should act (C. E. Harris, 2007). The primary truth in natural law is that humans should do whatever promotes the fulfillment of human nature. To find out about human nature, one observes behavior to identify the goals that humans pursue because those goals reflect the foundation of our human nature. Therefore, for Aquinas, the goals are the "natural inclinations" that all human beings have in common.

According to C. E. Harris (2007), human inclinations are divided into two groups: biological values and human values. Biological values are composed of two values, life and procreation (C. E. Harris, 2007). A basic natural inclination is to preserve and maintain one's self. Natural law is based on the view that individuals have an obligation to maintain their health and a right to defend themselves. As a consequence, suicide and murder are unethical. Procreation is a biological value in natural law; it is considered unethical/immoral to use artificial contraception or engage in homosexuality. A second inclination, human values, is composed of pursuing knowledge and sociability. Humans have a natural tendency to seek knowledge of the world and of God. Any hindering of the pursuit of knowledge of the world or God is not considered ethical. Humans also have an inclination to seek relationships with others through friendship and love—sociability. Anything that interferes with the sociability inclination is considered wrong.

Two additional qualifying principles guide moral decision making from a natural law perspective (C. E. Harris, 2007). The two principles are forfeiture and double effect. Forfeiture states that one gives up his or her own rights when he or she threatens the rights of others. Any person who threatens the life of an innocent person (one who has not threatened anyone's life) forfeits his or her own right to life. This principle justifies acts of self-defense for individuals and allows state actions such as capital punishment and defensive war. It also justifies forfeiture of liberty if one engages in such behavior as killing another person or stealing another's possessions; the result is imprisonment or death.

Based on the principle of double effect, an action must meet four criteria to be considered a violation of a fundamental value (C. E. Harris, 2007). It is morally permissible to perform an action that has two possible effects, one good and one bad. The following criteria are relevant in determining whether an outcome is moral based on double effect (C. E. Harris, 2007): (a) The act itself must be morally permissible; (b) the bad effect of the act must be unavoidable to achieve the good effect; (c) the bad effect must not be the means of producing the good effect, but only a side effect; and (d) the good effect must be at least as morally desirable as the bad effect is morally undesirable. C. E. Harris (2007) concluded that if all four conditions are not met, then the act is immoral or unethical. An example in counseling is when the counselor is confronted with determining whether to break confidentiality because a client states he has gotten overly physical with his child. The act must be permissible (state laws allow it). Second, hearing about child abuse is not something the counselor can ignore; it is unavoidable. Disclosing events of a counseling session to inform legal authorities of possible child abuse does not maintain confidentiality. Last, the good effect of protecting the child outweighs the bad effect of breaking confidentiality.

Table 13.2 Summary of Natural Law Ethical Concepts

Concept	Definition/Description
Free will	Humans have free will and can decide on courses of action, whether ethical actions or not.
Biological values	
Life	Humans have a natural inclination to preserve life; suicide and murder are wrong.
Procreation	Engaging in activities that do not promote procreation, for example, contraception and homosexuality, is unethical.
Human values	
Sociability	Humans seek connections with others and promote positive relationships with others. Engaging in conflict is wrong.
Knowledge	Humans have a desire to understand the world and to understand God. Interfering with seeking knowledge is unethical.

Concept	Definition/Description
Principle of forfeiture	One gives up the right to life if he or she takes another life. One gives up the right to freedom (e.g., goes to prison) is he or she threatens others. One can defend oneself if threatened, and this is one instance wherein the biological value of promoting life can be violated ethically.
Principle of double effect	There may be two choices of action with one good and one bad possible outcome. One may still make the choice even though there can be a bad outcome. Four criteria for ethical action include the following: The act must be morally permissible, the bad effect is unavoidable to achieve the good effect, the bad effect is a side effect, and the good effect must equal the bad effect.

UTILITARIAN ETHICS

Utilitarian theory originated during the 18th century. Shanahan and Wang (2003) summarized many of the contributing factors in the development of utilitarian theory. These include the impact of the Industrial Revolution, which focused on economics and a cost-benefit analysis. The theory has affected many aspects of our lives including state and federal laws as well as professional codes of ethics. C. E. Harris (2007) stated that "utilitarianism is one of the most powerful and persuasive traditions of moral thought in our culture" (p. 121). One of the early contributors to utilitarian theory was David Hume in the mid-1700s (Shanahan & Wang, 2003). Hume proposed many of the basic concepts of utilitarian theory. He believed morals influenced human behavior, and he believed that humans are naturally kind. Also, Hume believed that humans sympathize with others, which affects their ethical behavior. Jeremy Betham was a follower of Hume, and he formally inscribed Hume's ideas about utilitarian theory (Shanahan & Wang, 2003). Betham's views were affected by his personal background in economics and government. Betham believed that pleasure and pain influence human behavior and human decision making. His basic view of ethics was that good or bad is a consequence of the difference in the amount of pleasure or pain involved in courses of action for all individuals involved (Shanahan & Wang, 2003). Second, Betham believed that good or pleasure as an outcome for all affected by a circumstance could be quantified. He was one of the first to introduce a method to quantify ethical choice. Specific amounts of pleasure could be attached to particular actions for an individual affected by the decision, and a total amount of pleasure could be calculated for everyone affected (Shanahan & Wang, 2003). Betham proposed the principle of utility, which states that one pursues actions that promote happiness or pleasure.

John Stuart Mill was another proponent of utilitarian theory, and he was influenced by Betham's views. Mill was informally trained at home and studied Greek and Latin. He read Betham's work and studied logic, which affected his views. Mill wrote on topics similar to those Betham addressed, focusing on government, economics, and ethics (Shanahan & Wang, 2003). Mill concluded that "happiness is the sole end of human action, and the promotion of it the test by which to judge of all human conduct; from whence it necessarily follows that it must be the criterion of morality" (Mill, 1863, Chapter 4).

Major Concepts

A basic premise of utilitarian theory is that humans seek out happiness and pleasure. Mill suggested that some human pleasures may be categorized hierarchically. One example of a higher pleasure is the use of the intellect. Reading an interesting and challenging book may result in new knowledge versus the satisfaction one obtains from sexual or physical desires that benefit only a few. Promoting use of the intellect is more ethical than pursuing one's own physical pleasures.

C. E. Harris (2007) noted that an evaluation of whether an act is moral is based on a determination of the utility of the act. According to Harris, utility is defined as "preference or desire satisfaction" (p. 122). He further suggested that preferences or desires can be determined hierarchically. The hierarchy may be stated in the following manner: "1) preferences whose satisfaction contributes to the preferences of others; 2) preferences whose satisfaction is neutral with respect to the preference satisfaction of others, 3) preferences whose satisfaction decreases the preference satisfaction of others" (C. E. Harris, 2007, p. 123). Another important perspective in utilitarian theory is the importance of happiness. Harris noted that utility is connected to happiness. Utilitarian theory proposes that fostering the happiness of others is the most important goal, whereas one may promote the satisfaction or happiness of oneself at the same time. A second type of happiness is happiness for the self when it has no impact on others: a neutral act. Finally, the least desirable type of happiness is happiness for the self that decreases the satisfaction of others and consequently has the least utility.

As has been mentioned, one of the goals or indicators of utilitarian ethics is promoting happiness, particularly in others. The Greatest Happiness Principle (GHP) provides a basis for considering ethical behavior. Knapp (1999) provided a good definition of the ultimate goal of utilitarian theory, stating, "The purpose of ethics is to engender the greatest amount of happiness for the greatest number of people. The sole moral duty is to produce as much pleasure as possible (positive utilitarianism) or to decrease as much pain as possible (negative utilitarianism)" (p. 384). Rachels (1998) further clarified the GHP, stating, "Each person's happiness counts the same" (p. 102). Utilitarian theory also is based on the belief that the needs of nonhumans or animals are relevant in considering ethical decisions.

C. E. Harris (2007) has developed an approach to quantify the utility of an act. Harris proposes assigning values to those affected by an ethical decision. First, one identifies the number of persons affected by an act. Second, values are assigned to units of utility per person. Below is an example based on Harris's model to quantify utility.

> Jennifer has a grandmother who is 83 years old, and she always had a good relationship with her grandmother while she was growing up. The grandmother is becoming more dependent on others to function. She lives alone but relies on family members to help her with paying bills and maintaining her household. Jennifer tries to help her grandmother at least 4 days a week despite living more than 20 miles away. Her brother lives only a few miles away, and he helps out about the same amount of time each week as Jennifer. He talks to the grandmother about things such as her will and what he may inherit when she is deceased. In fact, he asks the grandmother for money when he comes, saying it takes his time and gas to come to her to help. Jennifer cannot believe this is what he asks the grandmother. She is debating whether she should bring up this issue with her grandmother. Based on a utilitarian perspective and an assessment of utility, the following assessment illustrates the Harris model.

Action	*Number of People Affected*	*Utility per Person*	*Total*
1 (tell grandmother)	1 (Jennifer)	70	
	1 (brother)	10	
	1 (grandmother)	50	130
2 (do not tell grandmother)	1 (Jennifer)	10	
	1 (brother)	50	
	1 (grandmother)	10	70

The following interpretation is based on the C. E. Harris (2007) model. Action 1 receives a utility of 70 for Jennifer, 10 for her brother, and 50 for her grandmother. Utility scores are determined by attaching a value to each person's happiness if the act is carried out. Action 1, informing her grandmother that she feels her brother is taking advantage, receives an overall value of 130. Action 2, not informing the grandmother, receives a total value of 70. The brother would be happier, and the grandmother would not know of the grandson's intentions. The assignment of utility is somewhat arbitrary and not as mathematical as Harris proposed.

Utilitarian theorists have identified two types of utilitarian theory: act utilitarianism and rule utilitarianism (C. E. Harris, 2007). Act utilitarianism is based primarily on an assessment of the specific circumstance(s) that occur, most often a one-time event. The above example of Jennifer's ethical dilemma illustrates act utilitarianism. A determination of the more ethical action is based solely on the specific circumstances of the two acts considered. The outcome has little impact on future ethical decisions that affect others aside from the three individuals involved.

Rule utilitarianism is based on the view that general rules determine ethical behavior. There are choices of actions that result in the most utility across many circumstances, not just one. C. E. Harris (2007) described rule utilitarianism: "Rules or actions are right insofar as they promote utility and wrong insofar as they promote disutility" (p. 126). Moldoveanu and Stevenson (1998) proposed that rule utilitarianism based on GHP is "the rule embodied by an action, and asks about the global utility consequences of acting in accordance with that rule, given what we know about how everyone else usually acts" (p. 723). Rules that protect those from minority groups from discrimination follow rule utilitarianism (Knapp, 1999). For example, rule utilitarianism may be a foundation for rules against discriminating against minority groups in hiring practices. Although not as many benefit from rules to protect minorities from job discrimination, such rules benefit everyone because they protect a smaller group from discrimination. The conclusion of rule utilitarianism may be that the long-term benefit of having such protections is good for society and promotes fairness that can be used as a rule or model for all such decisions (see Table 13.3).

Table 13.3 Summary of Utilitarian Ethical Concepts

Ethical Concept	Definition/Description
Utility	An act is moral based on a determination of the utility of the act. It is the satisfaction of any preference a person has.
Happiness	Fostering the happiness of others is the most important goal. According to the Greatest Happiness Principle, the purpose of ethics is to engender the greatest amount of happiness for the greatest number of people.
Rule utilitarianism	General rules govern ethical behavior and promote the most utility across many circumstances.
Act utilitarianism	This requires an evaluation of a specific circumstance, a one-time event, for utility and happiness.

RESPECT FOR PERSONS ETHICS

One of the originators of respect for persons ethics was Immanuel Kant, who wrote several books outlining his moral theories, such as the *Fundamental Principles of the Metaphysic of Morals* (Shanahan & Wang, 2003). There have been alterations of his original ideas, but many of the underlying principles still apply. The central focus of the ethics of respect for persons is that there is equal respect for every human. The ethics of respect for persons is associated with Christian and Judaic views. Respect for persons has been categorized as a deontological perspective based on a duty or obligation (Shanahan & Wang, 2003).

The goal of equal treatment of all humans is found within the view that reason must be demanded of all rational beings, that it is a duty. In practice what this means is that moral perspectives are more often based on universal principles than on individual needs (Singer, 1993). Specifically, discovering a universal ethic or standard is a goal of this perspective. Individuals may seek ethical principles that are not self-focused by asking if a choice of actions would meet the approval of most individuals. C. E. Harris (2007) suggested there are universal principles on which most humans can agree. Specifically, Harris stated the following moral standard: "An action is right if you can consent to everyone adopting the moral rule presupposed by the action" (p. 155). There are several ways to determine whether a universal principle fits this standard. The Christian example may be found in Luke 6:31, which states, "Do unto others as you would have them do to you." Such a perspective provides an example of the source of a possible universal principle. Kant's ethical theory is based on the view that normal adults are autonomous and they have the capacity to be self-governing in moral decisions (Schneewind, 1992).

Major Concepts

C. E. Harris (2007) suggested several methods to determine whether a moral action is based on a universal principle. One approach was the "self-defeating test." The question Harris offered based on the self-defeating test was, "Can I consent to others' acting simultaneously according to the same rule I use without undermining my own ability to act in accordance with it?" (p. 155). There are common examples in everyday Western life that can be found even in our laws and customs. There are specific laws about stealing someone's car or taking someone's money. It is easy to see that such laws meet the criteria of the self-defeating test: Can I consent to another's stealing my car? We certainly do not want others taking our cars.

A second moral principle cited by C. E. Harris (2007) is the means-end principle. The specific moral standard states, "Those actions are right that treat human beings, whether you or another person, as an end and not simply as a means" (p. 160). Treating someone as an end is demonstrated when everyone is treated equally and respectfully. Treating another as a means to meeting one's own needs violates the means-end principle. Harris noted that there are a number of social/business circumstances/transactions wherein others are treated as a means versus an end. When you go into a convenience store, you are there typically to purchase something for your own needs, and the clerk is there to sell you something. Each may be treating the other as a means to benefit himself or herself. You want a product and are not necessarily concerned about the welfare of the clerk, and the clerk wants to be paid for doing his or her job. However, it is hoped that you treat the clerk respectfully (you probably have seen circumstances in which this was not true), but your primary purpose likely is to get the product. There is a forfeiture component of respect for persons that states that if one treats another as a means, he or she forfeits his or her right to freedom and his or her own well-being (C. E. Harris, 2007).

There are several other methods of evaluating the means-end test. One is the negative test, which states, according to C. E. Harris (2007), "Does the action override my own or others' freedom or well-being?" (p. 164). Concretely this means that I may seek to meet my own needs but cannot affect the freedom or well-being of others at the same time. I may want a new car, and so I begin talking to my neighbor who is a car salesperson. I did not care to talk to her previously, but I want to get information from her about when sales are offered and how to negotiate with another car salesperson. I am treating the neighbor as a means and not an end. Once I gather enough information from her and I buy my car, I return to ignoring her. Recall that a basic premise of respect for persons is that human are autonomous and self-governing. Humans have the capacity for self-governance but at the same time have an obligation to act in a certain way, morally, treating others with respect and not as a means to get what they want (C. E. Harris, 2007).

Respect for persons differentiates a hypothetical imperative and a categorical imperative. A hypothetical imperative is any action founded on acts that are personal or subjective. Schneewind (1992) clarified that the imperative is hypothetical because "the necessity of action it imposes is conditional. You ought to do a certain act if you will [attain] a certain end" (p. 319). The imperative is a personal interpretation and may have a goal of acting based on achieving a specific end. Kant did not believe such a perspective was ethical because he felt decisions should be based on universal principles that are not personal.

The basis of Kant's concept of the categorical imperative begins with his insistence that our actions possess moral worth only when we do our duty. Kant described the categorical imperative:

> Act only according to that maxim [subjective plan of action] through which you can at the same time will that it should become a universal law. . . . Act as if the maxim of your action were to become through your will a universal law of nature. (Kant, 1953/1785, pp. 88–89)

Key to determining whether an act is based on a categorical imperative is that it is based on a universal law of nature. Kant further explained the categorical imperative, stating, "Act in such a way that you always treat humanity, whether in your own person or in the person of another, never simply as a means, but always at the same time as an end" (Kant, 1953/1785, p. 96). What this statement refers to is treating others primarily as an end (with respect), whereas there is acceptance that one may involve the use of the person as a means to achieve the end. It is important to understand that many laws and professional codes of ethics are founded on universal principles and that we as part of society respect and follow them (see Table 13.4).

Table 13.4   Summary of Respect for Persons Ethical Concepts

Ethical Concept	Definition/Description
Hypothetical imperative	Decisions are based on personal interpretation and designed to achieve a certain end.
Categorical imperative	Acts are consistent with a universal law, for example, do not kill another. As a universal law or principle, treat others with respect.
Negative test	An important question is whether one consents to others' acting simultaneously or the same toward him or her.
Means-end principle	Treating someone as an end is demonstrated through everyone's being treated equally and respectfully. Treating another as a means to meet one's own needs violates the means-end principle.

FEMININE/FEMINIST ETHICS

We have discussed Lawrence Kohlberg's theory of moral and ethical development. He assumed that perspectives on care, friendships, and relationships would represent personal views and not ethical or moral principles (Cockburn, 2005).

Gilligan (1982), one of the originators of feminist/feminine ethics, argued that such a view limited how women interpreted the world and what was important ethically. Feminist ethics essentially consists of several views, and they have been identified as falling into feminist ethics and feminine ethics. Feminist ethics is focused on interpreting ethical acts according to promoting equal rights and ceasing domination of women. Feminine ethics is focused on the relevance of care, or the ethic of care. Women in feminine ethics interpret acts according to how the ethic of care is enacted. The creation of feminine ethics was a reaction to a point against a more psychoanalytic view that women were inferior to men in regard to moral or ethical development (Tong, 1998).

Major Concepts

Feminine ethics is more broadly associated with the ethic of care, whereas feminist ethics is associated with the ethic of justice. We start with feminine ethics and a discussion of the ethics of care. Gilligan (1982) introduced the feminine perspective and proposed that more traditional Western ethical theories such as virtue ethics and utilitarian ethics were male dominated and were founded on principles of justice. She argued that such views devalued women's ethical perspectives, which are more focused on the importance of relationships and the ethic of care. The ethic of care is founded on relationships and responsibilities. Gilligan noted the understanding that there is a difference in moral or ethical perspectives between men and women.

Peterson and Seligman (2004) described the concept of care as a compassionate identification of how to address another's needs. More specific elements of care include the following: care is contextual, care emphasizes the importance of emotions, and care focuses on maintaining relationships. The context of care is defined in terms of how much care is needed based on the context. For example, the amount of care needed for a 3-year-old is different than the amount of care needed for a 17-year-old. Emotions are important because they provide the person with a reference for addressing ethical issues and form the basis of bonds or attachments. The element of care focused on maintaining relationships may be understood as involving the establishment of specific long-term relationships such as mother-child relationships. There is a stronger connection and a stronger emphasis on care and an ethic of care for these types of relationships. It has been proposed that men and women reason differently when considering ethical or moral issues (Grimshaw, 1993). Nodding (2003) also contributed to an understanding of the ethics of care. She proposed that the ethic of care is not a theory or perspective that is inferior to reasoning but in fact is better than the ethic of justice. Chadrow (1978) cited how the psychoanalytic perspective supports the perspective that women are predisposed to a care orientation compared to men. Held (1987) concluded that mothers develop an understanding that relationships are about cooperation, community, and serving others' needs. In practice the ethic of care may be understood as incorporating consideration of relationships and the importance of relationships over other issues such as justice. Based on this perspective a mother may choose to give more attention to a 3-year-old than to a 16-year-old because of the context of need. A 5-year-old child needs more care than does a 17-year-old, generally. This is not based on a perspective of justice that might suggest there should be approximately equal time. Conversely, the 17-year-old may receive more money to spend than a 5-year-old may. These are rather simplistic examples, but they illustrate the relevance of the ethic of care. Women understand such need for care and make decisions accordingly.

The feminist approach is considerably different from the feminine approach to ethics. The focus in the feminist approach is on power and an effort to achieve justice and equality. In essence, the feminist approach operates within the traditional view, focusing on justice and reasoning. The feminist view promotes the equality of women and advocates for justice. The feminist perspective is more focused on reducing oppression, specifically oppression of women. The intent of feminist ethics is to develop a gender-free perspective and sensitivity to discovering oppression, which in this theory is unethical. The feminist perspective of ethics has been expanded to include many oppressed groups such as those that are oppressed due to sexual preference (Jagose, 2009). Feminists do not agree with the ethic of care perspective and believe it promotes the status quo and does not reduce oppression. Ross (1989) concluded that a feminine approach reinforces a view of women as primarily nurturing and less powerful than men. Another important point is that not all ethical situations can be interpreted in terms of the parent-child relationship.

Several researchers have found that women actually use a justice perspective in ethical thinking, which is in conflict with the feminine argument that care is more important than justice in women's ethical decision making (Blasi, 1980; Rest, 1986; Steward & Sprinthall, 1994). Through reasoning and recognition of oppression, a feminist approach can identify situations that are theoretically unethical because of the oppression of women or a particular vulnerable group. Cummings (2000) suggested that women entering counseling bring in issues that involve oppression. If this is true, then awareness and assessment of such oppression is an ethical issue in working with women and girls (see Table 13.5).

| Table 13.5 | Summary of Feminist/Feminine Ethical Concepts |

Ethical Concept	Definition/Description
Ethic of care	Compassionately identify how to address another's needs as well as develop a strong ethic of care and attachment between mother and child.
Justice and equality	Develop a gender-free perspective and sensitivity to discovering oppression, which is unethical. Equality and justice or fairness are found in ethical acts and situations.

The Case of Carol: Multicultural Competence

Carol is a 42-year-old White woman who lives in a major Midwestern city. She attended public schools, and she is the second oldest of five children. Carol grew up in a working-class family. She graduated from high school and was an average student. Carol's parents divorced when she was 10 years old. She keeps in contact with both parents. Both parents and all siblings are alive and live within 100 miles of her. Carol was raised a Catholic but converted to the Wiccan Way (witchcraft or "the craft," also called neopaganism) at the age of 35. She worked as a factory worker for more than 10 years (with some intermittent layoffs between jobs) and most recently has been unemployed due to mental health problems.

Carol initially presented with the following symptoms more than 20 years ago: anxiety and depression with feelings of helplessness. She has had no remarkable medical problems. She has been diagnosed with major depressive disorder (according to the *Diagnostic and Statistical Manual of Mental Disorders*). She was first hospitalized more than 20 years ago and was placed on medication for depression. She has had two subsequent hospitalizations, neither lasting for more than 2 weeks. The most recent hospitalization was more than 8 years ago. She has been stable for the past 8 years. She did have one pregnancy, and it resulted in an abortion; her family pushed for this outcome. Carol practices the Wiccan Way and is a strong believer in her spirituality. Carol attends a day program for those with severe mental illness. She lives in an apartment with one other woman, Susan. In addition to attending the day program, she has seen a counselor at a community mental health center on a biweekly basis. Her original counselor left the agency, and Carol has been assigned a new counselor, Robert.

The counselor, Robert, is a 25-year-old White man who has worked as a mental health counselor since his graduation from a master's program in mental health counseling. He was born and raised in a small Midwestern town. He attended a conservative

Protestant church, and he still attends church on a regular basis. Robert grew up in a middle-class family. He still lives in a small town and commutes to the larger city to complete his internship experience. Robert was raised in a family with a mother and father and an older brother. He is married and has no children. He attended a public university for both his undergraduate and graduate degrees.

Robert's supervisor, Alice, has been working for the mental health center for 6 years and is a licensed social worker. Alice is a White 47-year-old woman who is married and has three children. She lives in the suburbs of the larger Midwestern city. She grew up in the area. Her family of origin was upper middle class, and Alice attended a private university for both her master's and her bachelor's degrees. Alice's family attended a Unitarian church. Alice started in the agency providing therapy to a wide range of clients including those with severe mental illness. She was promoted to supervisor 2 years ago and sees only a few clients while serving as a supervisor. She was promoted because she maintained her paperwork, met regular quotas for client contact, and represented the mental health center well in interacting with other agencies.

We have identified relevant elements of the horizon based on the case of Carol, and they include the ethical dilemma; the client's, counselor's, and supervisor's respective values, race, gender, and personal history; the counseling agency's policies; local, state, and federal laws that apply; professional knowledge; geographic region; professional ethical codes; and ethical theories.

Ethical Dilemma

Robert met with Carol for the first time, and she discussed her mental illness. She described her personal history, which included her thoughts about her religious beliefs—the Wiccan Way or the craft. She talked about her creative power and the craft. She also talked about her belief that Christianity holds animosity toward witchcraft and her rejection of Christian attempts to restrict the freedom of other ways of religious practice, for example, neopaganism. Carol discussed how she influenced two other members of the day program she attends to come to services.

Robert was unsure of which direction to take in addressing this issue. His personal values, which are conservative, hold that such religious practices are immoral. His initial inclination was to discuss how immoral it would be to engage in such a religion. He also was concerned about Carol's influencing others to follow this type of immoral religion. However, he reserved expressing this until he had further time to think about the direction of the counseling. Thus, one ethical issue is whether Robert should focus counseling on what he perceives as an evil religious practice, witchcraft. Recall one of the major ethical issues cited in Chapter 8 is multicultural competence, which includes acceptance of others' values and beliefs. Another major ethical issue is autonomy of the client.

Robert: The Counselor's Personal Values, Race, Gender, Personal Ethical Identity, and Personal History

A second part of the horizon in ethical decision making is the counselor and his or her personal values, race, gender, personal history, and so forth. Robert brings to the counseling sessions conservative religious values. He was raised in a Baptist church, and he feels it is a sin for anyone to engage in religious practices such as worshiping pagan gods and practicing witchcraft. Robert grew up in a middle-class family where his mother and father were nurturing and active in his life. Robert completed the Defining Issues Test and was in the conventional stage, which stresses adherence to laws and authority. He believes he should follow what his community supports, and it does not believe in alternative religions.

Carol: The Client's Personal Values, Race, Gender, and Personal History

Carol lives with another woman, Susan, in a two-bedroom duplex in a working-class neighborhood in a large Midwestern city (more than 300,000 residents). Susan, who also practices the Wiccan Way, is Carol's best friend, and they attend services on a regular basis. Susan first introduced Carol to the Wiccan Way. Carol believes in the creative power of the universe and relates to Wicca, which is an earth-centered religion. She rejects the religion of her family of origin, Catholicism, and believes that Christians seek to suppress the religious practices of her chosen religion. She is suspicious of those who practice Christianity, particularly those who are more conservative. Carol attends services, participates in the casting of a circle (the consecration of a sacred space), and participates in casting spells, singing, and so forth. Carol talks about her religious beliefs to others at the day program, and two have attended Wicca services with her and Susan.

The Supervisor and Agency: Personal Values, Race, Gender, and Personal History

Alice, the supervisor, grew up in the suburbs of the urban area where she works. She grew up in an upper-middle-class family, and she attended a Unitarian church. She is a White woman with a family, a spouse, and three children. She attends church on a regular basis. She considers herself liberal and open-minded with regard to religious practices and choices.

Research on supervisory relationships has examined the role of the gender of the supervisor and supervisee (Wester, Vogel, & Archer, 2004). It has been noted that male supervisees present a defensive style when working with female supervisors (Wester et al., 2004).

Professional Codes of Ethics

Walden, Herlihy, and Ashton (2003) stated,

> A defining characteristic of a professional organization is the formulation of a code or system of standards that prescribes acceptable professional behaviors for the members of that group. The establishment of a code of ethics signifies the maturation of a profession. (p. 106)

Counseling is a relatively young profession, but there are well-established professional codes. Hadjistavropoulos, Malloy, Sharpe, Green, and Fuchs-Lacelle (2002) also provided insight into the relevance of professional ethics, stating, "A primary purpose of a code of ethics is to assist members of an organization in making consistent choices when faced with ethical dilemmas" (p. 254). There are several professional codes that potentially apply to the ethical dilemma faced by Robert. The following American Counseling Association codes may apply:

> C.2.a, Professional Competence: Boundaries of Competence—Counselors practice only within the boundaries of their competence, based on their education, training, supervised experience, state and national professional credentials, and appropriate professional experience. Counselors gain knowledge, personal awareness, sensitivity, and skills pertinent to working with a diverse client population.

> F.11.c, Roles and Relationships Between Counselor Educators and Students: Multicultural/Diversity Competence—Counselor educators actively infuse multicultural/diversity competency in their training and supervision practices. They actively train students to gain awareness, knowledge, and skills in the competencies of multicultural practice. Counselor educators include case examples, role-plays, discussion questions, and other classroom activities that promote and represent various cultural perspectives. (American Counseling Association, 2005)

Professional Knowledge

Robert was trained in a traditional, monocultural training program, where typically one course in multiculturalism is completed (Sue, Arredondo, & McDavis, 1992). Training in multiculturalism is not integrated across courses in this type of model. Is religion a culture? Falcov (1988) defined culture as "those sets of shared world views and adaptive behaviors derived from simultaneous membership in a variety of contexts: ecological settings (rural, urban, suburban), religious background, etc." (p. 336). Chi-Ying Chung and Bemak (2002) stated, "One major problem in working across cultures is the tendency for counselors to impose their cultural values on clients, which may occur in a conscious or unconscious level" (p. 159).

Sue et al. (1992) stated, "The profession of counseling oftentimes reflects the values of the larger society," which results in its being the "handmaiden of the status quo and transmitters of society's values" (p. 66). With regard to cross-cultural competence, Sue et al. stated, "a culturally skilled counselor is one who is actively in the process of becoming aware of his or her own assumptions about human behavior, values, biases, preconceived notions, personal limitations" (p. 67). Furthermore, Sue et al. concluded that "a culturally skilled counselor is one who actively attempts to understand the world-view of his or her culturally different client without negative judgments" (p. 67). Eriksen, Marston, and Korte (2002) suggested that to maintain ethical practice, counselors should understand the beliefs and values of clients based on religious views.

Another area of knowledge relevant in this horizon is an understanding of how to assess and counsel clients about religious beliefs (Hathaway, Scott, & Garvey, 2004). Hathaway et al. (2004) noted the importance of religiousness and adaptive mental health functioning. Religion may give the client a sense of meaning and promote hope and optimism (Hathaway et al., 2004). Also, Hathaway et al. noted that the *Diagnostic and Statistical Manual of Mental Disorders* (fourth edition, text revision; American Psychiatric Association, 2000) includes categories of mental health problems that focus on religious beliefs and practices, specifically found in V codes. V codes typically involve issues about relationships but also address concerns such as conversion to a new religion.

A third area that is relevant in understanding the horizon of this ethical dilemma is the history of treatment of those who have followed the religion of the Wiccan Way (Barstow, 1994; Bever, 2002). For example, more than 50,000 individuals were put to death for witchcraft in Europe during the Middle Ages (Barstow, 1994). In addition, Houser and Ham (2004) suggested that religion may be considered a minority status and result in the loss of power and influence in society. Those following the Wiccan Way have faced more recent discrimination including loss of jobs and loss of custody of children (Blummer, 2000; Merriam, Courtenay, & Baumgartner, 2003).

Geographic Region

Geographic region can play a role in this case because both urban and rural personal experiences apply. Also, the counseling services are provided in an urban setting. Researchers have noted the unique characteristics of those living and growing up in urban and rural environments (Sears, Evans, & Perry, 1998; Silk, Sessa, Morris, Steinberg, & Avenevoli, 2004). Researchers have studied the development or lack of development of collective efficacy (Ford & Beveridge, 2004; Sampson, 2002). Sampson (2002) defined neighborhood collective efficacy as "an emphasis on shared beliefs in neighbors' con-joint capability for action to achieve an intended effect, and hence an active sense of engagement on the part of residents" (p. 224). Ford and Beveridge (2004) concluded that collective efficacy "emphasizes shared expectations and mutual trust among neighborhood residents and promotes an agentic sense of cohesion" (p. 27). The client, Carol, grew up in an urban environment and experienced little connection to her community or neighborhood. She felt little support from her neighborhood. Currently she lives in a working-class neighborhood with little cohesion or sense of community or neighborhood collective efficacy.

Local, State, and Federal Laws

The First Amendment to the U.S. Constitution protects the right to religious freedom. Also, recent hate law legislation has made it illegal to act violently against others due to religious beliefs (Levin, 2002). The First Amendment states,

> Congress shall make no law respecting an establishment of religion or prohibiting the free exercise thereof; or abridging the freedom of speech, or of the press; or the right of the people to peaceably assemble, and to petition the Government for a redress of grievances.

The First Amendment does not indicate which religious beliefs or lack of beliefs are acceptable or covered; that is, all beliefs are protected.

Ethical Theory: Utilitarianism

There are several individuals who were potentially affected by this ethical dilemma, including Carol's roommate, those she knows who practice witchcraft, and possibly those at the day program. So Robert decided to use utilitarian theory as one source in ethical decision making. There are other theories that may be relevant, such as Native American ethics.

The use of utilitarian ethics in practice is well accepted in counseling and psychology (Henry, 1996; Knapp, 1999). Henry (1996) identified several underlying principles of the American Counseling Association's professional code of ethics, and utilitarianism provides a foundation based on the greatest good and the importance of assessing the consequences of an action. Knapp (1999) suggested that utilitarianism may help professionals in four ways in practice. It can "(a) identify and justify the underlying moral principles on which their ethics codes are based, (b) assist them in ethical decision-making, (c) encourage moral behavior, and (d) evaluate the culpability of their colleagues who are accused of ethics violations" (p. 383). Knapp further noted that "many standards of the APA [American Psychological Association] Code of Conduct appear to be based on rule utilitarianism" (p. 390). However, Knapp stated that the use of act utilitarianism provides the professional with a foundation for ethical decision making when professional codes are less clear about a circumstance or when codes conflict.

The basic concepts of utilitarian theory that potentially apply to this ethical dilemma include the GHP, utility, the consequentialist principle, rule utilitarianism, and act utilitarianism. The GHP may apply because the intent of using this theory is to determine the amount of happiness or benefit for all involved. Utility is relevant to account for how each decision may affect all involved. Ultimately, the outcome is what matters in this theory, which is the consequentialist principle. Using this principle, the ethical issue may be interpreted as how each decision ultimately affects those involved, without regard for their intentions. Applying both rule utilitarianism and act utilitarianism allows for an understanding of how each perspective may help in understanding the ethical dilemma, from either an individual or a societal perspective.

Source: Adapted from Houser, Wilczenski, and Ham (2006). Reprinted with permission.

The Case of Mark: A Question of Counselor Competence

Carefully read the case of Mark. Information is provided about an ethical dilemma, the counselor's values and personal ethical identity, the client's personal values, and the supervisor's personal values. Generate information about elements of the hermeneutic model: professional codes that may apply, geographic region, and professional literature that is relevant. Choose an ethical theory or theories to apply (Western theory or theories presented in this chapter), and summarize your ethical decision based on the hermeneutic model. Be sure to gather information about relevant codes of ethics that apply, laws and statutes that apply, and professional literature that applies. Also, interpret the impact of the counselor's professional ethical identity and development on the case. How would your own professional identity and development affect such a case?

A gay man in his mid-20s, Mark entered counseling because of a court order as a consequence of driving while under the influence of alcohol. He is employed as an accountant with a restaurant franchise. Mark was raised in a Catholic religious tradition within his family of origin, but because of that church's position on homosexuality and gay marriage, he no longer attends services. Andrew, the counselor, is 25 years old. For the past 6 months, Andrew has been employed in a community counseling agency where his caseload consists primarily of clients with substance abuse problems.

Initially, Mark discusses his concerns about his DUI. Mark states that he does not usually drink to excess and that it was just his bad luck to have been arrested. Andrew has heard similar stories from other clients in the past and feels comfortable dealing with these issues. During the third counseling session, however, Mark begins to talk about conflicts with his spouse, and Andrew assumes he is referring to a female partner. When Mark names his partner Bill, Andrew realizes that Mark is involved in a gay relationship. Mark reports that he has been drinking lately because of conflicts with his partner and concerns about his sexual orientation. He reports that his relationship with Bill is his first gay relationship. Now Mark questions whether he is gay and wonders if he acted too impulsively in marrying Bill.

The counselor in this case does not have experience working with gay and lesbian clients, nor does he know about homosexual issues. He leaves the counseling session feeling uncomfortable and unsure of which steps he should take.

Potential relevant elements of the horizon based on the case of Mark include the ethical dilemma; the client's, counselor's, and supervisor's respective values, race, gender, and personal history; counseling agency policies; local, state, and federal laws that apply; professional knowledge; geographic region; professional ethical codes; and theories of virtue ethics.

Ethical Dilemma

Andrew feels that he can deal with Mark's drinking problem. His initial treatment plan would be to help Mark stop drinking. However, Andrew has no experience dealing with issues presented by gay or lesbian clients and does not know how to address issues surrounding Mark's gay relationship and sexual orientation.

The ethical question for Andrew is whether he is competent to address Mark's sexual orientation. He must decide whether to retain this client on his caseload or to request that Mark be reassigned to another counselor. Andrew is concerned about how a request to transfer a client will be viewed by his supervisor because he is a relatively new counselor at the agency and does not want to appear to be incompetent or unwilling to accept challenging cases.

The Counselor's Personal Values, Race, Gender, and Personal History

Andrew is an effective substance abuse and mental health counselor, but he has no experience counseling gay and lesbian clients. Currently, Andrew is involved in a heterosexual relationship; he has been married for 2 years and has a 1-year-old son. He is the sole financial support for his family. Andrew was raised in a rural community. He attended a small high school and then attended a small state college where he majored in mental health counseling. Andrew decided to specialize in substance abuse treatment during his counseling graduate program where his career focus was influenced by the work of a professor whom he admired. Andrew completed the Defining Issues Test and discovered he fell into the conventional stage of moral development, following authority and social norms.

Through his religious affiliation, Andrew is aware of the Catholic Medical Association's ([CMA's] 2000) position on homosexuality, and he personally opposes same-sex marriage. The CMA's position is that there is no compelling evidence that same-sex attraction is genetic but that it results from unfortunate childhood experiences or other psychological problems. From this point of view, therapy is directed at uncovering the root cause of the emotional trauma that gave rise to the same-sex attraction and turns to spirituality in the healing process. Although Andrew does not openly acknowledge his religious views among professional colleagues and supervisors, he privately agrees with the CMA's diagnostic and treatment recommendations. He assumes that taking a natural law point of view on homosexuality is appropriate in this case because of the client's Catholic religious upbringing.

The Client's Personal Values, Race, Gender, and Personal History

Mark was married to Bill 4 months ago in the state of Massachusetts. Although his family of origin is Catholic, Mark no longer practices Catholicism but participates at the Unitarian church that his partner attends. Mark's parents disapprove of his marriage and have let it be known to Mark that although he is welcome to attend family gatherings, his partner is not. His two siblings live out of state and maintain friendly though infrequent contact with Mark.

His gay relationship with Bill was Mark's first sexual experience. He occasionally dated girls during high school and college. Throughout his adolescence and early adulthood, he tended to be a loner. Bill befriended Mark after they were introduced by a mutual acquaintance, and they found that they had many common interests. Within the gay community, Mark found social acceptance and companionship. Although Mark was reluctant, Bill insisted that they marry as soon as same-sex marriage became legal in Massachusetts. Mark acquiesced out of fear of losing the relationship. Since his marriage, Mark has felt increasingly isolated at work and distant from his family of origin. His relationship with Bill is now strained, and Mark and Bill argue frequently.

Mark notes a recent shift in public opinion in the United States away from liberal political views and tolerant attitudes toward diversity to a more conservative orientation and religious fundamentalism. Religious fundamentalism and authoritarianism are associated with negative attitudes toward homosexuality (Heaven & Oxman, 1999; Hunsberger, Owusu, & Duck, 1999). Mark is concerned that he will face increasing societal discrimination as a married gay man and wonders if it is already affecting his professional relationships at work. He feels that his coworkers were somewhat more accepting of him prior to his marriage. Mark now questions his sexual identity and why he entered into a gay relationship. Because of mounting interpersonal pressures with his partner, family, and coworkers, Mark finally admits that he has been drinking excessively.

The Supervisor's Personal Values, Race, Gender, and Personal History

The supervisor, Tony, is married with two children. He is Catholic but attends Mass irregularly and does not agree with some of the Church's positions on contemporary issues such as birth control. There are gay members of Tony's immediate and extended family, and he, his parents, and his relatives feel that they are quite tolerant of diversity. Tony favors civil unions for gay and lesbian couples but is opposed to same-sex marriage.

Source: Adapted from Houser, Wilczenski, and Ham (2006). Reprinted with permission.

Use Figure 13.1 to identify relevant elements of the horizon. Fill in the appropriate elements to help with your understanding and ethical decision.

Figure 13.1 Ethical Dilemma

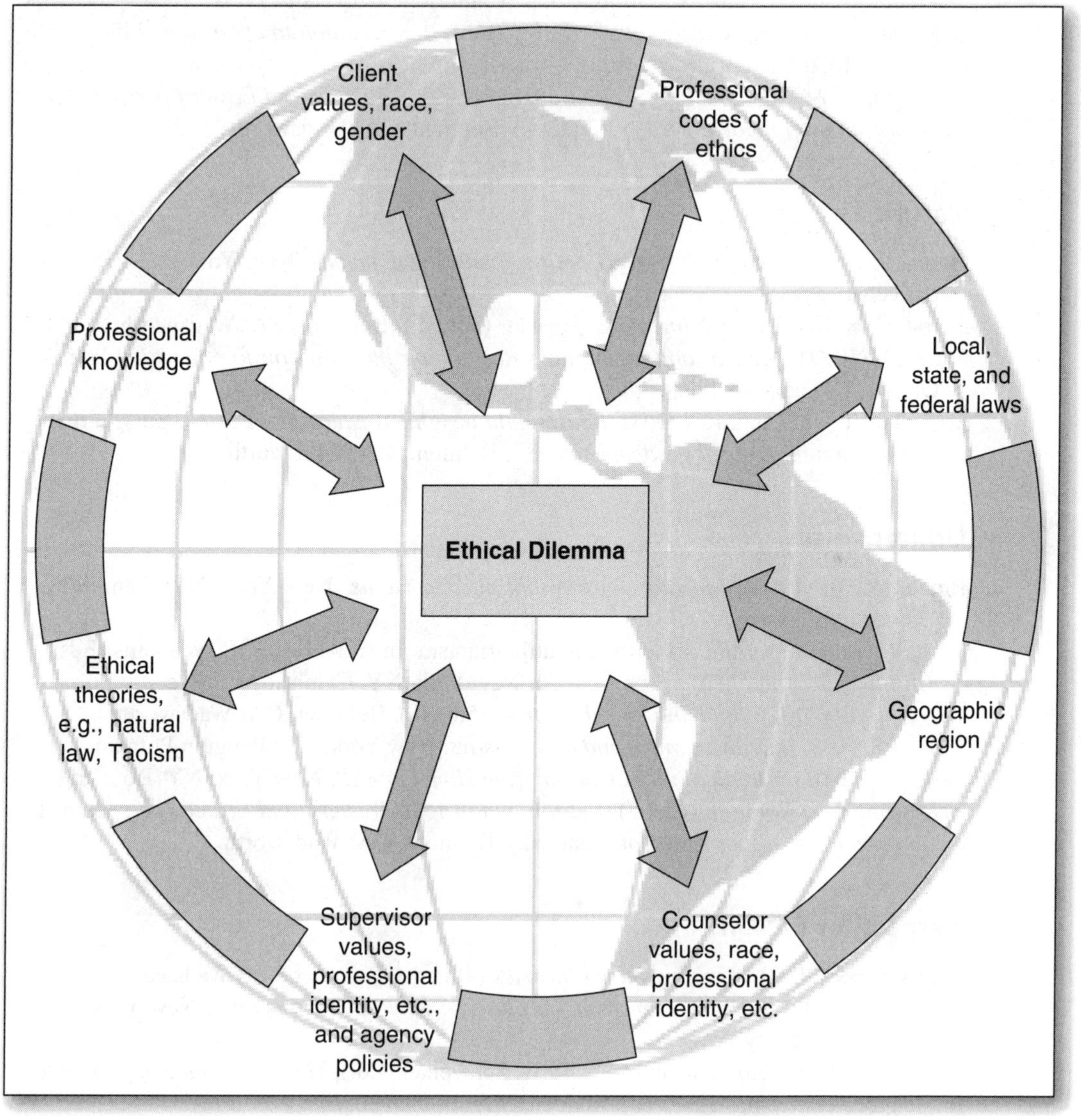

Additional Recommended Readings

Virtue Ethics

Harris, C. E. (2007). *Applying moral theories* (5th ed.). Belmont, CA: Thompson-Wadsworth.

Hursthouse, R. (2003). Virtue ethics. In E. N. Zalta (Ed.), *The Stanford encyclopedia of philosophy.* Retrieved from http://plato.stanford.edu/archives/fall2003/entries/ethics-virtue/

Hutchinson, D. S. (1995). Ethics. In J. Barnes (Ed.), *The Cambridge companion to Aristotle* (pp. 195–232). Cambridge, UK: Cambridge University Press.

Pence, G. (1993). Virtue theory. In P. Singer (Ed.), *A companion to ethics* (pp. 249–258). Malden, MA: Blackwell.

Shanahan, T., & Wang, R. (2003). *Reason and insight: Western and Eastern perspectives on the pursuit of moral wisdom* (2nd ed.). Belmont, CA: Wadsworth.

Natural Law

Finnis, J. (1998). *Aquinas: Moral, political and legal theory.* New York, NY: Oxford University Press.

Harris, C. E. (2007). *Applying moral theories* (5th ed.). Belmont, CA: Wadsworth.

Porter, J. (1999). *Natural and divine law: Reclaiming the tradition for Christian ethics.* Ottawa, Canada: Novalis.

Shanahan, T., & Wang, R. (2003). *Reason and insight: Western and Eastern perspectives on the pursuit of moral wisdom* (2nd ed.). Belmont, CA: Wadsworth.

Utilitarianism

Brandt, R. B. (1992). *Morality, utilitarianism, and rights.* New York, NY: Cambridge University Press.

Hare, R. M. (1982). Ethical theory and utilitarianism. In A. K. Sen & B. Williams (Eds.), *Utilitarianism and beyond* (pp. 23–38). New York, NY: Cambridge University Press.

Harris, C. E. (2007). *Applying moral theories* (5th ed.). Belmont, CA: Wadsworth.

Mill, J. S. (1987). *Utilitarianism and other essays.* New York, NY: Penguin Putnam.

Rosen, F. (2003). *Classical utilitarianism from Hume to Mill.* New York, NY: Routledge.

Shanahan, T., & Wang, R. (2003). *Reason and insight: Western and Eastern perspectives on the pursuit of moral wisdom* (2nd ed.). Belmont, CA: Wadsworth.

Respect for Persons

Harris, C. E. (2002). *Applying moral theories* (4th ed.). Belmont, CA: Wadsworth.

Hill, T. E. (2000). *Respect, pluralism, and justice: Kantian perspectives.* New York, NY: Oxford University Press.

Ilesanmi, S. O. (2005). Human rights. In W. Schweiker (Ed.), *The Blackwell companion to religious ethics* (pp. 501–510). Malden, MA: Blackwell.

Kellenberger, J. (1995). *Relationship morality.* University Park, PA: Penn State University Press.

O'Neill, O. (1993). Kantian ethics. In P. Singer (Ed.), *A companion to ethics* (pp. 175– 185). Malden, MA: Blackwell.

Roberts, L. W., & Dyer, A. R. (2004). *Concise guide to ethics in mental health care.* Arlington, VA: American Psychiatric.

Shanahan, T., & Wang, R. (2003). *Reason and insight: Western and Eastern perspectives on the pursuit of moral wisdom.* Belmont, CA: Wadsworth.

Sullivan, R. J. (1994). *An introduction to Kant's ethics.* New York, NY: Cambridge University Press.

Feminine/Feminist Ethics

Clement, G. (1996). *Care, autonomy, and justice.* Boulder, CO: Westview.

Lindemann, H. (2005). *An invitation to feminist ethics.* Columbus, OH: McGraw-Hill.

Moore, M. (1999). The ethics of care and justice. *Women and Politics, 20*(2), 1–16.

Nodding, N. (2003). *Caring: A feminine approach to ethics and moral education* (2nd ed.). Berkeley: University of California Press.

Tong, R. (2003). Feminist ethics. In E. N. Zalta (Ed.), *The Stanford encyclopedia of philosophy.* Retrieved from http://plato.stanford.edu/archives/win2003/entries/feminism-ethics/

Chapter 14

EASTERN THEORIES OF ETHICS

CHAPTER OBJECTIVES

- Acquire an understanding of Confucian ethics and relevant concepts
- Acqurie an understanding of Taoist ethics and relevant concepts
- Acquire an understanding of Hindu ethics and relevant concepts
- Acquire an understanding of Buddist ethics and relevant concepts

This section focuses on Eastern ethical theories. We include in our discussion the following theories: Confucianism, Taoism, Hinduism, and Buddhism. Confucius was the primary originator of Confucianism, which began in China centuries ago. The theory is founded on making ethical decisions from rituals and practices. We also present Taoism (Daoism); the primary contributor to this theory was Laozi, who was a Chinese contemporary of Confucius (Shanahan & Wang, 2003). The foundation of the theory is an intuitive seeking of balance in one's life. Shanahan and Wang (2003) noted that Hinduism is the oldest historically recorded philosophical view, dating back to 2500 BCE. The search for truth is a primary focus of Hinduism. Also, ethics in Hinduism may be understood as including virtues such as humility, patience, and honoring others. Buddhism is founded on the primary belief in finding the "middle way." Buddhism, an older philosophy that was developed around 500 BCE, was created in response to the perceived limitations of Hinduism (Shanahan & Wang, 2003). Siddhartha Gautama, later called the Buddha, was a major contributor to this theory. A key feature of the theory is the belief in suffering as a natural and expected human experience. The focus is on understanding suffering and achieving the middle way to overcome suffering.

CONFUCIAN ETHICS

Confucianism is considered one of the three main sources of ethical thinking in Asian cultures; the other two are Buddhism and Hinduism. The history of Confucianism dates back more than 2,000 years. Confucianism is focused on developing desired virtues established through obligations to others (Shanahan & Wang, 2003). Confucius lived during the Zhou dynasty from 551 to 479 BCE. Confucius is Latin for the Chinese name Kong Fuzi or Master Kong (Yao, 2000). Confucius's father died when Confucius was 3, and he was raised by his mother (Shanahan & Wang, 2003). Chinese consider Confucius the "first teacher" (C. Hansen, 1992; H. Smith, 1991). Confucius became a teacher and had more than 3,000 students (Yao, 2000). Confucius sought out jobs in government, but he was too honest and questioned governmental officials' actions. Consequently he held only lower-level positions. Confucius's personal history influenced his attitudes and ethical perspectives, which support a positive, respectful relationship between rulers and the common people. He concluded that not following traditions and rituals created confusion and chaos.

H. Smith (1991) described Confucius: "Confucius was undoubtedly one of the world's greatest teachers. Prepared to instruct in history, poetry, government, propriety, mathematics, music, divination, and sports, he was, in the manner of Socrates, a one-man university" (p. 156). Key principles in understanding Confucianism are rituals, tradition, and respect for social order. He encouraged acceptance of respect for political rulers, but at the same time, as Smith noted, he also promoted democratic attitudes and supported fair treatment of common people by rulers/leaders.

H. Smith (1991) noted that while Confucius was living, he was a well-respected teacher but that he did not receive any acceptance beyond this role. Several generations after his death, he was still perceived to be the mentor (H. Smith, 1991). Smith suggested that it is unclear exactly what contributed to the dramatic increase in his influence after his death. However, Smith hypothesized that Confucianism highlighted the importance of family as well as a process or structure to bring individuals together and develop a society that is predictable and reduces chaos. Consequently, Chinese society embraced Confucianism because of its simplicity and its functional nature.

Confucianism has typically been associated with China, but it has been accepted in other Asian countries as well. Yum (1988) noted that Confucianism has been accepted in both Korea and Japan. Yum stated, "Confucianism was institutionalized and propagated both through formal curricula of the educational system and through the selection process of government officials" (p. 376). Oldstone-Moore (2002) included Vietnam as a country that also was greatly influenced by Confucianism.

The foundation of this theory is that we learn our social roles through life experiences and literature; it includes life through models (Yao, 2000). Confucius proposed that humans seek a well-ordered society. A well-ordered society may be achieved through understanding one's social role and understanding others' roles. Yao (2000) concluded that "the vitality of Confucianism can be generated through learning and education" (p. 30).

Major Concepts

Several major concepts have been identified as important in understanding Confucian ethics (Houser, Wilczenski, & Ham, 2006). Oldstone-Moore (2002) identified *Li* is an important concept in Confucian ethics; it is described as standards of acceptable social behavior. The actual interpretation of Li involves understanding appropriate use of ritual, etiquette, manners, and ceremonies. The acquisition and understanding of Li is obtained through models that provide information about acceptable social behavior; typically the models are elders. A concept related to Li is seeking the mean (*chun yung*) or the middle way, which is a balance of extremes (H. Smith, 1991). Overindulging is a violation of the mean, violating the middle way. According to Smith (1991), Confucius suggested there are five basic relationships or social roles in which Li is achieved: parents and children, husband and wife, elder sibling and younger sibling, elder friend and younger friend, and ruler and subject. The ideal social role behavior for parents is to express love and caring toward their children. Children in return should express respect and obedience for their parents, which is a correct demonstration of Li. The Li, or social role, for elder siblings in interacting with younger siblings is to be gentle toward younger siblings; conversely, younger siblings should show respect for elder siblings. The Li for husbands is to be good to their wives, and wives should be good at listening to their husbands. Younger friends should defer to elder friends, and elder friends should be considerate of younger friends. Leaders should be benevolent to followers, and followers should show corresponding loyalty. According to Li, there is a special position in society for elders. Tweed and Lehman (2002) quoted Confucius as saying, "To honor those higher than ourselves is the highest expression of a sense of justice" (p. 95). Confucius concluded that virtue is obtained by observing and learning from people who are models of virtue. Understanding of rituals provides additional information about how to achieve Li. Rituals provide clarity for Li in a society and for the expected social behaviors, for example, a wedding ceremony where specific social roles may be demonstrated.

Ren is another important concept in Confucian theory and is defined as the ideal relationship between human beings (Oldstone-Moore, 2002; H. Smith, 1991).

Goodness, benevolence, and love between humans are characteristics of the concept of Ren. Ren also has been described with the term *human heartedness*. H. Smith (1991) suggested that Ren is both respect for oneself and a feeling of humanity toward others. Ren is a sense of the dignity of and respect for humans. Smith concluded that Ren may be understood as similar to the "silver rule," stating, "Do not do unto others what you would not want others to do unto you" (p. 173).

There are two ways to manifest Ren: through reciprocity (*shu*) and through sincerity (*zhong*). Reciprocity may be manifested through the silver rule. The consideration of another individual's reaction to a situation or action is the basis of reciprocity (Oldstone-Moore, 2002). Zhong is demonstrated through sincerity in expressing feeling and is consistent with one's actions (Oldstone-Moore, 2002).

Mencius was another proponent of Confucian thinking (Shanahan & Wang, 2003). He lived several hundred years after Confucius, and he observed that other schools of thought had abandoned many concepts of Confucius's original theory. Mencius believed that humans are born with an instinctive morality and what he called seeds of wisdom for growth. Instinctive morality is demonstrated through inclinations to behave that are illustrated in the *Xin,* or heart mind. Xin is similar to Western views of conscience. Mencius concluded that seeds of instinctive morality include empathy and sympathy (commiseration), or the virtue of humanity; ability to feel shame; respect and deference to superiors and modesty; and the ability to know right from wrong (Shanahan & Wang, 2003). The development of such instinctive seeds can be hindered through deprivation and also through events that affect normal development. Events that may hinder development are political, social, economic, and psychological conditions. These instinctive seeds may not develop if we do not attend to or focus on their development. Table 14.1 contains a summary of Confucian ethical concepts.

TAOIST ETHICS

The three major philosophical thoughts in China are Buddhism, Taoism, and Confucianism (Robinet, 1997). Taoism was first introduced about 500 BCE with Laozi. Many philosophers have suggested that Taoism developed as a reaction against Confucianism (Kohn, 2001). Taoists believe that Confucian ways of living resulted in a disruption in the natural order of human nature and, most important, the natural order of things. The model for early Taoists was the farmer and his life, or an agrarian orientation. Taoism is thought to be simple and was in harmony with nature. According to Taoism, farmers are aware of the natural rhythms of nature. Taoism does have a religious orientation and is based to some degree on goals of immortality.

Table 14.1	Summary of Confucian Ethical Concepts
Concept	*Definition/Description*
Li	Standards of acceptable social behavior
Middle way	Involves the balance of extremes—no overindulging in material activities such as eating or drinking
Ren	Ideal human relationship, representative of benevolence and love between humans
Seeds of instinctive morality	Empathy and sympathy, ability to feel shame, deference to superiors, and ability to know right from wrong

Laozi, who was referred to as the old master, presented his major written description of Taoism in the *Tao Te Ching* (Classic of the Way and Its Power). One problem with discussing major concepts in Taoism is that writings about Taoism were presented as short, disjointed commentaries.

Major Concepts

There are several important concepts in understanding Taoism: Tao, yin and yang, the harmony of opposites and relativity, simplicity, reversal and cyclicity, and nonaction (Shanahan & Wang, 2003). Tao is interpreted as a way or a path that is true and desirable to follow. A concrete definition of Tao is theoretically impossible primarily because it can be discovered only through analogies and metaphors (Shanahan & Wang, 2003). The way, or Tao, must be experienced before one can fully understand it. A common experience may help explain Tao. You are trying to find a location you have been before; however, you cannot remember exactly the direction. You search for clues by walking or driving and discover the right direction. You have the feeling or intuition of finding your way and knowing it is the right way.

Two other concepts that are closely related are yin and yang. Most have heard of these concepts and may have a vague idea of their definitions. *Yin and yang* refers to the interaction of opposites. The yin is considered the receptive and weaker aspect of the union between yin and yang. It has been interpreted as negative and destructive. The opposite of yin is yang, which has been associated with adjectives such as *strong, positive,* and *constructive.* Neither yin nor yang is believed to be good or bad by itself. The negative of yin or yang comes from an extreme of either, which can create problems. There needs to be a balance between yin and yang.

Harmony of opposites and relativity are two important concepts in Taoism. They refer to the reality that life and events have opposites. Experiencing the opposite provides an opportunity to comprehend the opposite. Understanding that something is done fast requires that something is done slowly. The second step in understanding opposites is the concept of relativity. Relativity is based on the idea that opposites are relative, which is based on a person's perceptions and the context of the situation. For example, if someone from Alabama visited Boston in the spring and the temperature were 45 degrees, he or she might find it cold. However, if someone from Minnesota visited, he or she might find it comfortable. The context and perception (relativity) influence conclusions. The concept of relativity in Tao states that there are no absolutes but that everything is relative, including ethics and morals. According to the *I Ching* (Book of Changes), simplicity states that the way of heaven and earth is simple. Taoism is based on the simple life; a farmer is used as an example. The farmer follows the natural flow of nature. He or she understands the change of seasons and bases decisions on this flow, on simplicity.

Reversal is an interesting process wherein two competing forces interact and the perceived weaker force dominates the stronger force through persistence. Reversal is an achieved process, with the weaker force overcoming the stronger force and consequently becoming the stronger force. The process continues, and the weaker force again overcomes the stronger force through persistence, eventually becoming the stronger force. Cyclicity is the process of changing from weak to strong. Shanahan and Wang (2003) gave an example of reversal and proposed that water and stone are examples of reversal and cyclicity. Water initially is viewed as weak, and a stone is viewed as strong; however, with persistence, water pressure wears away the stone. The water is now stronger than the stone because it wears away the stone. However, the water may not maintain its force; it carves out a gorge in the stone and flows more slowly. Consequently the stone becomes stronger again. Understanding this process of change shows that nature is not static.

Nonaction, or *wu wei,* is another important concept in Taoism. Nonaction, according to Shanahan and Wang (2003), does not mean doing nothing; it refers to following nature and being natural, spontaneous, and harmonious with nature. Most important, nonaction may be understood as doing nothing to disrupt the natural course of events. Nonaction is accomplished only through not engaging in the pursuit of knowledge or not pursuing desires beyond what is necessary for basic needs for living. Knowledge provides individuals with information about what could be different and may lead to an analysis of what could be that changes the natural flow. The desired practice based on Taoism is letting nature take its course. Attempting to fulfill desires that go beyond meeting one's needs violates the concept of nonaction. An illustration of a violation of wu wei is pressuring a client to change behavior when he or she is not ready. The primary goal of nonaction is to act spontaneously without forethought (see Table 14.2).

HINDU ETHICS

Hindu philosophical thinking may be traced back more than 5,000 years to 2500 BCE (Shattuck, 1999). Hinduism may be understood as a way of life and is noted to be one of the oldest religions. Early developments of Hinduism originated from several pagan religious perspectives. Shattuck (1999) described the origins of the word *Hindu,* which illustrate the context of the theory's development, and stated,

Table 14.2	Summary of Taoist Ethical Concepts
Concept	*Definition/Description*
Tao	The way that is desirable to follow—one has to discover the way based on the natural course of events
Yin	Weaker aspect of the union of yin and yang—may be associated with *destructive* or *cold*
Yang	Stronger part of the yin-yang union, represented as strong and positive—balance between yin and yang is necessary
Harmony of opposites	An understanding that there are two poles—if there is a good, then there is a bad; if there is a hot, then there must be a cold
Relativity	Opposites are influenced by relativity; perceptions of opposites are interpreted through the context—a climate that is considered warm is based on the context, for example, if one is in Alaska, a warm day may be 50 degrees, whereas if one is in Florida, a warm day may be 90 degrees
Simplicity	Seek simplicity and maintain a simple life—an example of a simple life is a farmer's
Reversal	Refers to two competing forces that interact; one dominates and one is weaker—reversal occurs when the weaker overcomes the stronger or dominant
Cyclicity	Involves the continuous cycle of the weaker's overcoming the stronger
Wu wei	Refers to nonaction or not interfering with the natural flow of events, for example, letting nature take its course

The term Hinduism is of recent origin, having been applied mostly by Westerners to denote the majority religion of India. Only groups that had clear non-Hindu identities, such as Jains, Buddists, Parsis, Muslims, Jews, and Christians were not included in the generic Hindu category. The use of a foreign designation derives from the fact that there is no corresponding word indigenous to South Asia. There, people generally define themselves according to local caste and community and, among these, there is no single scripture, deity, or religious teacher common to all that can be designated as the core of Hinduism. Yet, the very vagueness of the term makes it useful. This is because the word Hinduism comes from Hindu, a name used by medieval Muslims to refer to the people living around the Sindu (Indus) River. This then became an umbrella term for all the people residing in the Indian subcontinent. (p. 14)

There are three sources of information illustrating Hindu perspectives: the *Upanishads,* the *Bhagavad Gita,* and the Brahma sutras. The *Upanishads* and *Bhagavad Gita* focus on morality. Dharma is the primary concept in Hinduism, which focuses on ethics and duty. It is discussed in more detail under Major Concepts.

Major Concepts

Creel (1977) noted that *ethics* is a Western term, whereas in Sanskrit, there is no clear differentiation between religion and ethics or between philosophy and ethics. Consequently one question is whether the term *ethics* can be applied adequately to Hinduism. Despite there being such diversity in how Hinduism developed, one can identify major concepts in the theory (Doniger-O'Flaherty, 1990).

Dharma refers to seeking the truth and elevation to a higher level. Dharma provides information about how to behave as a woman or man. Cush, Robinson, and Robinson (2008) suggested that dharma involves "moral virtues to be practiced by all human beings" (p. 182). Dharma may also be described as referring to duty and righteousness. Radhakrishnan (1922) described dharma: "It stands for all those ideals and purposes, influences and institutions that shape the character of man both as individual and as a member of society. It is the law of right living" (p. 2). In addition, characteristics associated with dharma are honesty and respect for others. The ideal human is described as having truth, beauty, and goodness. The ideal human has such virtues as humility, a sense of calm in difficult circumstances, tranquility, control of anger, and moderation of pride (Radhakrishnan, 1922).

Ahimsa refers to not injuring or killing others. It is based on the concepts of benevolence, protection, and compassion (Cush et al., 2008). Ahimsa is also associated with protecting the sanctity of life, and this includes questions about the act of abortion. Ahimsa includes protecting one's own life, for example, not engaging in activities that are harmful to an individual such as smoking or overeating. Ahimsa goes beyond more aggressive acts of harming others such as murder and includes any form of harm to others.

Singh (2008) identified the seven major principles of Hindu ethics/morality: *Satya, Asteya, Aparigraha, Brahmacharya, Sauch, Santosh,* and *Swadhayay.* Satya refers to telling the truth. Asteya concerns not focusing on what others have or becoming overly interested in what others possess. Aparigraha occurs when one becomes focused on obtaining luxurious items; it involves overindulgence in seeking material possessions. Brahmacharya refers to following the natural flow of body and senses, being aware of sensations and needs. Sauch concerns maintaining cleanliness of both body and mind. The last moral principle is Swadhayay, which involves promoting self-learning and self-realization.

Other concepts important in understanding Hindu ethics are discovered through the three paths of liberation. Morgan (2001) suggested that Hindu ethics may be understood through the three paths of liberation: *Karma Marga* (the path of works), *Jnana Marga* (the path of knowledge), and *Bhakti Marga* (the path of loving devotion). Karma Marga concerns laws of the social system. Hinduism is an older religious perspective and is founded to some degree on the social/political systems that were connected to a caste system (Morgan, 2001). Ethical behavior is associated with expected behaviors based on one's caste status. There were four caste levels: Brahmins (scholars, priests, and teachers), Kshatriyas (warriors and enforcers of the law), vaishyas (bankers, businesspeople, and farm owners), and Shudras (laborers, service providers, and members of the peasant class). Ethical behavior is founded on acting in ways that are consistent with the expectations of one's caste. Jnana Marga involves acquiring certain characteristics, including tranquility, endurance, concentration, and seeking liberation. Focusing on Bhakti Marga is intended to achieve higher levels of consciousness and a better understanding of God (see Table 14.3).

BUDDHIST ETHICS

Buddhism has its roots in present-day India during the sixth and fourth centuries BCE. From this beginning, Buddhism spread across Asia and is currently the

Table 14.3	Summary of Hindu Ethical Concepts

Concept	Definition/Description
Dharma	Seeking the truth, involves how moral virtues are practiced, has been described as the law of right living
Ahimsa	Not injuring or killing others
Satya	Telling the truth
Asteya	Not becoming interested in others' possessions
Aparigraha	Overindulgence in seeking or pursuing material possessions
Brahmacharya	Following the natural flow of body and sensations, an awareness of one's sensations and needs
Sauch	Maintaining cleanliness of mind and body
Swadhayay	Promotion of self-learning and self-realization
Karma Marga	The path of works—acting within socially acceptable limits
Jnana Marga	The path of knowledge—seeking tranquility and liberation
Bhakti Marga	The path of loving devotion—a focus on achieving higher levels of understanding and an understanding of God

fourth-largest religion in the world. More recently, Buddhism has enjoyed an increasing following in the West, particularly since the latter part of the twentieth century. Over the course of this history there have been varieties of Buddhist thought, and common to these perspectives is the focus on the human experience, what it is to be human and how one can transcend this life (Burnouf, 2010; Mitchell, 2002; H. Smith & Novak, 2003). Unlike traditional Western religions, Buddhism does not frame its teaching around a supreme deity, nor does it make a clear distinction between theology and ethical philosophy. Buddhism sees the two as linked and makes few distinctions between them. Thus, to live a moral life is to live a spiritually fulfilling life. Both considerations come from the same source and same concerns (Keown, 2005).

Prior to Buddhism, the primary religion was Brahmanism, which itself is a predecessor to Hinduism. During the period when Buddhism became influential, there was increasing concern about the power of the high-caste priests and the focus on sacrifices, particularly of animals. Buddhism gained ground as a reaction against these traditions and practices. Leading this movement was Siddhartha Gautama, the son of a prominent family who was being groomed to take over his father's position in society. During his youth, Gautama became curious about life outside his familiar surroundings and began to explore different places and meet different types of people. He noted that people outside of the upper classes experienced much suffering. Indeed, life seemed to be characterized by despair. Only a holy man he encountered seemed at peace. Following these observations, Gautama committed his life to finding a way to solve the problem of suffering and despair as a primary feature of human existence. To this end he renounced his privileged lifestyle, left his wife and family, and began to live a spiritual life in the forest. This phase of his life is identified as the great renunciation, in which Gautama's life shifted away from that which was prescribed by his birth into a ruling family to a spiritual life of his choosing (Burnouf, 2010; H. Smith & Novak, 2003).

After the Buddha's death, his followers attempted to identify his original teachings. Buddhism concludes that suffering, impermanence, and no-self are fundamental components. The primary premise of suffering and impermanence is that existence as a human involves pain, and existence gives rise to suffering. Impermanence was also viewed as a condition of human existence, consequently giving rise to desire. Human desires cause suffering because desire is transitory and ever changing (Goldstein & Kornfield, 1987; Mitchell, 2002; H. Smith & Novak, 2003; Tucci, Nakamura, & Reynolds, 1993). Impermanence is a consequence of human existence, with human beings and all aspects of human life being impermanent. Living with impermanence requires human beings to search for a way of deliverance, for enlightenment, that is beyond the transitory experiences of human existence (Goldstein & Kornfield, 1987; Tucci et al., 1993).

Major Concepts

The Middle Way

The Buddha noted the importance of traditions and focused on living a life of deprivation. As he confronted his suffering and nearing death, the Buddha had a revelation that there was a middle way in life that balanced self-indulgence and self-destruction. Following the middle way, he claimed, leads one to wisdom and truth and ultimately Nirvana or the pure state in which one is released from the suffering associated with life. Following these events, the Buddha focused his attention on exploring the ramifications of his insight about the middle way, and he sought out religious leaders to help him in the process. The end result of this study was the discovery of dharma or the natural order of life. Dharma has many meanings but carries the idea of the order that exists in the physical and moral world. This order is not divinely inspired but is a force to which even the gods must adhere. Understanding and following the natural order of life described by dharma leads to the good life and salvation. A failure to follow the natural order leads to suffering and endless rebirth (Burnouf, 2010; H. Smith & Novak, 2003).

It should be noted that suffering, as it is used in the Four Noble Truths, encompasses a range of emotions that have in common the disruption of peace and contentment. Thus, suffering can be the result of pain, disappointment, desire, and other emotions that are disruptive and lead one away from living in concert with the natural order of life (Shanahan & Wang, 2003; H. Smith & Novak, 2003).

The Four Noble Truths

The Four Noble Truths suggest that to become aware of the natural order in life one must first acknowledge that suffering is central to the human experience. In this view, suffering begins at birth and follows us throughout life. This fact of life is a given and must be considered if one is to lead a good life. The second Truth addresses the causes of suffering and focuses on desire. Desires can be for material things, for relationships, or for life itself. The Buddha noted that if one desires something, the end result is suffering because desires are not permanent, lead to more desires, and leave one unfulfilled. The third of the Four Noble Truths pivots off the second by noting that the way to end suffering is to end desire. According to this view, if desire is driving suffering, then one must avoid desire. The solution provided in the fourth Noble Truth is to follow the middle way. That is, one should not avoid suffering through a total detachment from life that in the extreme form is suicide. However, like the Buddha found in his own life, one must confront life and work at finding the middle way. The Buddha helped us in this process by laying out the Eightfold Path. The fourth of the Four Noble Truths, the Eightfold Path, is a set of considerations and actions one must take to achieve the middle way. These are practical steps the individual can take to hone in on the middle way; they include directives about the appropriate personal orientation one must assume, appropriate moral actions one should prioritize, and specific daily practices one must master to enter into the right state of mind. Following the Eightfold Path leads to Nirvana—the state in which one can break out of the endless cycle of birth, life, and death. This state is the equivalent of salvation because one is once and for all released from confronting suffering.

The Eightfold Path. The Eightfold Path is further subdivided into three levels. The first level is termed Insight and consists of the call to hold the right views and adopt the right resolve. Right views are demonstrated by adopting the Four Noble Truths as a guide to life. To adopt the Four Noble Truths as a governing perspective requires the individual to develop an appreciation of and commitment to exploring these Truths. Over time this commitment leads to wisdom and spiritual growth.

The right resolve, or right intention, suggests that one must focus on the right aspects of life, avoiding wrong desires and immoral acts, and instead attend to the spiritual, be peaceful, do no harm, and be a positive force for good.

The second division of the Eightfold Path is attention to moral thinking and actions. The three paths under this division include right speech, right action, and right livelihood. Right speech encompasses the need for an individual to use his or her words carefully and to not lie, be aggressive, be divisive, or waste time on idle chitchat. This path highlights the good and harm that words can create and calls on the individual to be consistent in words as he or she is in deeds. Similarly, right action attends to the impact of one's actions and requires individuals to avoid actions that are inconsistent with the Four Noble Truths, including the taking of another's life or another's property and behavior based on lust or other worldly desires. It also calls the individual to be merciful, helpful, and considerate of others. Finally, right livelihood requires one to avoid making a living in ways that might harm others. Typically included on the list of prohibited occupations are those that deal in arms; use people as commodities, as in slavery or prostitution; involve drugs or other substances that affect thinking and reduce inhibitions; and involve materials that could poison other people or animals. Due to the view that harming animals is not acceptable, occupations that raise animals for slaughter either on farms or in processing plants are also prohibited. Taken together, the moral paths lead one to act and speak in ways that promote the good and to avoid participating in occupations that affect the good in others.

The final division focuses attention on the right states of mind. Labeled meditation, this division comprises right effort, right mindfulness, and right meditation. Right effort is the call to focus one's energies on following the Eightfold Path and to minimize thoughts that attend to the difficulties of these efforts. Right mindfulness, the second of the meditational paths, directs one's attention to the important life consideration, not to be diverted by the trivial or—worse—thoughts that lead to greed, anxiety, and lust. Finally, right meditation is defined as the state of mind that allows one to focus full concentration on the Four Noble Truths and leads to an absence of suffering and associated desires. This ability to concentrate is furthered by one's development in the other paths; thus, one must have an understanding of the Noble Truths to know on what to focus. There are many traditional actions that can be employed to further the ability of the individual to concentrate, such as chanting and regulating the body through the control of breathing, among others.

Taken together, these divisions and paths operate as a guide for the individual's ethical and spiritual progress. As such, these paths and the actions they promote operate in much the same way as the virtues in the Western tradition. Earlier we described these virtues as leading the individual to follow actions and habits that ultimately support good character. Clearly the Eightfold Path has this goal as well. However, there are some significant differences. In Western virtue ethics, the focus is on the individual and the actions he or she must adopt to become a person who is and does good. It does not include the spiritual aspect of this process, which is left to theology to explore. Buddhism, by contrast, merges the two notions and provides a spiritual foundation for ethical thinking and action. Right action in the Buddhist tradition leads to good character and salvation (Burnouf, 2010; Keown, 2005; Mitchell, 2002; H. Smith & Novak, 2003).

Karma

The notion of Karma is often misunderstood to be a set of rewards and punishments meted out by God as a payback for good or bad deeds. Some also misconstrue Karma as synonymous with good or bad luck. Instead, Karma is best viewed as moral choices and actions that have objective results that are either positive or negative. In the Buddhist view, the outcomes of these actions have an effect on others; thus, good Karma is the result of a moral action that has a positive effect on others, and similarly bad Karma has a bad effect. However, also important in the Buddhist view of Karma is the effect of the moral action on the actor. One not only benefits others by moral actions but also benefits the self; over time the individual builds good Karma and offsets bad Karma. Therefore, each moral act becomes a part of the individual's character that has implications for this life and subsequent lives. In the Buddhist view, the cycle of birth, life, and death continue until one reaches Nirvana (by understanding the Four Noble Truths and following the Eightfold Path). Karma, then, is the accounting of each life and represents the progress one has made toward salvation (Keown, 2005).

The question of what constitutes good or bad moral actions in Buddhism has many similarities to that question in Western ethical traditions. In both systems, good acts are judged by a clear focus on the intentions of the actor and the outcomes of the actions on others. Specifically, in the Buddhist tradition, a good outcome that originates from a lucky event or some unintended action is not ethically good. Similarly, good intentions that are not matched with appropriate actions are deficient. More generally, actions that are motivated by benevolence, empathy, and a lack of concern for personal gain are good. Similarly, actions resulting from greed, anger, hatred, and delusional thinking are bad (Keown, 2005). Table 14.4 summarizes the Buddhist ethical concepts.

| Table 14.4 | Summary of Buddhist Ethical Concepts |

Concept	Definition/Description
Middle way	Balance of self-indulgence and self-destruction—following the middle way, not extremes, leads to gaining wisdom and understanding
Dharma	Following the natural order of things
Suffering	The result of pain, disappointment, desire, and other emotions that interfere with the natural order of life
Right view	Seeing things as they are, seeing that the world is impermanent and changes, expecting loss and suffering
Right intention	Focus on the right aspects of life and avoidance of wrong or immoral acts
Right speech	Not telling lies, engaging in slanderous speech, or expressing harsh words toward others
Right action	Not harming others, not stealing, and avoiding sexual misconduct
Right livelihood	Not engaging in certain professions, such as selling weapons or selling drugs, which violate right livelihood
Right effort	Mentally focusing on completion of tasks, not being distracted, showing discipline, focusing one's energies on following the Eightfold Path
Right mindfulness	Seeing things in full conscience and seeing things with clear perception, not focusing on excesses such as greed or lust
Right concentration	Development of natural consciousness, typically through meditation, clearing the mind, and focusing on the Four Noble Truths

The Case of Melissa: Minors' Rights and Confidentiality

Melissa is a 17-year-old Taiwanese girl who is a junior in high school. She lives with her mother and father in a medium-size city in the northwestern United States. She has an older brother who is a college student and lives away from home. She is a good student and is active in student government and sports in her high school. She is planning to attend college and expresses aspirations of becoming a veterinarian.

Melissa visits her school counselor and asks to talk about concerns she has about several peers who are having difficulty with some other girls. Donna, a 28-year-old White woman, is the school counselor, and she notes that Melissa is pleasant and sensitive. Donna has spoken to Melissa on other occasions about her career aspirations, so the counselor feels she has a positive relationship with this student. At a second meeting,

Melissa speaks about her friends and how they are getting along with another group. Then she asks Donna how an adolescent can go about getting an abortion. This is quite a change in the conversation, and Donna asks Melissa who is looking for an abortion. At first, Melissa states it is a friend, but after a few minutes she confirms it is herself and begins to cry. Melissa states she is 2 months pregnant and does not want to tell her parents. She has decided it would be best to get an abortion.

Donna thinks it would be a good idea to meet with Melissa and spend time discussing this decision. She explains that an adolescent can receive an abortion without the consent of her parents in the state in which they live, but Donna wants to discuss with Melissa whether she should include her parents in the decision. Donna wonders whether she should contact Melissa's parents and share this information with them. This is an important decision, and Donna thinks that she herself would want to know this about her daughter if she were the parent of such a child. Also, Donna is Catholic and does not believe in abortion. Donna knows that the primary decision she has to make is whether to contact the parents because her school has a policy of informing parents when issues arise with their children.

The elements of the horizon in this case potentially include the ethical dilemma; the counselor and her values, race, gender, personal history, and so forth; the client and her values, race, gender, personal history, and so forth; the supervisor and his values, race, gender, personal history, and so forth; agency policies; local, state, and federal laws that apply; professional codes of ethics; professional knowledge; geographic region; and ethical theories.

Ethical Dilemma

A few days after the meeting in which Melissa shared her secret about being pregnant, Donna set up another meeting. Donna had an opportunity to review the hermeneutic model of ethical decision making and come prepared to address the issue. Donna defined the ethical dilemma in terms of maintaining confidentiality with an adolescent. Furthermore, she noted that parental rights were an issue here. What do parents have a right to know about their child? Do parents have a right to know that their child is pregnant and is seeking an abortion? Taiwanese culture is collectivistic and family oriented. Expectations are that children represent the family honorably.

A critical value in the school in which Donna works is open communication and sharing information with parents. However, the school has not had a situation in which an adolescent chose to seek an abortion without parental consent, so this is a new dilemma for the counselor and the school. A secondary ethical issue is the personal values of the counselor that conflict with the primary choice of the client, that is, seeking an abortion. Donna is Catholic and strongly believes abortion is morally wrong. Can Donna provide counseling that is objective and free of her personal values?

Donna: The Counselor's Personal Values, Race, Gender, Personal History, and Professional Ethical Identity

Donna is single and lives with her roommate in an apartment in a small town in Oregon. The school where she is employed as a counselor is in the community where she lives. She grew up in a small town not too far from where she now resides. Her parents were supportive and caring of her and her brother, who is 2 years younger. She received her undergraduate degree in psychology at a small, private, Catholic college and her master's degree in school counseling from a state university. She took a course in ethics and uses the hermeneutic model of ethical decision making in her practice. Donna completed the Defining Issues Test and found that she fell into the postconventional stage of development, which emphasizes the social contract. She believes in a responsibility to others and the need to adhere to basic principles of the Constitution.

She has been employed as a school counselor for the past 4 years. She likes the school and the students. Her colleagues are pleasant and share feedback openly. The administration is supportive of the school counseling program and recognizes the importance of good counseling services. Donna was raised as a Catholic and attended both a Catholic high school and a Catholic undergraduate institution. She holds strong beliefs in her faith and describes herself as living her religion. She does not believe in abortion and is prolife.

Melissa: The Client's Personal Values, Race, Gender, and Personal History

Melissa is a B-plus student, and she is active in student government. She also participates in various sports in her high school. She attends church regularly and is planning to attend college. Melissa began dating when she was 15, and during the past year, she has been dating a senior at her high school. He is planning on furthering his education and was recently accepted into a prestigious private college.

Melissa reportedly gets along well with her parents. Her mother, in particular, has encouraged her to excel in school and pursue a college degree. She knows her parents would not agree to an abortion. She also knows they would be very upset if they knew that she had gotten pregnant. Melissa believes that her pregnancy would not only disappoint her parents but also prevent her from attending college.

David: The Supervisor's Values, Race, Gender, and Personal History

David, Donna's supervisor, is the director of guidance at the school. He is a 48-year-old White man. He has been employed in the school for more than 20 years, and he has fostered relationships between parents and the school that he feels are effective.

He supports his counselors in sharing information with parents if the students in question are at risk of serious harm. He is prochoice and believes that women should be able to decide for themselves whether to have abortions. He grew up in the 1970s when the Supreme Court decision to legalize abortion was hotly debated.

Professional Codes of Ethics

Donna completed a review of the American School Counselor Association's professional codes, and she found that several professional codes potentially applied to this situation. These include the following codes:

> A.1 Responsibilities to students. The professional counselor: a) has a primary obligation to the counselee who is to be treated with respect as a unique individual; b) is concerned with the educational, career, emotional, and behavioral needs and encourages the maximum development of each counselee; c) refrains from consciously encouraging the counselee's acceptance of values, lifestyles, plans, decisions, and beliefs that represent the counselor's personal orientation.

> A.2 Confidentiality. The professional school counselor: b) keeps information confidential unless disclosure is required to prevent clear and imminent danger to the counselee or others or when legal requirements demand that confidential information be revealed. Counselors will consult with other professionals when in doubt as to the validity of an exception. (American School Counselor Association, 2010)

Professional Knowledge

Donna reviewed the professional literature addressing an adolescent's right to confidentiality in obtaining an abortion. She also reviewed research on the impact on an adolescent of obtaining an abortion versus that of carrying a pregnancy to term. She found that approximately 350,000 girls younger than 18 become pregnant each year, and 31% of those have abortions (American Civil Liberties Union, 2001). In addition, 61% of pregnant adolescents who choose abortion decide to discuss the decision with their parents, whereas 39% decide not to discuss the issue with their parents, instead pursuing an abortion without parental consent (American Civil Liberties Union, 2001).

There have been considerable research and writing on the issue of adolescents' having the right to choose to obtain abortions without informing their parents (Gardner, Scherer, & Tester, 1989; Griffin-Carlson & Schwanenflugel, 1998; Gruber & Anderson, 1990; Melton, 1990; Worthington et al., 1989). For example, Worthington et al. (1989) discussed adolescents' ability to make competent decisions about choosing abortions. They suggest that in general, based on psychological research, adolescents show less ability to make competent decisions than do adults. However, there appears to be an association with age; younger adolescents do not make as good decisions as older adolescents, that is, those younger than 15 make worse decisions than those 16 and older (Liebowitz, Eisen, & Chow, 1984). Other researchers have found no difference in adolescent versus adult decision making about whether to obtain abortions (Blum & Resnick, 1982). However, Gardner et al. (1989) suggested that not enough is known about adolescent decision making to conclude whether adolescents are competent to make decisions such as whether to pursue abortions.

The American Academy of Pediatrics (1996) noted that minors have the right to obtain abortions without parental consent despite state laws that require parental consent. The U.S. Supreme Court has concluded that states must provide for judicial bypass if state laws require parental consent to obtain abortions. Judicial bypass allows adolescents to petition courts to request abortions without parental consent. The decision is made based on an assessment of an adolescent's capacity to make an informed decision.

Donna also reviewed the professional literature on adolescent pregnancy and abortion. R. Wang, Wang, and Hsu (2003) noted that the pregnancy rate among adolescents in Taiwan is lower than the rate in the United States, but it is still considered an issue. The United States has the highest adolescent pregnancy rate among developed countries (Griffin-Carlson & Schwanenflugel, 1998). Melissa grew up in the United States and is likely influenced by both cultures.

Stone (1990) concluded that prochoice advocates believe that choosing abortion is the least costly and safest choice when there is an unwanted pregnancy. Adler, Ozer, and Tschann (2003) further stated that "abortion itself carries relatively few medical risks, especially compared with the risks of childbearing" (p. 212). In addition, researchers have found few negative psychological problems associated with adolescents' choosing abortion (Zabin, Hirsch, & Emerson, 1989). Other researchers have found a significant impact on adolescents who become parents (Milan et al., 2004). Jaffee (2002) summarized many of the negative outcomes for teenage mothers, stating, "Compared with women who delay childbearing, they have lower incomes, less education, and more children. Women who first give birth as teens experience increased welfare dependency, higher unemployment, higher rates of depression, more marital instability" (p. 38). Research seems to support a negative association between adolescents' becoming mothers and their future successful adult functioning.

Geographic Region

Twenty states have parental consent laws for minors seeking abortions, whereas 16 require parental notification; that is, an adolescent can choose to have an abortion, but parents must be informed (Americans United for Life, 2003). Melissa lives in a northwestern state, Oregon, which does not have state parental involvement laws for minors seeking abortions. If she lived in another state that had such a law, her options would be more restricted, and she may have had to obtain a court bypass to receive an abortion without informing her parents. Melissa lives in a medium-size city, and because of this, even if the state did have a parental involvement law, her confidentiality would more than likely be maintained. However, if she lived in a smaller town and attempted to petition for a court bypass, she might have lost her privacy because many of those working in the court would know her and her family.

Local, State, and Federal laws

Parent involvement laws typically restrict adolescent access to abortion and require permission from one or both parents. However, the U.S. Supreme Court requires that there be a process for not involving the parents in cases wherein states have parental involvement laws, and this is accomplished through judicial bypass of parental involvement (Adler et al., 2003). So if an adolescent decides not to include her parents in her decision to seek an abortion, she must petition the court to bypass parental involvement. The court must decide whether the adolescent is competent to make the decision. The court's decision is not whether the adolescent should have the abortion but whether she is competent to make the decision by herself without parental involvement. Finally, the U.S. Court of Appeals affirmed that adolescents have the right to obtain abortions without parental consent, even in states that require it, if no means of bypassing this requirement (e.g., a court bypass) is available (see http://www.romingerlegal.com/sixthcircuit/opinions/01a0286p-06.htm).

Ethical Theory

Melissa is Taiwanese, so Donna decided to review and use Taoism as one ethical theory she wanted to apply to the situation. She found that three major concepts potentially applied to this ethical dilemma: Tao, yin and yang, and wu wei. Donna knew that Tao is defined as a way or a path that is true and desirable to follow. The way or Tao must be experienced to understand it. So Donna believed that the action or way to pursue would become clear through her interaction with Melissa. This would involve carefully listening to Melissa and respecting her perspective. In addition, Donna would need to place the decision in the context of the school environment and rules.

Donna recalled from her ethics course that *yin and yang* refers to the interaction of two opposites. These opposites include yin, which is the receptive and weaker aspect of the union and may be considered negative and destructive, and yang, which has been referred to as strong, positive, and constructive. In this dilemma, Melissa may be considered the yin, the weaker partner of the union when coming together (because she is an adolescent), and Donna may be considered the yang, the stronger partner of the union. Donna noted that the ideal relationship is a balance between yin and yang, not too much strength or dominance and not too little. To act ethically based on Taoism, Donna will want to be aware of the balance in the relationship; for example, how assertive or dominant should she become in encouraging Melissa to inform or herself acting to inform the parents?

Wu wei is another concept that may apply. Donna recalled it referred to nonaction and involved following nature and being natural, spontaneous, and harmonious with nature. The dilemma for Donna is discovering what is natural or spontaneous in this situation. Nonaction may be interpreted in this situation as not letting the adolescent decide naturally whether to contact the parents. In addition, the question becomes, How much information does Donna give or influence does Donna exert on Melissa if she follows wu wei?

Source: Adapted from Houser, Wilczenski, and Ham (2006). Reprinted with permission.

Questions for Further Reflection

1. Is there an Eastern theory or theories that fit more closely with your ethical view and perspective? If so, what is attractive about the theory or theories?

2. How important are the ethical theories in the hermeneutic model of ethical decision making?

3. Do you see similarities among the ethical theories? Are there similarities across Western and Eastern theories? Do you think you would come to the same conclusion if you used each theory with an ethical dilemma?

The Case of Shi-Jiuan: Conflict Between Laws and Client Worldviews

Carefully read the case of Shi-Jiuan. Information is provided about an ethical dilemma, the counselor's values and personal ethical identity, the client's personal values, and the supervisor's personal values. Generate information for elements of the hermeneutic model: professional codes that may apply, geographic region, and professional literature that is relevant. Choose an ethical theory or theories to apply (one of the Eastern theories presented in this chapter), and summarize your ethical decision based on the hermeneutic model. Be sure to gather information about relevant codes of ethics that apply, laws and statutes that apply, and professional literature that applies.

Shi-Jiuan is a 33-year-old woman who emigrated from Hong Kong to the United States 3 years ago. She is Chinese. She is married, and her spouse, also Chinese, holds a graduate degree in electrical engineering and works in a large corporation in New York City. The couple has two children: a 12-year-old daughter and a son who is 9. Shi-Jiuan was diagnosed with depression and has been coming to counseling for the past 2 months. She initially reported fatigue, memory loss, irritability, and sleep disturbances. Zoloft was prescribed for her, and she has been on this medication for 2 months. She states that the medication has helped and she feels less fatigue and irritability.

Another complaint, along with her depression, is that she misses her homeland, Hong Kong, and that she is having difficulty with her children in maintaining cultural values—that is, Confucian values such as respect for one's elders—and retaining many of their Chinese views and traditions. Shi-Jiuan is the oldest of three children, and she grew up in a traditional Chinese family. She and her husband, who grew up in similar environments, were socialized into traditional Confucian values and beliefs, including respect for elders, loyalty to family, and respect for the social order. Shi-Jiuan's and her husband's families valued education, and the couple have attempted to instill the importance of education in their children.

Shi-Jiuan has seen the same counselor for the past 2 months on a biweekly basis to monitor her medication and provide counseling. The counselor, Joan, is a White, middle-aged, 42-year-old mother of one. Counselor and client have developed a good relationship despite the initial hesitance Shi-Jiuan expressed about seeing a counselor. She feels it is a sign of weakness to see a counselor and to discuss personal feelings outside the family. She states she feels ashamed that she has to receive such help but acknowledges counseling is helpful to her. Shi-Jiuan describes her marital relationship as that of a woman in a traditional Chinese family, with the husband being dominant and her primary role being caretaker of the children.

After 2 months of counseling, Shi-Jiuan presents a new issue in the counseling session. She is discussing her frustrations about some of the behaviors of her children, particularly her daughter. Her daughter has shown some disrespect and talked back to her. Shi-Jiuan states that she has slapped her daughter on the face when the daughter has talked back. Joan, the counselor, listens to Shi-Jiuan's account of the face-slapping incidents and asks her about the response of her daughter to this type of discipline. Shi-Jiuan states that the daughter has become more compliant since the slapping. Shi-Jiuan recalls seeing her brother slapped when she was growing up and how she learned to become more respectful of elders. Joan notes that she is a mandated reporter of child abuse and decides she must review the situation carefully to make an important decision at this juncture in counseling.

The relevant elements of the horizon based on the case of Shi-Jiuan include the ethical dilemma; the counselor and her values, race, gender, personal history, and so forth; the client and her values, race, gender, personal history, and so forth; the supervisor and his values, race, gender, personal history, and so forth; agency policies; local, state, and federal laws that apply; professional codes of ethics; professional knowledge; geographic region; and ethical theories.

Ethical Dilemma

Joan must decide which course of action to take: Should she continue working with Shi-Jiuan and attempt to address her parenting actions, or should she submit a report of child abuse to the New York Office of Children and Family Services? As a counselor, Joan is a mandated reporter according to New York State law (New York Office of Children & Family Services, 2002). Joan has worked with many Asian clients and families previously and knows that an authoritarian parenting style is typical and that corporal punishment is used on a frequent basis. Joan believes she has developed a good but still tentative relationship with Shi-Jiuan. The counselor is concerned that if she reports the abuse, even though it is anonymous, Shi-Jiuan will deduce who filed the report because she probably has not talked about slapping her daughter with anyone else, and she may withdraw from treatment. If the client withdraws from treatment, she may stop taking her medication; in addition, Joan would lose an opportunity to work with her on her parenting skills. Alternatively, how severe is the physical abuse, and what damage has it done to the 12-year-old adolescent? Last, Joan is a mandated reporter, and failure to report child abuse is a Class A misdemeanor and subject to criminal penalties. Joan believes in following the law but also believes in broader ethical principles that influence her decision making. Joan knows her supervisor, Greg, has very strong feelings about reporting child abuse because he worked for the Office of Children and Family Services prior to coming to the counseling agency.

Joan: The Counselor's Personal Values, Race, Gender, and Personal History

Joan grew up in a middle-class family where discipline was person centered and resulted in no physical punishment. She is the oldest of three children, and she did not see any of her siblings receive any corporal punishment. Joan used verbal praise, feedback, removal of problem stimuli, and time-outs to educate her son, now 18, about expected prosocial behaviors and never used physical punishment. Her spouse shared her view of child rearing. She received her graduate training from a public university and took a course on behavioral theories that addressed parent training and behavioral principles. Joan took the Defining Issues Test and found she fit the criteria for the postconventional (social contract) stage.

Shi-Jiuan: The Client's Personal Values, Race, Gender, and Personal History

Shi-Jiuan is the oldest of three children; she has an older brother. Her mother and father worked hard and provided a comfortable living environment for her and her brother. Her parents expected their children to follow Confucian practices such as showing respect and obedience. Shi-Jiuan remembers seeing her brother being slapped for talking back to his mother. She always listened to her parents, and she was never slapped, but she knew it would happen if she was disrespectful. She married when she was 19, while her spouse was attending college. After graduating from engineering school, her spouse began working in Hong Kong. Shortly after, she became pregnant and had their first child, a daughter. Shi-Jiuan and her husband were disappointed that the child was not a boy, but she provided good care for their daughter. Her husband became involved in his work, and as a traditional Chinese mother, she cared for the child. They had a son 3 years later.

Then 3 years ago her husband's company acquired a major project in New York, so he took a position there, and the family moved there. Shi-Jiuan has never been employed outside the home; instead she has cared for the children. At first, her children did not want to come to New York, but since the move, they have done relatively well in school. Shi-Jiuan gets out of the house through shopping and parties with her husband's company. She is ambivalent about living in the United States and hopes to return to Hong Kong in the future. She misses the traditions and cultural opportunities in Hong Kong.

Greg: The Supervisor's Personal Values, Race, Gender, and Personal History

Greg, Joan's supervisor, is a 42-year-old African American man. He worked for 5 years for the New York State Office of Children and Family Services before coming to the mental health facility 6 years ago. He is married without children. During his master's program he was educated as a counselor, and he follows the same professional codes of ethics that Joan follows. At times when he was growing up, his parents disciplined him using corporal punishment.

Source: Adapted from Houser, Wilczenski, and Ham (2006). Reprinted with permission.

Use Figure 14.1 to identify relevant elements of the horizon. Fill in the appropriate elements to help with your understanding and ethical decision.

Figure 14.1 | Ethical Dilemma

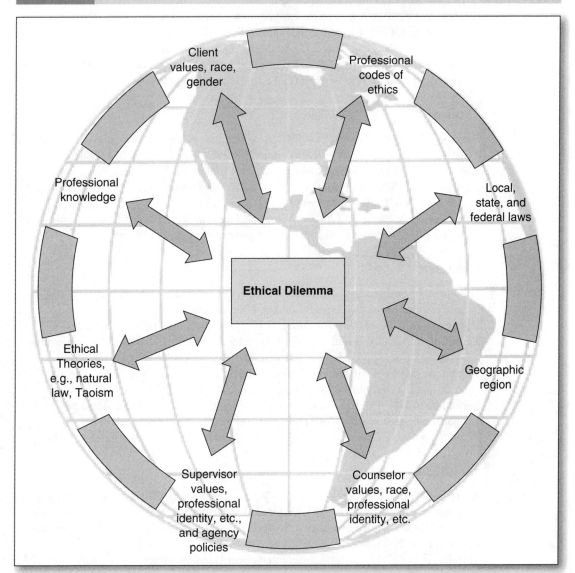

Figure 14.1   Ethical Dilemma

Additional Recommended Readings

Confucianism

Berling, J. A. (1982). Confucianism. *Focus on Asian Studies, 2*(1), 5–7. Retrieved from http://www.askasia.org/frclasrm/readings/r000004.htm

Csikszentmihalyi, M. (2005). Differentiations in Chinese ethics. In W. Schweiker (Ed.), *The Blackwell companion to religious ethics* (pp. 381–394). Malden, MA: Blackwell.

Hansen, C. (1993). Classical Chinese ethics. In P. Singer (Ed.), *A companion to ethics* (pp. 69–81). Malden, MA: Blackwell.

Ivanhoe, P. J. (2002). *Ethics in the Confucian tradition.* Indianapolis, IN: Hackett.

Mollgaard, E. (2005). Chinese ethics? In W. Schweiker (Ed.), *The Blackwell companion to religious ethics* (pp. 368–373). Malden, MA: Blackwell.

Shanahan, T., & Wang, R. (2003). *Reason and insight: Western and Eastern perspectives on the pursuit of moral wisdom* (2nd ed.). Belmont, CA: Wadsworth.

Taoism

Berkson, M. (2005). Trajectories of Chinese religious ethics. In W. Schweiker (Ed.), *The Blackwell companion to religious ethics* (pp. 395–405). Malden, MA: Blackwell.

Kohn, L. (2001). *Daoism and Chinese culture.* Cambridge, MA: Three Pines Press.

Lagerwey, J. (1987). *Taoist ritual in Chinese society and history.* New York, NY: Macmillan.

Miller, J. (2003). *Daoism: A short introduction.* Oxford, UK: Oneworld.

Shanahan, T., & Wang, R. (2003). *Reason and insight: Western and Eastern perspectives on the pursuit of moral wisdom* (2nd ed.). Belmont, CA: Wadsworth.

Hinduism

Bilimoria, P., Prabhu, J., & Sharma, A. (Eds.). (2004). *Indian ethics: Classical traditions and contemporary challenges.* London, UK: Ashgate.

Klostermaier, K. K. (2000). *Hinduism: A short introduction.* Oxford, UK: Oneworld.

Perrett, R. W. (2005). Hindu ethics? In W. Schweiker (Ed.), *The Blackwell companion to religious ethics* (pp. 323–329). Malden, MA: Blackwell.

Prabhu, J. (2005). Trajectories of Hindu ethics. In W. Schweiker (Ed.), *The Blackwell companion to religious ethics* (pp. 355–367). Malden, MA: Blackwell.

Sarkar, K. (1912). *The Hindu system of moral science.* Calcutta, India: Majudar.

Shanahan, T., & Wang, R. (2003). *Reason and insight: Western and Eastern perspectives on the pursuit of moral wisdom* (2nd ed.). Belmont, CA: Wadsworth.

Buddhism

Carter, J. R. (2005). Buddhist ethics? In W. Schweiker (Ed.), *The Blackwell companion to religious ethics* (pp. 278–285). Malden, MA: Blackwell.

Harvey, P. (2000). *An introduction to Buddhist ethics: Foundations, values, and issues.* New York, NY: Cambridge University Press.

Kasulis, T. P. (2005). Cultural differentiation in Buddhist ethics. In W. Schweiker (Ed.), *The Blackwell companion to religious ethics* (pp. 297–312). Malden, MA: Blackwell.

Keown, D. (2000). *Contemporary Buddhist ethics.* London, UK: Curzon Press.

Keown, D. (2005). *Buddhist ethics: A very short introduction.* Oxford, UK: Oxford University Press.

Keown, D. (2005). Origins of Buddhist ethics. In W. Schweiker (Ed.), *The Blackwell companion to religious ethics* (pp. 286–296). Malden, MA: Blackwell.

Shanahan, T., & Wang, R. (2003). *Reason and insight: Western and Eastern perspectives on the pursuit of moral wisdom* (2nd ed.). Belmont, CA: Wadsworth.

Singh, A. K. (2008, October 19). *Dharma—The universal law of morality.* Retrieved from http://ezinearticles.com/?Dharma---The-Universal-Law-of-Morality&id=1597760

Chapter 15

MIDDLE EASTERN ETHICAL THEORIES

CHAPTER OBJECTIVES

- Acquire an understanding of Islamic ethics and relevant concepts
- Acquire an understanding of Judaic ethics and relevant concepts

This section of the book is focused on Middle Eastern theories of ethics; it includes the presentation of the ethical theories of Judaism and Islam. Islam has a long history, and Islamic ethics is tied to religious beliefs. Islamic ethics is more of an absolutism theory rather than a moral relativism approach (C. E. Harris, 2007). As is the case in many of the other ethical theories, there is a connection between Jewish ethical behavior and Judaic religious beliefs. Dorff (2000) noted the key foundation in Judaism and its ethics is a linkage between the individual, family, and community. Judaic ethics is founded on the belief that humans have a responsibility to repair the world. Repair of the world is accomplished through finding cures for disease, promoting peace, and taking responsibility for the care of others in the family, the community, and all of humanity.

ISLAMIC ETHICS

Islam has a long history dating back more than 1,400 years. The term *Islam* is Arabic, meaning "submission to God," and it is supported by derivatives of earlier interpretations of the meaning of *Islam* including concepts of "peace" (Belt, 2002). The primary contributor to Islam was the Prophet Muhammad ibu Abd

Allah, who was born in Mecca in 570 CE. After his father died when he was 6 years old, he lived with his grandfather until the grandfather passed away and then went to live with his uncle. Belt (2002) described the first insight Muhammad experienced:

> At about age 40 Muhammad retreated to a cave in the mountains outside Mecca to meditate. There, Muslims believe, he was visited by the archangel Gabriel, who began reciting to him the Word of God. Until his death 23 years later, Muhammad passed along these revelations to a growing band of followers, including many who wrote down the words or committed them to memory. (p. 78)

After Muhammad's death these writings were used in the composition of the Qur'an (frequently referred to as the Koran in English).

Initially, Muhammad experienced considerable struggle to gain acceptance. He introduced his ideas in Mecca and after 10 years moved to Medina. He had been invited to Medina and eventually governed that city. Consequently, he acquired numerous followers in Medina. After several years, he decided to return to Mecca with a small army and he successfully conquered Mecca after three battles (Gale Group, 2002). Muhammad died in 632 CE. Belt (2002) noted that Islam was well established at the time of Muhammad's death in the Arabian Peninsula. After Muhammad's death, several caliphs further consolidated followers of Islam (Esposito, 1999). Islam's influence expanded but at times also contracted in some geographic locations due to wars and peoples' being conquered (Haddad, 1999). Islam continued in the Middle East, parts of North Africa, and eastern Europe, for example, Romania and Bulgaria. The prevalence of Islam more recently has increased in the West. In the United States, the practice of Islam has increased significantly during the past 20 years both from immigration and conversion. For example, there has been a significant increase by African Americans in adopting Islamic thought, belief, and religion in the United States (Carter & Rashidi, 2003; Gomez, 1994; Haddad, 1991). It has been projected that Islam will become the second-largest religious group in the United States (U.S. Department of State, n.d.).

Major Concepts

One of the major writers on Muslim ethics was Abd al-Jabbar (Hourani, 1971). A first step in understanding Islamic ethics is the consideration of knowledge, which is defined as "an intellectual content corresponding to reality in the manner of truth, and an emotional state of satisfaction and tranquility" (Hourani, 1971, p. 13).

Knowledge can be achieved through introspection, or finding knowledge and truth within oneself. Referring to introspection, Hourani (1971) stated, "There is no clearer or stronger evidence of truth than what is learned in this way" (p. 21). Knowledge or knowing, according to Hourani, is based on the following general truths: that doing wrong is always evil, that humans usually act in their own interest, and that humans believe what they perceive. Referring to knowledge, Hourani concluded that

> the knowledge of general truths is not innate, prior to any evidence; it is drawn out from particular experiences, in which it is learned by a direct apprehension like that of geometry, where we learn through but not from physical diagrams. (p. 22)

So the conclusion is that Islamic ethics and knowledge, or knowing what is ethical, are clear and specific. Islam is a theory based not on moral relativism but on moral absolutism; there is a right way to interpret an ethical issue. Hourani (1971) noted that truths are generally acknowledged by every rational person.

Islamic ethics differentiates five major classes of ethics and/or acts: evil or forbidden acts, undesirable acts, neutral acts, desirable acts, and good or required acts. Forbidden acts may be defined as "disgraceful, shameful or bad acts" (Hourani, 1971). Essentially, forbidden acts cause harm to others or oneself. Hourani (1971) stated, "Pain is evil in itself, that is, when it is simply useless suffering" (p. 32); then pain is considered evil. The exception is an act that is based on retribution or is deserved by the recipient; that act is not evil. A forbidden act may be defined as an outcome that causes pain regardless of the individual's intent. One may not intentionally try to inflict pain, but it does occur; if the person experiencing the pain does not deserve it, then it is considered undesirable. Undesirable acts are those that can be avoided if one attends to them, but they generally do not involve direct action on the part of the individual. An act is also unethical if a person acts to hurt others or self or if a person lets an event happen that injures others.

Neutral acts are those that have no impact on others. Someone can go into the woods and scream loudly, and it does not harm anyone. It is considered a neutral act as long as it does not harm others and there is not a positive outcome. If someone screams in a department store and it upsets others, then it becomes an undesirable act.

Desirable acts are those that one can perform, creating a positive outcome. Such acts are not obligations on the part of the actor but can improve or promote happiness. A worker's entering the office and saying hello to others with a smile may promote good feelings and may be considered good. It is not required, but it is a desirable act.

Good or required acts are those that potentially help others or remove harm. For example, not killing others (unless there is a good reason) is considered a required act. Hourani (1971) stated, "Good is objective, like evil; subjectivism is to be rejected" (p. 103). Again, this is an illustration of a moral absolutist position. There are four components of good: justice, benefit, truthfulness, and willing good (Hourani, 1971). Justice concerns engaging in socially good actions to help or injure others. Injury may be just if the recipient is deserving of it. Benefit, according to Hourani, is whatever brings pleasure. Truthfulness is considered good if it brings about pleasure and does not inflict pain. However, if truthfulness hurts someone who is undeserving of pain, then it is considered evil. The solution is not to tell a mistruth but to remain silent or avoid stating a mistruth (Hourani, 1971). The will for good is based on the intent of the actor; it refers to motivation or intent. Having the intention to bring about benefit is considered good, but not all intentions are good if pain and suffering occur as a result of an intended good act. So a counselor can have a good intent, for example, wanting to help a client, but if the counselor does not have the skills to be helpful and tries to help anyway, the counselor's efforts become an undesirable act. The outcome may be harmful, and therefore the act would be evil. Table 15.1 summarizes Islamic ethical concepts.

Table 15.1 Summary of Islamic Ethical Concepts

Concept	Definition/Description
Evil or forbidden acts	These types of acts cause harm to others or to oneself. An example is driving under the influence of alcohol.
Undesirable acts	These are acts that can be avoided if one focuses on them, but they generally do not involve a direct action on the part of the individual. An act is also unethical if a person acts to hurt others or self or if a person lets an event happen that injures others. An example is seeing a wet floor and not doing anything to clean it up, resulting in someone's falling and hurting himself or herself.
Neutral acts	These are acts that have no impact on others. Watching and enjoying an orchestra has no impact on others if one is alone.
Desirable acts	If one performs an act that creates a positive outcome, then the act is good. Such acts are not obligations on the part of the actor but can improve or promote happiness. Taking the time to talk to a clerk at a store may show interest and caring, and this may make the clerk happy; however, it is not required.
Good or required acts	These are acts that possibly help others or remove harm. One example is not killing others (unless there is a good reason—then it becomes a required act). There are four components of good: justice, benefit, truthfulness, and willing good.

JUDAIC ETHICS

Judaic ethics is founded on several sources including the Torah. Specific reference to ethical behavior may be found in sections referred to as *halacha* and *mitzvoth*. Kinzbrunner (2004) noted that there are 248 references to positive things humans should do and 365 references to acts that should be avoided. Another source of Judaic ethics is the Talmud. Both the Torah and the Talmud provide the foundation of Judaic ethics. Judaic ethics may be traced back to 250 BCE and early writings that were included in the Hebrew Bible and later in the Talmud (Green, 2005). There may be slightly different interpretations of ethics, similar to other ethical perspectives, due to the perspectives of various Jewish sects (Kinzbrunner, 2004). According to Kinzbrunner, these different perspectives may be found in orthodox, conservative, reform, reconstructionist, and unaffiliated traditions. Dorff's (2003) discussion of Judaic ethics and definition of classical Jewish morals involve a careful review of a particular ethical issue and exploration of Jewish views and traditions to determine what is moral.

Major Concepts

Major concepts presented in the Talmud focus on five prohibitions relevant to Judaic ethics: blasphemy, idolatry, destruction of human life, inappropriate sexual acts (adultery, incest, homosexuality, and bestiality), and robbery (Green, 2005; Kinzbrunner, 2004). Telling the truth is a moral act; lying is considered unethical. Engaging in inappropriate sexual acts such as adultery and homosexuality does not promote natural order. Robbery is an unethical act. Leviticus 19:13 states, "Do not oppress your neighbor and do not rob him." Destruction of human life is considered a significant violation of Judaic ethics (Kinzbrunner, 2004). Deuteronomy 30:19 states, "I call heaven and earth to witness against you today, that I have set before you life and death, blessing and curse. Therefore choose life, that you and your offspring may live" (Kinzbrunner, 2004). The key in this statement is the injunction to choose life, and this may be expanded to include choosing life for self, others, and animals—all living things.

Judaic ethics also may be understood through major broad perspectives. One such perspective is family, community, and the importance of these two entities. Liebman and Fishman (2000) suggested that the family is an essential component in Judaic life and acts of morality. Dorff (2003) also noted the importance of the family and particularly the marital relationship. The marital relationship is the foundation of the family; Jewish laws hold that sexual relations between spouses are necessary and abuse of a spouse is not acceptable. Dorff stated that "the family creates, educates, and supports the next generation" (2003, p. 27). It has been noted that one of the first commandments in the Torah is to "be fruitful" and multiply. So families have an ethical/moral responsibility to procreate and establish a family focused on preparing the next generation. Parents are encouraged to monitor what children learn and ensure it is adequate and is consistent with Jewish tradition.

Education is another ethical obligation. Adults and children should engage in educational activities. Dorff (2003) suggested that education and learning are lifelong activities. Knowledge should be obtained not only from religious texts but from other sources so one becomes aware and makes the best decisions. The only limitation is that gathering knowledge from different sources and disciplines must be done through an integration of principles derived from the Torah.

According to Dorff (2003), the community is second only to the family in importance. The community provides the environment and opportunities for acting ethically. This includes opportunities for learning (through synagogues or other resources such as universities). Community responsibility is another element of Judaic ethics, and Dorff (2000) proposed that social action is a component of the Jewish identity. Responsibility to the community is not voluntary but is a covenant with God. Dorff (2003) suggested that the three elements just mentioned are essential to achieving the Jewish mission, which is social action and repairing the world. Consequently, Dorff proposed that "human beings are to help God in that task as God's agents and partners in the ongoing repair of the world" (2003, p. 31). The duty to repair society includes such activities as finding cures for diseases, finding solutions to social problems, and teaching morality and understanding. A concept from virtue ethics, beneficence, fits into social action. Judaic ethics suggests that humans have a responsibility to help others, the family, the community, and the world. One interpretation of beneficence is repairing the world, which involves reducing the pain others experience. Repairing the world may be achieved through assisting with resolution of social problems or discovering medicines to cure disease. See Table 15.2 for a summary of Judaic ethical concepts.

Table 15.2 Summary of Judaic Ethical Concepts

Concept	Definition/Description
Five prohibitions	Avoid blasphemy, idolatry, destruction of human life, and inappropriate sexual acts (adultery, incest, homosexuality, and bestiality).
Family and community	Families have an ethical/moral responsibility to procreate and establish families focused on preparing the next generation.

Concept	Definition/Description
Education	Education and learning are lifelong activities. Knowledge should be obtained not only from religious texts but from other sources so one becomes aware and makes the best decisions.
Community responsibility/ social responsibility	One has a duty to repair society. This may involve finding solutions to social problems, conducting medical research, and so forth to reduce the pain of others.

The Case of Ahmed: A Mandated Client

Ahmed is a 24-year-old man of Middle Eastern descent who has entered counseling as a mandated client. He was charged with assault and battery against his spouse, and he was found guilty. As part of his sentence he must attend individual and group counseling focusing on anger management.

Ahmed has a history of aggressive acts. He would often get into physical fights with his brothers when they were adolescents. During his college years, he was arrested for assaulting another student when they had an unpleasant verbal exchange. Most recently, he acknowledges, he becomes angry at his spouse about different issues, primarily about money and family finances. The incident that resulted in his physically attacking his spouse involved her spending money on items he felt were unnecessary. His wife told him that she worked and had a right to buy whatever she wanted. Ahmed felt his wife was being disrespectful of him because he thought they could not afford the items she purchased. He admitted hitting her several times. His wife then called the police, and Ahmed was arrested. Ahmed was found guilty of assault and battery and mandated to obtain counseling for anger management or go to jail. With counseling, his 2-year sentence was reduced to probation. After the incident he and his spouse decided to remain together to try to work through this situation.

Ahmed attends an anger management group in a local mental health agency. The group meets for 2 hours weekly, and this will last for 16 weeks. The group focuses on psychoeducational and insight-oriented approaches. Typically, psychoeducational information is provided in the first couple of sessions, and the remaining sessions are process oriented and self-reflective. Session participants are informed when the session begins that the agency policy is that any potential threats of violence will require the counselors to contact the client's spouse and give him or her a warning. Clients sign releases of information acknowledging that they have been informed and give permission to disclose if necessary.

Ahmed attends the first three sessions but does not participate in any significant way. During the fourth session, the group focuses on the triggers that set up the anger and aggression for group members. Ahmed describes a recent trigger for him, that is, his spouse's spending money on things he felt she did not need. Then, during the second part of the session, Ahmed states he would still physically assault his spouse if she overspent. He says that his spouse would argue with him about her expenditures. He feels it is his obligation to correct his spouse's behavior. The group is led by two counselors, Jeremy and Sally. Jeremy and Sally are pleased that Ahmed participates in the fourth session, but they are concerned about his continued belief in aggressive acts toward his spouse. They do not want to hinder the continued participation of Ahmed in future groups, but they feel they need to consider breaching confidentiality and inform the spouse of the threat.

Relevant elements of the horizon include the ethical dilemma; the counselors and their respective values, race, gender, personal history, and so forth; the client and his values, race, gender, personal history, and so forth; the supervisor and her values, race, gender, personal history, and so forth; agency policies; local, state, and federal laws that apply; professional codes of ethics; professional knowledge; geographic region; and ethical theories.

Ethical Dilemma

Jeremy and Sally must decide whether to break confidentiality and contact Ahmed's spouse about the potential threat of violence. The fact that he signed a release of information prior to beginning the group sessions gave them legal authority to do so, but they also think that such a breach of confidentiality may hinder his participation and honesty in future anger group sessions. Their possible courses of action are (a) to contact Ahmed's spouse and share the information that he expressed violent thought toward her and (b) to not share the threat of violence with his spouse and work with Ahmed in the group sessions to address his anger. Several issues need to be considered in the decision. What if they do not inform the spouse and she is physically abused? What responsibility do they have in tacitly allowing this aggressive behavior? Another issue is that Ahmed may become more aggressive if his spouse confronts him with information she receives from the counselors. Alternatively, Ahmed may be more open to treatment in the group if he feels accepted and can express himself without negative consequences. This may result in more openness to treatment and ultimately better management of his anger. Jeremy and Sally disagree about whether to break confidentiality. Jeremy is looking at what principles apply to breaking confidentiality (e.g., fidelity, beneficence), whereas Sally wants to follow agency policy and state law. Jeremy and Sally decide to use the hermeneutic approach to making this decision; this will include a consultation with the agency director and their supervisor, Cheryl.

Jeremy and Sally: The Counselors' Respective Personal Values, Race, Gender, and Personal History

Jeremy is an African American man in his early 30s who is married without children. He is a practicing Muslim, and so is his spouse. He lives in a suburban community of middle-income families. He grew up in a middle-class family, and both parents were teachers. While growing up he attended a Christian church; then he converted to Islam in his early 20s. He is the oldest of three boys. His parents provided a good model for a marital relationship; they rarely argued, and he never observed any aggressive acts on the parts of his parents toward each other or toward his siblings or himself.

Jeremy attended a small, private, liberal arts college and earned a degree in psychology. He furthered his education with a master's degree in mental health counseling at another small, private college. During his training program, Jeremy took the Defining Issues Test and discovered he emphasized postconventional strategies in his moral thinking. He considers himself highly principled, and he considers rules important in acting ethically. However, he believes in openness in attempting to understand an ethical course of action; each situation may be different. Jeremy has been a practicing counselor for more than 5 years. He is licensed by the state as a counselor and is a member of the American Counseling Association, so he follows the American Counseling Association's code of ethics.

Sally is a 40-year-old divorced White woman. She lives with her two children, ages 15 and 17, in the urban community where the counseling center is located. She and her older brother grew up in a working-class family. The family was not particularly religious, but on occasion she did attend a Protestant church. Her mother and father argued frequently, and she observed their conflicts. At times, her father became physically abusive toward her mother, but they did not divorce. She attended college and obtained her bachelor's degree in social psychology. She met her husband in college, and they married after graduation.

Sally divorced as a consequence of an abusive relationship with her husband. She lived with physical abuse for the first 8 years of their marriage. She then sought help to get out of the abusive relationship and lived in a shelter for a period of time with her children. After the divorce, she decided to return to school while working to support her two children. She attended a local urban university for her master's degree in community counseling. She completed an internship in the same counseling center where she works now. Sally completed the Defining Issues Test and discovered that she emphasizes conventional moral thinking. She became involved in the anger management groups, working with men who engage in violence against their partners. Sally has become an advocate for women in abusive relationships and is passionate about her work. She graduated with her master's degree 2 years ago and began working in the counseling center full-time. She sees clients individually and runs several groups focusing on anger management and abused women.

Ahmed: The Client's Personal Values, Race, Gender, and Personal History

Ahmed was born and grew up in the United States. His father and mother entered the United States in the 1970s, and they received master's degrees in engineering and education, respectively. He is the oldest of his siblings; he has two younger brothers. He attended college but did not complete a degree. Ahmed currently works in construction as a laborer. He has been married for 3 years and has no children.

Ahmed recalls that his parents were emotionally distant. He observed his father physically abusing his mother on a relatively frequent basis. His father would not hit his mother on the face or head, but he hit her on the arms, back, or stomach. Ahmed was teased in school for his Middle Eastern complexion, and he fought back. He was expelled from school on two occasions as a consequence for fighting. He also would get into fistfights with his two brothers on occasion. Even though Ahmed was the oldest, his middle brother was larger than him and picked on him at times. Ahmed was an average student in school and graduated with an undistinguished academic record. He attended a public university for 1 year before dropping out and getting a job in construction. He liked construction work because the pay was good.

He began dating women only in his late teens, and he found it hard to find another Muslim even though he lived in a relatively large Muslim community. After attending college he met his spouse, and after a short courtship they decided to marry. He was physically aggressive toward his spouse early in their relationship, and after dating for only a few months he twisted her arm when she was teasing him about his dark complexion.

After they were married, the couple lived in an apartment and seemed to have enough money to meet their monthly expenses. Currently, Ahmed lives in an apartment with his spouse in a large urban area in the Midwest. He is a practicing Muslim and is planning a pilgrimage to Mecca in the next few years. He attends a mosque in his community. His spouse also is Muslim and is of Middle Eastern descent. She works as a clerical staff member in an insurance agency. Because Ahmed views his role as a man as the head of the household, he believes it is his responsibility to limit what he considers his spouse's excessive spending. Ahmed manages the household funds and feels pressure to manage the money well.

Cheryl: The Supervisor's Values, Race, and Personal History

Cheryl is the agency director and the supervisor for Jeremy and Sally. She is a 46-year-old White woman who has been married for 5 years. This is her second marriage. Her first marriage ended in divorce from a man who was physically and psychologically abusive. She was married to her first husband for 5 years, and she had two children with him.

Cheryl raised the children alone and remarried when they were adults. She received her master's degree in social work 10 years ago and began working in an agency providing services to abused women. After 4 years in this agency, she became the director of the current community agency, which provides counseling services primarily to abused women and their abusive partners.

Agency Values

The agency is committed to reducing physical and psychological abuse of spousal partners, particularly abuse of women. Its staff members have developed policies that are designed to protect abused partners, for example, informed consent that gives permission to disclose potential violence to a spouse and break confidentiality.

Professional Codes of Ethics

A number of professional codes potentially apply to this case. Jeremy and Sally decided to use the codes from the Association for Specialists in Group Work. Relevant codes include the following:

A.6 Professional Disclosure Statement—Group workers have a professional disclosure statement which includes information on confidentiality and exceptions to confidentiality.

A.7.b Group and member preparation—Group workers facilitate informed consent. Group workers provide in oral and written form to prospective members; the professional disclosure statement; group purpose and goals; group participation expectations including voluntary and involuntary membership . . . procedures for mandated groups.

A.7.d Group member preparation—Group workers define confidentiality and its limit. (Association for Specialists in Group Work, 2007)

Professional Knowledge

Estimates of the number of individuals who are victims of violence by partners or former partners range from approximately 1 million to 4 million a year, with 85% of these victims being women (Hassouneh-Phillips, 2001; Rennison & Welchans, 2002). Many theorists and researchers studying violence and spousal abuse suggest that a social learning theory model is the best approach to understanding the problem (Bevan & Higgins, 2002; Rosenbaum & Leisring, 2003). Social learning theory is based on a view that behaviors are learned through exposure and modeling. So observing a parent's abusing another parent may result in intergenerational transmission of violence (Bevan & Higgins, 2002; Margolin, Gordis, Medina, & Oliver, 2003).

Ahmed reportedly observed his father's physically abusing his mother when he was a child. Bevan and Higgins (2002) stated that social learning theory suggests that children identify with their parents, particularly the parent of the same sex as the child. When a child observes aggression by a parent, and the child later identifies with the aggressor, the aggression may be repeated. Thus, Ahmed had a model for aggressive acts from his father, and this aggression appears to have been passed on to Ahmed in his relationship with his spouse. Researchers also have found a strong connection between adult spousal abuse and witnessing spousal violence during childhood (Cappell & Heiner, 1990). Bevan and Higgins also found a strong association between observing family violence during childhood and physical spousal abuse. Rosenbaum and Leisring (2003) noted that domestic violence is "about power and control" (p. 7), and Ahmed sought control over his spouse's spending habits.

Both group leaders, Jeremy and Sally, are concerned about whether Ahmed will continue active participation in treatment if they break confidentiality. A concept that focuses on the process of counseling that may be relevant here is the therapeutic alliance (Bordin, 1979). The three important components of the therapeutic alliance, according to Bordin (1979), are mutual liking, attachment, and trust between the client and therapist. Researchers have found that the therapeutic alliance is an important variable in treatment outcome (Brown & O'Leary, 2000). If the group leaders break confidentiality, what impact will this have on the therapeutic alliance? Will Ahmed trust the group leaders and continue sharing his thoughts and feelings?

Researchers have found that self-esteem among Muslim men and women is associated with support for physical abuse of partners (Ali & Toner, 2001). More specifically, Ali and Toner (2001) found that Muslim men with low self-esteem were more likely to support physical abuse of spouses. Also, Muslim men expressed more supportive attitudes toward physically abusing partners than did Muslim women.

The recidivism rate of abusive partners is about 40% within a 5-year period (Shepard, 1992). There have been several attempts to develop a method for assessing the danger that an offender will return to physically abusing his or her spouse (Kropp, Hart, Webster, & Eaves, 1999; Stuart & Campbell, 1989). However, results are mixed in predicting significant harm to a spouse as a consequence of recidivism (Hilton, Harris, & Rice, 2001). So based on the literature, it is difficult to predict significant harm to Ahmed's spouse if he relapses into violent acts.

Geographic Region

Geographic region can play a role in this case because of some characteristics of urban settings. Ahmed lives in an urban area, and the counseling center is located in an urban area. Researchers have noted the different characteristics of those living and growing up in urban and rural environments (Sears, Evans, & Perry, 1998; Silk, Sessa, Morris,

Steinberg, & Avenevoli, 2004). Urban researchers studied the development or lack of development of collective efficacy (Ford & Beveridge, 2004; Sampson, 2002). Sampson (2002) defined neighborhood collective efficacy as "an emphasis on shared beliefs in neighbors' conjoint capability for action to achieve an intended effect, and hence an active sense of engagement on the part of residents" (p. 224). Ford and Beveridge (2004) concluded that collective efficacy "emphasizes shared expectations and mutual trust among neighborhood residents and promotes an agentic sense of cohesion" (p. 54). The client, Ahmed, lives in an urban area and may not feel close to his neighbors; however, his belonging to the Muslim community may make up for any lack of connection to his physical community. The concept of *ummah* (Kelly, 1984) refers to a particular community that is instituted by Islamic teaching and practice. Islam encourages the development of bonds by the moral and social codes espoused. Islam also has been described as "a community of believers which transcend tribal difference" (Kelly, 1984, p. 164).

Local, State, and Federal Laws

Waller (1995), in describing federal and state laws governing confidentiality, stated that they are "a crazy quilt of federal and state constitutional, statutory, regulatory and case law" (p. 44). The surgeon general's report on mental health observes that there are no national standards governing confidentiality (Satcher, 1999). The report also notes the significant differences in state laws on confidentiality. However, there appear to be some similarities that may apply to the case of Ahmed. It has been suggested that each state has identified exceptions to confidentiality (Satcher, 1999). One obvious exception is if the client gives informed consent to release information. This is the case with Ahmed, but it may be more complex than simply a record of release. The circumstances of how the release was obtained are relevant. Beauchamp and Childress (1989) suggested that informed consent involves free choice. Ahmed was mandated into counseling, and if he did not comply, he could have been surrendered to the court and sent to jail for his remaining sentence. Therefore, an important consideration is how the consent was obtained. Did Ahmed have a free choice to sign the release? If he did not have free choice, then his signature on the consent form may be considered invalid.

Another exception to maintaining confidentiality is based on a court decision, *Tarasoff v. Regents of the University of California* (1976). The *Tarasoff* case involved a client, Prosenjit Poddar, who was being seen in the student services office at the University of California, Berkeley. He expressed a threat toward a woman, Tatiana Tarasoff, in a counseling session with a psychologist, Dr. Moore. The intended victim, Tatiana Tarasoff, was out of the country at the time of the threat; she was in Brazil. However, Dr. Moore concluded that Mr. Poddar was a serious threat and needed psychiatric hospitalization, and he contacted the campus police to detain Mr. Poddar for an evaluation. Dr. Moore also informed his supervisor of the threat and the actions he took. The campus police initially did detain Mr. Poddar and determined that he was not a danger, so they released him. Upon returning from Brazil, Ms. Tarasoff was killed by Mr. Poddar.

The parents of Tatiana Tarasoff filed a lawsuit against Dr. Moore, the campus police, and the university. Ultimately, the California Supreme Court ruled in favor of the parents against the university. The court determined that Dr. Moore was responsible for accurately determining the level of dangerousness of his client and taking appropriate action, including warning the intended target or victim, or the family in this case since Ms. Tarasoff was away. Thus, duty to warn the intended victim of a threat requires that a counselor contact an intended victim. There are two conditions of duty to warn: First, there must be a specified target, not a general threat against humanity, and second, the individual making the threat must be able to carry out the threat. For example, an incarcerated individual serving a 20-year sentence who threatens to harm a relative when he or she gets out of prison may not be considered a threat; however, if the person makes the threat closer to the time of release, then duty to warn is in effect.

The question in the case of Ahmed is the level of potential harm and a clinical judgment about whether he intends to act on his threat. This is always the issue with duty to warn—the responsibility of the counselor to determine the seriousness of the threat and to assess the dangerousness of the individual making the threat.

Ethical Theory: Islam

Jeremy and Sally decided to use Islamic ethics in their ethical decision making because Islam is the worldview of the client (see Chapter 13). Islamic ethics defines five major classes of acts: forbidden acts, undesirable acts, neutral acts, desirable acts, and required acts. More specifically, good or required acts potentially help others or remove harm. For example, rescuing a drowning person if you can swim well is a good and required act. Also, there are four components of good: justice, benefit, truthfulness, and willing good (Hourani, 1971). Justice refers to performing socially good acts to bring about help or, alternatively, to bring about injury if the recipient is deserving of it. Benefit accordingly refers to acts that bring pleasure (Hourani, 1971). Truthfulness is considered good if it brings about pleasure and does not inflict pain (Hourani, 1971). Conversely, if truthfulness hurts someone who is undeserving of pain, then it is considered undesirable. The solution is not to tell a mistruth but to remain silent or avoid speaking such a mistruth (Hourani, 1971). The will for good is based on an evaluation of the intent of the actor, and it refers to motivation or intent. Having the intention to bring about benefit is considered good; however, not all good intentions remain good if pain and suffering occur as the result of an intended good act. One can have a good intent, for example, a counselor's wanting to help a client get better, but if the counselor does not have the skills to be helpful and tries to help anyway, the counselor's action may become an undesirable act. If the outcome were harmful, the act would be undesirable.

Source: Adapted from Houser, Wilczenski, and Ham (2006). Reprinted with permission.

Questions for Further Reflection

1. What do you imagine you would say to Ahmed's spouse to explain the potential threat of violence made toward her?

2. What suggestions would you give Sally and Jeremy about working with Ahmed and dealing with him in future group counseling sessions?

3. What impact might their moral stages of development and professional ethical identities have on the group leaders, Sally and Jeremy (they are in different stages of moral development)?

4. Which other ethical theories would you apply?

5. What would be your ethical decision in this case using a hermeneutical model?

The Case of Ariel: Counselor Competence and Minor Informed Consent

Carefully read the case of Ariel. Information is provided about an ethical dilemma, the counselor's values and personal ethical identity, the client's personal values, and the supervisor's personal values. Generate information for elements of the hermeneutic model: professional codes that may apply, geographic region, and professional literature that is relevant. Choose an ethical theory or theories to apply (Islamic or Judaic ethics presented in this chapter), and summarize your ethical decision based on the hermeneutic model. Be sure to gather information about relevant codes of ethics that apply, laws and statutes that apply, and professional literature that applies. Finally, reflect on and incorporate into your analysis how your personal ethical identity could affect your interaction with such a client and a similar ethical dilemma. How would your own personal ethical identity and ethical development affect your ethical decisions in this case?

Ariel, a severely depressed 17-year-old adolescent boy who was born in Israel, seeks counseling at a college counseling center. He is assigned to see a White female counselor, Karla. Ariel has been in the United States for a short time and is experiencing new academic and personal adjustment challenges. He shares an apartment with one other student and has frequent contact with a sponsoring Israeli family living in the vicinity.

Ariel, a 1st-year medical student at a prestigious university, was referred for counseling by one of his professors. Ariel is not sleeping well, has lost weight, and seems unmotivated in class. Ariel explains that he does not find the traditional American diet healthy, so he believes his weight loss is associated with the lack of kosher food. Ariel knows that there are expectations for high academic achievement from his family and professors, and he is very concerned that if his parents are informed of his difficulties, they will be disappointed in him or blame him for his problems.

The counselor, Karla, feels that in addition to counseling, Ariel would benefit from a holistic approach including nutrition and use of reiki (a spiritual treatment typically involving touch). Ariel is resistant to the alternative treatments and refuses treatment. Karla interprets this as his being resistant. Karla shares her counseling efforts and strategies with her supervisor, Dr. Smith, during a supervision session. He listens to her description of the case and decides to use a hermeneutic ethical decision-making approach to help Karla understand the case and determine the course of counseling.

The relevant elements of the horizon based on the case of Ariel include the ethical dilemma; the client's, counselor's, and supervisor's respective values, race, gender, and personal history; counseling agency policies; local, state, and federal laws that apply; professional knowledge; geographic region; professional ethical codes; and relevant ethical theories.

Ethical Dilemma

Rather than using alternative treatments such as nutrition and reiki, Ariel prefers to seek traditional medical treatment, seeing a psychiatrist. Karla's initial impression is that Ariel is defensive and resistant. Ariel agrees to continue in counseling but not to pursue alternative treatments. Moreover, he does not want his parents notified by the counselor because he is concerned that a call will alarm his parents about his mental health. In seeking counseling, he already sees himself as disappointing his family. Karla is concerned that if she informs Ariel's parents about his seeking mental health counseling, he will drop out. She questions whether it would be best to not contact Ariel's parents, as he requested. Karla believes she is knowledgeable about the use of alternative treatments, and she does not believe in the sole use of medication in treating depression. Karla is searching for universal principles to guide her ethical decision making.

Dr. Smith questions whether Karla should seek informed consent from Ariel's parents. Ariel is considered a minor in the United States, and states require parental consent for medical and psychological treatment. Second, Dr. Smith questions Karla's competence in aggressively pursuing the use of use of alternative treatments such as reiki.

Karla: The Counselor's Personal Values, Race, Gender, and Personal History

Karla attended a progressive mental health counseling graduate program in the midwestern United States. She learned holistic approaches to mental health treatment and found them to be effective. Although she interned in clinics that served diverse populations, she had no experience working with recent immigrants. Now Karla occasionally has international students in her caseload at the college counseling center, where she has worked for the past 5 years. She assumes that Ariel is experiencing culture shock and misses his family. She is concerned about his reports of eating and sleeping disturbances.

Karla recalls her own difficult adjustment when she left home and entered college. The first semester, she felt homesick and overwhelmed with depression. Karla visited the college counseling center to obtain antidepressant medication, and the staff offered alternative counseling treatments such as nutrition, which helped her immensely. She perceives her own past college experience as comparable to Ariel's, and she feels that the same treatment is a reasonable approach for him. Karla completed the Defining Issues Test and found that she emphasized postconventional moral strategies and a tendency to focus on universal principles to determine courses of action.

Ariel: The Client's Personal Values, Race, Gender, and Personal History

Ariel is the oldest of three children, and he knows his parents are having difficulty supporting his education in the United States. Ariel was born in Israel and attends a synagogue regularly in the United States. Ariel has always excelled in school, particularly in science, and was granted a full scholarship to study medicine in the United States. Ariel has expressed during his counseling sessions both acculturative stress (stress related to entering a new and unfamiliar culture) and feelings of guilt about leaving behind family members in Israel. He does not want to create more problems and stress for his family by letting them know he is having mental health problems.

Dr. Smith: The Supervisor's Personal Values, Race, Gender, and Personal History

Dr. Smith is the director of the college counseling center. His work is primarily administrative, and he is responsible for the fiscal management of the center. A student sued the center for incompetent treatment in the past, and the lawsuit was settled out of court. Because of the lawsuit against one of the center's counselors, Dr. Smith has started to closely supervise the work of staff members. The counselors are often angry with him because his supervision sessions emphasize legal liability and how to protect the center and avoid another lawsuit. Many counselors see him as more concerned about legal issues and as placing the welfare of the counseling center above that of the clients.

Source: Adapted from Houser, Wilczenski, and Ham (2006). Reprinted with permission.

Use Figure 15.1 to identify relevant elements of the horizon. Fill in the appropriate elements to help with your understanding and ethical decision.

Figure 15.1   Ethical Dilemma

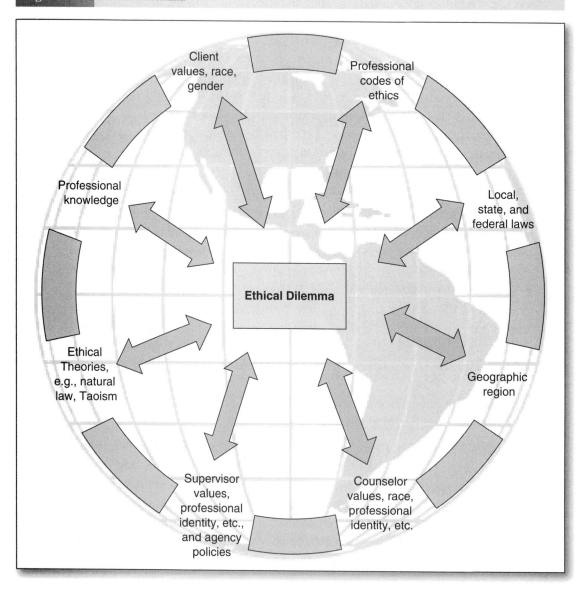

Additional Recommended Readings

Islam

Carter, D., & Rashidi, A. (2003). Theoretical model of psychotherapy: Eastern Asian-Islamic women mental illness. *Health Care for Women International, 24*(5), 399–413.

Denny, F. M. (2005). Muslim ethical trajectories in the contemporary period. In W. Schweiker (Ed.), *The Blackwell companion to religious ethics* (pp. 268–277). Malden, MA: Blackwell.

Esposito, J. (1999). *The Islamic threat: Myth or reality?* (3rd ed.). New York, NY: Oxford University Press.

Hourani, G. F. (1985). *Reason and tradition in Islamic ethics.* New York, NY: Cambridge University Press.

Moosa, E. (2005). Muslim ethics? In W. Schweiker (Ed.), *The Blackwell companion to religious ethics* (pp. 237–243). Malden, MA: Blackwell.

Nanji, A. (1993). Islamic ethics. In P. Singer (Ed.), *A companion to ethics* (pp. 106–118). Malden, MA: Blackwell.

Reinhart, A. K. (1983). Islamic law as Islamic ethics? *Journal of Religious Ethics, 11,* 186–203.

Reinhart, A. K. (2005). Origins of Islamic ethics: Foundations and constructions. In W. Schweiker (Ed.), *The Blackwell companion to religious ethics* (pp. 244–253). Malden, MA: Blackwell.

Safi, O. (Ed.). (2003). *Progressive Muslims: On justice, gender, and pluralism.* Oxford, UK: Oneworld.

Judaism

Dorff, E. N. (2003). *Love your neighbor and yourself: A Jewish approach to modern personal ethics.* Philadelphia, PA: Jewish Publication Society.

Dorff, E. N., & Newman, L. E. (1995). *Contemporary Jewish ethics and morality: A reader.* New York, NY: Oxford University Press.

Green, R. M. (2005). Foundations of Jewish ethics. In W. Schweiker (Ed.), *The Blackwell companion to religious ethics* (pp. 166–175). Malden, MA: Blackwell.

Kellner, M. (1993). Jewish ethics. In P. Singer (Ed.), *A companion to ethics* (pp. 82–90). Malden, MA: Blackwell.

Novak, D. (1998). *Natural law in Judaism.* New York, NY: Cambridge University Press.

Putnam, H. (2005). Jewish ethics? In W. Schweiker (Ed.), *The Blackwell companion to religious ethics* (pp. 159–165). Malden, MA: Blackwell.

Sherwin, B. L. (2000). *Jewish ethics for the twenty-first century: Living in the image of God.* Syracuse, NY: Syracuse University Press.

Chapter 16

Native American, Hispanic/ Latino, and African Ethics

In this chapter we discuss Native American, African, and Hispanic or Latino ethics. These theories are not quite as well organized because of the multitude of influences on their development. However, they all have consistencies and common threads that provide insight into ethical and moral behavior. Native American ethics is complex primarily because of the number of Native American tribes in the United States; there are more than 400 tribes and other indigenous populations such as Hawaiians and Alaskan Eskimos. There are a number of influences on Latin American ethics, which makes the theory complex. These influences include natural law (Christianity), African ethics, Judaic ethics, and the beliefs of indigenous people, for example, Aztecs and Mayans (Zea, Mason, & Murguia, 2000). There are numerous groups composing Hispanic/Latino categories such as Cuban, Puerto Rican, and Mexican, which affects the development of common ethical concepts. African ethics may be understood as incorporating a three-dimensional community and promotes interpersonal relations. The three communities are the living, the dead, and the not yet born (Bujo, 2005). The idea is that all three communities are interconnected cosmically and influence each other. Consequently, acting ethically involves taking into account each community and how it will be affected by certain acts. Also, there is a strong connection between humans and the rest of nature, including plants and animals. Africans are associated with those whose origins are in the sub-Saharan continent or Africa. Africans as a whole are composed of groups from various tribes and groups from Africa with various influences and characteristics that may influence ethics and morality. Examples of some of the larger groups are Nilotic, Swahili, and Bushmen or San.

NATIVE AMERICAN ETHICS

Native Americans are identified as indigenous people who were residents of the United States before Europeans entered the Americas. The definition includes indigenous people of both Hawaii and Alaska along with American Indians. Estimates of the number of those who identify as Native American—that is, American Indian, Alaskan Native, and Hawaiian Native—range from 2.5 million to 5 million (Gone, 2004; U.S. Census Bureau, 2000). This compares with more than 112 million Native Americans prior to the entrance of Europeans into the Native Americans' world in 1492 (Gone, 2004; Sioui, 1995). Diseases were primarily responsible for the significant decrease in the Native American population both on the U.S. mainland and in Hawaii. More recently there have been increases in Native American populations (U.S. Census Bureau, 2010). There has been more than an 18% increase in Native American and Alaskan populations since 2000 and more than a 35% increase in Native Hawaiian and Pacific Islander.

American Indians, Alaskan Natives, and Hawaiian Natives share similar histories despite not sharing similar geographical space. American Indians have a history of more than 10,000 years in the Americas (Freuchen, 1957; C. Taylor, 1997). Native Americans have a longer history without contact with Europeans and Whites than contact with them. Approximately 1,500 years ago, Americans Indians first were introduced to White Europeans. Alaskan Natives entered the Americas reportedly through the Bering Strait from Europe between 5000 and 3500 BCE. The Vikings were believed to be the first Europeans to come in contact with Alaskan Natives beginning in the 10th century CE. More frequent contact began in the 1800s with the introduction of missionaries and whaling ships to Native Americans (Freuchen, 1957).

Similar to American Indians on the American continents, Hawaiian Natives lived on the islands for more than 1,400 years before foreigners entered their world (Kuykendall & Day, 1967). Hawaiians are believed to have originated from the western islands of Indonesia. Hawaii was discovered by Captain Cook in the late 1700s. Both Native Hawaiians and American Indians valued living intertwined with nature. An introduction to Native American ethics begins with understanding the perspective that everything in the universe is connected. Several symbolic representations have been offered to illustrate this connection. One view is that the universe is a great circle that is continuous (Lombardi & Lombardi, 1982; Marshall, 2001). Lombardi and Lombardi (1982), in describing the interconnectedness, noted,

> The perspective of the universe as the Great Circle becomes charged with a truth that is more than a physical fact, yet not merely a metaphysical concept. The chain of interdependence becomes sacred. The exchange of life-giving power transforms every commonplace act into a ritual and faith and solidarity. (p. 11)

Bopp, Bopp, Brown, and Lane (1985) identified the "Sacred Tree" as a symbol of connections within the universe. They described the Sacred Tree:

> For all people on the earth, the Creator has planted a Sacred Tree under which they may gather, and there find healing, power, wisdom and security. The roots of this tree spread deep into the body of Mother Earth. Its branches reach upward like hands praying to Father Sky. The fruits of this tree are the good things the Creator has given to the people: teachings that show the path to love, compassion, generosity, patience, wisdom, justice, courage, respect, humility and many other wonderful gifts. (p. 7)

A related connection in understanding Native American ethics is the strong relationship between Native Americans and the environment. Bopp et al. (1985) referred to "Mother Earth" and "Father Sky" as a way to illustrate this connection. Bopp et al., in addition, used the symbol of a wheel, which is round, or a circle to demonstrate the connections in the universe. The "Medicine Wheel" represents the universe, and one model incorporates four aspects of human nature (Bopp et al., 1985). The four components of human nature represented on the medicine wheel are the mental, physical, emotional, and spiritual. Humans seek to discover a balance of these four dimensions of human nature.

The medicine wheel is another approach to understanding the universe and human nature and can be found in the "Gifts of the Four Directions." These directions provide for the development of a person's nature; that is, the mental, emotional, physical, and spiritual.

Major Concepts

Native American ethics, as was noted earlier, is not as coherent as other ethical theories because there are so many groups represented, that is, more than 400 American Indian tribes. There are several sources that provide insight into Native American ethical concepts (Bopp et al., 1985; Bopp, Lane, Brown, & Bopp, 1989;

Cohen, 2003; Lombardi & Lombardi, 1982). We will present the most common concepts that compose Native American ethics. Fowler (2009) noted the importance of words in American Indian life, including moral life. Momaday (1987) described how words are valued in American Indian lives, stating,

> The American Indian has a highly developed oral tradition. It is in the nature of oral tradition that it remains relatively constant. One who has only oral traditions thinks of language in this way: my words exist at the level of my voice. If I do not speak with care my words become wasted. (p. 400)

He further explained the ethical or moral nature of words: "If I do not listen with care, words are lost. If I do not remember carefully, the very purpose of words is frustrated. This respect for words suggests an inherent morality" (p. 400). One can see how listening to others and carefully monitoring one's speech are relevant to acting morally. Listening to others promotes a deeper understanding and therefore fewer problems or miscommunications that may result in unethical behavior.

A concept related to the value of words is truthfulness (Bopp et al., 1985; T. Cooper, 1998). Native American ethics is founded on the perspective that one should not tell mistruths, even socially acceptable mistruths. An example of a mistruth is telling someone his or her clothes look wonderful when they do not. Telling the truth in this theory demonstrates being respectful. Marshall (2001) described truth as something that is not easily identified. He stated,

> Truth can, at times, hide so well that we can't find it to save ourselves, or it disguises itself so skillfully that we walk over it without knowing. And in the next instance it becomes plain as day, whether we want it to or not. (p. 119)

Marshall (2001) described truth in the context of physical reality: "Reality is what is, first and foremost in our physical world. . . . Truth is the result of trials and errors of life, the lessons we have learned" (p. 120). Truth can be confused and seen as an illusion, and it is the individual's responsibility to attempt to find the truth and not be misled by an illusion. It requires an openness to the realities of the physical world and an openness to discovery.

According to Bopp et al. (1985), a major concept in Native American ethics is respect or esteem for other people and/or nature. T. Cooper (1998) noted that respect or esteem is demonstrated through not putting anyone down, not taking another's possessions, protecting the natural environment, and not criticizing others. Another element of the concept of respect for another person is respect for elders (T. Cooper, 1998), which involves not offending or disrespecting an elder. Marshall (2001) noted the attitude of the Lakota, an American Indian tribe, toward elders: "Among us the old ones are the best models for how we should live our lives" (p. 1). Bopp et al. concluded, "Special respect should be given to elders, parents, teachers and community leaders" (p. 76). Bopp et al. proposed that respect is demonstrated as "treat[ing] every person, from the tiniest child to the oldest elder with respect at all times" (p. 76).

Serving others and not seeking to fulfill one's own personal needs are other important concepts in Native American ethics. Bopp et al. (1989) described the concept of serving others: "Do not fill yourself with personal affairs, but remember the meaning of life is only known in serving others" (p. 21). Serving others is composed of two elements: sacrifice and generosity. Sacrifice means giving up something you value and is not simply giving. An example may be donating money or time and thereby creating a burden. A related concept is generosity, which involves freely giving both time and money.

Another major concept, according to Bopp et al. (1989), is pursuing moderation in one's life. Engaging is excesses is perceived to be unethical; this is in contradiction to moderation. Bopp et al. (1985) discussed the medicine wheel and how moderation may be violated.

The Medicine Wheel teaches us that we have four aspects to our nature: the physical, the mental, the emotional, and the spiritual. Each of these aspects must be equally developed in a healthy well-balanced individual through the development of volition (i.e., will). (p. 12)

Based on the medicine wheel, one needs to find a balance among the four aspects—physical, mental, emotional, and spiritual—to make a moral decision. We have free will and make choices about whether to overindulge in one aspect, which may lead to problems and not understanding the truth about an ethical dilemma. See Table 16.1 for a summary of concepts in Native American ethics.

Table 16.1   Summary of Concepts in Native American Ethics

Ethical Concept	*Definition/Description*
Value of words	Pursuing truthfulness, listening to others, and speaking carefully
Respect for others and environment	Demonstrating respect in the broadest sense, not stealing from others, and honoring and not criticizing elders
Moderation	Pursing a balance between the four components of humans: physical, mental, emotional, and spiritual
Serving others	Serving others through sacrifice and generosity

HISPANIC/LATINO ETHICS

It has been noted that Hispanic/Latino ethics is interpreted through an emphasis on the social, which includes communities, families, and social institutions (Garcia, 1997). Garcia described the moral/ethical understanding of Hispanic/Latino ethics as "closely tied to our being members of well-defined ethnic groups. Group life, especially when it is defined by ethnicity and race, is a basic reality that shapes our conception of self and morality" (p. 16). Hispanics and Latinos are not a homogeneous group and are composed of a number of different groups. *Hispanic* is more closely associated with a cultural heritage from Spain, whereas *Latino* is more closely associated with those whose origins are in Latin America. *Latin American* typically includes those from countries that were influenced by Spain, including South American, Central American, and Caribbean countries. *Latino* includes those who are indigenous people such as descendants of Mayan and Aztec culture.

Major Concepts

One of the major concepts and ethical perspectives in Hispanic/Latino ethics is the importance of the family (Reese, 2001). *Familismo* has been defined in terms of a strong connection to the nuclear family and extended family members (Castillo & Cano, 2007; Castillo, Perez, Castillo, & Ghosheh, 2010). Guilamo-Ramos et al. (2007) defined familismo as "the attachment, loyalty, and reciprocity that characterize relationships among members of a nuclear family and among extended family members, including significant nonfamily individuals who play a key role in the upbringing of children" (p. 19). Family members have responsibilities to the family, and these are influenced to a large extent by the gender and role of the respective family members. Women and mothers have the responsibility of focusing on primary care and nurturance in the family (Castillo et al., 2010). The importance of the family in ethics is demonstrated through respect for elders; respect for elders particularly includes parents (Reese, 2001). Respect for elders also includes showing respect for older siblings. The major emphasis in Hispanic/Latino ethics is the emphasis on respect within the family, *respeto*. It is not unusual for older children to take on parenting roles with younger children, and younger children are expected to show respect for this arrangement. Respect for elders extends to all who are older, and this ethic is communicated to children early in family life (Reese, 2001).

The importance of social responsibility and caring for others is an important ethical concept. Guilamo-Ramos et al. (2007) described this social responsibility, stating, "Latino collectivism may express greater concern for family values and family well-being than for individual opportunities" (p. 19). Binderle and Montoya (2008) further explained the collective perspective from a Hispanic/Latino view, stating, "Collectivists emphasize relationships, obligation to in-groups and the subsuming of personal interests and needs to the good of the group or community" (p. 148). Key in this concept is the minimizing of individual interests and the emphasizing of actions to promote the welfare of the group.

Another ethical concept in this theory is machismo for male Latinos, which has been associated with both negative and positive characteristics. The negative characteristics of machismo, it has been noted, are sexism, chauvinism, and hypermasculinity (Arciniega, Anderson, Tovar-Blank, & Tracey, 2008). A word that represents the positive aspect of machismo is *caballerismo,* which refers to masculine chivalry (Arciniega et al., 2008). Positive aspects of machismo and caballerismo involve acts of protecting the family and a sense of responsibility. Also, caballerismo includes the characteristics of being sincere and assertive. The concept has been described as being a gentleman and being family centered (Estrada, Rigali-Oiler, Arciniega, & Tracey, 2011). Acting ethically from a Latino perspective is based on caballerismo and is associated with the male gender role.

Marianismo refers to the desired characteristics of female Latinas. Moral behavior is associated with gender roles in Latino ethics. These characteristics may be understood as virtues; Latinas are expected to be virtuous, humble, and spiritually superior to men and boys (Castillo & Cano, 2010). Gil and Vazquez (1996) noted that marianismo encompasses a sense of duty and expressions of caring for others. The moral practice of marianismo is caring for one's family and providing nurturance to members. Castillo and Cano (2010) identified characteristics of marianismo and found that it includes serving as a family pillar and remaining a virgin until marriage. These are both moral actions. The concept of marianismo includes being subordinate to others, particularly male partners, and attempting to maintain harmony in the family.

Simpatia refers to maintaining harmony and avoiding controversy or conflict (Guilamo-Ramos et al., 2007). Ways to demonstrate simpatia are being polite and being agreeable. It also may be expressed by respectful behavior. It is important to reduce conflict through interpersonal connections and cooperation with others. Table 16.2 summarizes concepts in Hispanic/Latino ethics.

Table 16.2 Summary of Concepts in Hispanic/Latino Ethics

Ethical Concept	Definition/Description
Familismo	Relationships among members of a nuclear family characterized by attachment, loyalty, and reciprocity
Machismo/caballerismo	Male gender role associated with acts of protecting the family and a sense of responsibility as well as sincerity and assertiveness
Marianismo	Female gender role associated with virtue, humility, and spirituality as well as being family focused and providing care for members
Collectivism	Greater concern for the family and its well-being than for individual needs
Simpatia	Maintaining harmony and avoiding conflict

AFRICAN ETHICS

Similarly to other ethical theories presented here, African ethics is linked to religious perspectives (Gbadegesin, 2007). This theory too emphasizes a strong connection to nature and the universe. Gbadegesin (2007) noted that African ethics emphasizes the promotion of humanity and human nature. The ethical perspective suggests that morals come from God and that God gives humans the capacity to make ethical decisions. God passes along to humans this capacity to make right decisions and the ability to understand the difference between right and wrong (Gbadegesin, 2007). An additional element is that the transmission of morals to humans from God includes an understanding of how context and time account for determination of an ethical decision. Concretely this means that morals and ethics are relative from the African perspective.

Major Concepts

There are a number of concepts that are relevant in understanding African ethics. Similarly to some of the other theories we have discussed, African ethics considers "good character" an essential feature of ethics and morals (Gbadegesin, 2007). There is an underlying structure of African ethics that is consistent with the person's embodying a good person with a good character. Gbadegesin (2007) described this character with the Yoruba (West African) word *iwa,* which means "character and existence." Interestingly, the demonstration of character is essential, permeates the total person, and is not shown in just one or a few acts. Character is demonstrated through existence completed with the person's total entity.

Truthfulness is an important concept and is more than simply not telling a lie (Gbadegesin, 2007). The concept is linked to religious influence and the notion that those who are not truthful may be punished. Kirk-Greene (2001) pointed out that a lie can harm others, and a key aspect of African ethics is avoiding harming others. Trust involves keeping one's word and demonstrating trustworthiness through action. For example, if one has agreed to care for a child with a developmental disability, he or she must provide the care. Not doing so is considered not being truthful or honest, because the one who agreed to provide care did not keep his or her word.

A second important concept is industry, which involves completing acts and following through. Those illustrating industry show efforts in various ways through active work and completion of tasks. The perception and belief is that people who are not industrious do not take responsibility for their families and communities and thus are not moral. Moderation, as in many other theories we have discussed, is a foundation of moral and ethical principles. This translates into moderation in basic human desires such as eating, drinking (alcohol), and sexual activities. Gbadegesin (2007) noted that not acting in moderation may result in loss of dignity. Another major concept in African ethics is generosity. Generosity involves giving time, effort, and money to others (family, friends, and the community). Sacrifice is considered essential in demonstrating generosity. One needs to commit to sacrifice to help others. This means not only giving to others but doing so in such a way that it has an impact on the giver.

Patience is another concept in acting ethically, and it involves behaving toward others without extreme responses (Gbadegesin, 2007). Extreme responses may include acting with urgency or overexcitement. Temperance promotes a more positive response to others and shows good moral character. Another ethical concept in African ethics is respect for elders (Gbadegesin, 2007). Elders are held in high esteem and hold a certain level of wisdom. Consequently, respecting elders who can share their wisdom is ethical and moral. Elders have lived a long time and thus deserve respect. Also, if one does not respect an elder, he or she may be cursed by the elder; elders are thought to hold certain powers that can bring about negative consequences (Gbadegesin, 2007). The last concept is respect for community, which is founded on the belief that everyone is part of a community and therefore has a responsibility to the community (Gbadegesin, 2007). Children are brought into the community, and the community is responsible to them. All members are responsible to each other for promoting everyone's growth and development. Responsibility to the community involves not doing anything to harm any member. This includes not committing murder in the community and not taking advantage of other community members. Omonzejele (2005) described the relevance of respect for the community, stating, "African ethics is based on communal living. It fuses the society into one big whole. In traditional African society there is no 'me' but 'us' no 'my' but 'ours'" (p. 1). Mbiti (1969) noted that behaving in a way that is not harmful to others in the community is showing respect. See Table 16.3 for a summary of African ethical concepts.

Table 16.3   Summary of African Ethical Concepts

Ethical Concept	Definition/Description
Truthfulness	A lie can harm others: family, friends, and the community.
Industry	Individuals show effort in the completion of tasks. People who are not industrious do not take responsibility for their families and communities and thus are not moral.
Moderation	Moderation must be observed in basic human desires such as eating, drinking (alcohol), and sexual activities.
Generosity	Generosity involves giving time, effort, and money to others (family, friends, and the community).
Patience	One should act in moderation toward others and not act with urgency or be overexcited in interacting with others.
Respect for elders	Elders are held in high esteem and hold a certain level of wisdom.
Respect for community	Everyone is part of a community and therefore has a responsibility to the community.

The Case of David: Supervisor-Supervisee Conflict

David is a mental health counselor in Oregon. He is of American Indian descent, and he has worked as a mental health counselor for the past 2 years. His primary caseload is with clients who have severe mental illness and who are American Indians. David has fairly frequent conflicts with his supervisor about what the supervisor considers sharing too much information or sharing information that the clients theoretically cannot handle. For example, David has given feedback to clients that they were not being responsible in changing their lives despite having severe mental illness. David's supervisor has indicated that he feels such feedback is not helpful because members of this population cannot always control their behaviors.

David recently was assigned a new client, Sarah, who is a 28-year-old Native American woman diagnosed with schizophrenia. She has been inconsistent in attending a day program for those with severe mental illness and has come into counseling sessions with bruises on her arms. Sarah lives with her family—her parents and several siblings. David suspects someone in the family is physically abusing her. He wants to comply with a state law that protects those with disabilities, including those with mental illness, from abuse. David asks the client how she received the bruises on her arms, and Sarah answers that she fell.

David informs his supervisor, Dennis, about the situation with his client and his concern about abuse. The supervisor states that he would be reluctant to report any abuse without further information. Dennis believes doing so will jeopardize David's relationship with the client and the family. Dennis suggests that David not file a report of potential abuse but gather more information.

The potentially relevant elements of the horizon include the ethical dilemma; the counselor and his values, race, gender, personal history, and so forth; the client and her values, race, gender, personal history, and so forth; the supervisor and his values, race, gender, personal history, and so forth; agency policies; local, state, and federal laws that apply; professional codes of ethics; professional knowledge; geographic region; and ethical theories.

Ethical Dilemma

One dilemma for David is whether to break the confidentiality of the counseling sessions and report the suspected abuse of his client. A second ethical dilemma is whether he should ignore his supervisor's recommendation and make the report. The information from the client is not absolutely clear, and David can only suspect abuse. Disclosure to an outside source may affect the family and the client, who may decide to withdraw from counseling services. Typically, physical abuse of those with disabilities does not involve the counselor's monitoring for abuse as carefully as does abuse of children. David believes in honest disclosure to his clients, and if he were to report suspected abuse, he would share with his client that he had done so.

David has had frequent disagreements with his supervisor about honest disclosure to clients. David guides his ethical behavior from a principled perspective and respects agency policies and his supervisor's perspective, but he tries to see the underlying principles of any decisions. His supervisor, Dennis, believes that sharing information that the client can handle is the criterion for disclosure. David likes working with this agency and enjoys the clients with whom he works. He is concerned that his supervisor may use such conflicts to fire him from his position. In addition, David believes he should be respectful of his supervisor and follow his recommendations.

David: The Counselor's Personal Values, Race, Gender, and Personal History

David is 25 years old and lives in a medium-size city. He grew up on a reservation in western Oregon, and his parents educated him about the traditions and customs of his ancestors. He spent his first 18 years on the reservation and thus feels proud of his heritage.

Currently, David is single and lives in an apartment with a roommate. He continues to practice the traditions and customs of his heritage. He shows honor and respect to his parents, and he returns to the reservation frequently to visit his family and provide service to the community. David attended a public university for his bachelor's and master's degrees. His master's degree is in mental health counseling. During his training, he completed an internship working with those who had severe mental illness. Consequently, he decided to pursue employment working with this population. In addition, he feels it is necessary to work with Native Americans because of his own heritage and understanding of the population. He also feels a responsibility to his community to work with this population. David completed the Defining Issues Test and discovered he fell into the postconventional stage, emphasizing universal ethical principles. He follows laws and professional codes, but he believes in universal ethical principles that are considered beyond laws and codes.

Sarah: The Client's Personal Values, Race, Gender, and Personal History

Sarah received the diagnosis of schizophrenia when she was 22. She had been working in a clerical staff person in a dentist's office. She lives with her family, which includes her mother, father, and two younger siblings. Her family moved off a reservation in eastern Oregon before she was born. The family still observes Native American traditions and customs, and they return to the reservation frequently to see relatives and participate in community activities.

Sarah was a below-average student in school, and upon graduation she started a clerical job. She moved from job to job and did not stay long in any position. She reports having difficulty getting along with coworkers. After her initial hospitalization with psychosis, she attempted to return to work but felt coworkers were talking about her, so she quit her job again. The family was unhappy with Sarah's decision to leave her job because she was expected to contribute financially to the family.

Dennis: The Supervisor's Personal Values, Race, Gender, and Personal History

Dennis is a 48-year-old White man who is married without children. He grew up in a small family of four and has an older sister. Dennis lived a rather comfortable and protected childhood. He and his spouse were married after they graduated from college more than 20 years ago. Dennis grew up in the midwestern part of the United States. He did not have much contact with Native Americans until he took a position in the agency where he now works. He started practicing as a counselor more than 15 years ago and became a supervisor 10 years ago.

He has become more aware of Native American culture during his time living in Oregon. Over the years, he has had several clients who were Native American, and Dennis felt he got along well with them. The agency where he works is a mental health center that provides services to a wide range of clients and backgrounds. The primary ethnic and racial groups served are Native Americans, Asian Americans, and Whites.

Professional Codes of Ethics

A number of American Counseling Association professional codes of ethics may apply to the ethical dilemma:

> A.l.a Welfare of those served by counselors: Primary responsibility—The primary responsibility of counselors is to respect the dignity and to promote the welfare of clients.

> C.2.a Professional competence: Boundaries of competence—Counselors practice only within the boundaries of their competence, based on their education, training, supervised experience, state and national professional credentials, and appropriate professional experience. Counselors gain knowledge, personal awareness, sensitivity, and skills pertinent to working with a diverse client population.

> D.l.b Relationships with colleagues, employers, and employees: Forming relationship—Counselors work to develop and strengthen interdisciplinary relations with colleagues from other disciplines with which they work.

> D.l.e Relationships with colleagues, employers, and employees: Establishing professional and ethical obligations—Counselors who are members of interdisciplinary teams clarify professional and ethical obligations of the team as a whole and of its individual members. When a team decision raises ethical concerns, counselors first attempt to resolve the concern within the team. If they cannot reach resolution among team members, counselors pursue other avenues to address their concerns consistent with client well-being. (American Counseling Association, 2005)

Professional Knowledge

David determined that several areas of professional knowledge were possibly relevant and should be considered in understanding his ethical dilemma: supervisor-supervisee relationship, supervisor competence, and physical abuse of those with disabilities.

First, David discovered that there have been attempts to understand the supervisor-supervisee relationship based on the working alliance (Bordin, 1983), a concept also used to understand the client-counselor relationship (White & Queener, 2003). Berlin (1983) proposed that the working alliance consists of three components: bonds, goals, and tasks. Bonds are emotional bonds and feelings of attachment. This component does not appear to be directly relevant to David's ethical dilemma. Goals concern the supervisor's and supervisee's agreeing on goals, both those of clients and those of supervision. David and Dennis do not share the same goals for the client. David wants to promote more client responsibility and ensure the safety of the client. Dennis wants to maintain confidentiality and protect client rights. Tasks are the activities of the supervision or the activities of working with clients, for example, the interventions to reach the goals. David and Dennis also disagree on tasks. David wants to contact an outside agency to assist in the protection of the client from abuse. Dennis wants to use agency or counselor resources to monitor any suspected abuse.

Next, David reviewed the professional literature addressing supervisor competence. Muratori (2001) suggests that the inability of the supervisor to perform certain supervisory functions and roles is indicative of supervisor impairment. She stated that these supervisory functions are addressed by the Association for Counselor Education and Supervision (I. Bernard & Goodyear, 1998):

> (a) monitoring client welfare; (b) encouraging compliance with relevant legal, ethical, and professional standards for clinical practice; (c) monitoring clinical performance and professional development of supervisees; and (d) evaluating and certifying current performance and potential of supervisees for academic, screening, placement, employment, and credentialing purposes. (p. 306)

Function b—encouraging compliance with relevant legal, ethical, and professional standards—is potentially relevant and may be an example of Dennis's not performing adequately.

The third knowledge area that may apply is abuse of those with disabilities. There is a dearth of research about abuse of those with disabilities (Calderbank, 2000). Several authors have suggested that abuse of those with disabilities is founded on a power and control relationship (Hendey & Pascall, 1998). Furthermore, Hendey and Pascall (1998) suggested that issues of control and power are linked to personal caregiving for those with disabilities. They found that women with disabilities are more vulnerable to abuse than are men. An individual providing personal care for an adult with a disability usually does so in private, and therefore the community may not become aware of abuse as readily as it does with children, who attend school.

Geographic Region

The mental health agency where David works is located in western Oregon, close to a large American Indian reservation. David was raised on a reservation in eastern Oregon. Sarah's family lived on a reservation in eastern Oregon prior to her birth, and the whole family still returns to participate in tribal community activities. Several writers have noted the uniqueness of the American Indian reservation (Pandey, Zhan, & Collier-Tenison, 2004; Yurkovich, Clairmont, & Grandbois, 2002). Yurkovich et al. (2002) concluded that the mental health system is not well prepared to address the needs of American Indian groups.

David knows the American Indian culture intimately from growing up on a reservation. However, Pandey et al. (2004) observed that "American Indian communities differ in size, extent of geographic remoteness, economic opportunities, levels of welfare dependency, and structure of social services" (p. 94). In addition, Yurkovich et al. (2002) advised using caution in assuming an understanding of others based on similarity, which may result in a cultural blind spot: believing that if a person is similar to you in appearance and behavior, there are few other differences.

Local, State, and Federal Laws

Oregon has a state law for the protection of people with disabilities who are abused, the Elder and Disabled Persons Abuse Protection Act. As with child abuse, there are mandated reporters, professionals who are mandated by law to report abuse. A state worker will investigate a claim of abuse and can ask the court for a protection order on behalf of a victim. The Elder and Disabled Persons Abuse Protection Act defines abuse as

> conduct, within the last six months, that has caused physical injury. It can be physical injury inflicted on purpose or as a result of neglect, abandonment, or desertion of the victim when the abuser was supposed to be taking care of the victim in some way. Abuse also means the use of intimidating or harassing language threatening serious physical or emotional harm.

Ethical Theory: Native American Ethics

David and his client share similar backgrounds and values in Native American ethics, so this is one theory that potentially applies. Several concepts from Native American ethics potentially apply to this dilemma. These include respect for elders and respect for others, truthfulness, serving others, and taking responsibility for one's actions. The first dilemma, whether to break confidentiality and report suspected abuse, may involve being truthful. David values being truthful, and if he does not disclose the suspected abuse to the appropriate agency, then he may not be acting truthfully. Also, if he does decide to break confidentiality and report the suspected abuse, he feels he should also disclose such an action to the client, which would be a truthful act.

David also values taking responsibility for his actions. This means making difficult decisions about breaking confidentiality and reporting suspected abuse. Breaking confidentiality may result in the client's not continuing counseling, and David must decide whether he wants to take this risk.

David also agrees with Native American ethics and the concept of serving others. Will he be serving others if he breaks confidentiality and reports the suspected abuse? Will he be serving his agency by breaking confidentiality, possibly resulting in the Native American community's not using this service in the future? Showing respect for elders and others is another concept that possibly applies. David's supervisor, Dennis, disagrees with him about reporting the suspected abuse in the case of Sarah. Should David ignore his value of respect for others (reporting suspected abuse) because of his belief that he should respect his elders, that is, his supervisor?

Source: Adapted from Houser, Wilczenski, and Ham (2006). Reprinted with permission.

Questions for Further Reflection

1. Are there any circumstances that warrant ignoring a supervisor's recommendations?

2. What impact does a counselor's and client's sharing of the same racial background have on ethical decision making?

3. Do you think the supervisor behaved ethically based on a hermeneutic model?

4. How might David's level of ethical development and his professional ethical identity affect his decision?

The Case of Berice: Use of Culturally Sensitive Assessment Methods

Carefully read the case of Berice. Information is provided about an ethical dilemma, the counselor's values and personal ethical identity, the client's personal values, and the supervisor's personal values. Generate information for elements of the hermeneutic model: professional codes that may apply, geographic region, and professional literature that is relevant. Choose an ethical theory or theories to apply (Native American, Hispanic/Latino, or African ethics presented in this chapter), and summarize your ethical decision based on the hermeneutic model. Be sure to gather information about relevant codes of ethics that apply, laws and statutes that apply, and professional literature that applies. Finally, reflect on and incorporate into your analysis how your personal ethical identity could affect your interaction with such a client and a similar ethical dilemma. How would your own personal ethical identity and ethical development affect your ethical decisions in this case?

Berice is a 35-year-old married Jamaican man who sustained a closed-head injury approximately 6 months ago. He fell off a ladder while painting a friend's house. He was employed by a painting company at the time of the injury, but the injury did not occur on the job. He was knocked unconscious and was discovered by his friend, who called an ambulance. He was taken to a hospital and was admitted. He regained consciousness after a few hours. He was diagnosed with a moderate head injury, based on the Glasgow Coma Scale. Residual effects of the head injury include difficulty in concentration, mild memory loss, sudden mood swings from happy to sad, and anger that is either unprovoked or inconsistent with the circumstances of the situation.

Berice entered the United States approximately 2 years ago. His brother, who is a U.S. citizen, owned the painting company, and this brother sponsored him.

After the injury Berice was able to return to work, but he was unsteady on a ladder, and the company did not want to risk further injury. His family noted how the residual side effects affected his relationships with others. Berice would forget what he was talking about, and he was emotionally unpredictable. A relative of Berice informed him that he may be eligible for services at the state vocational offices. He decided to visit an office and apply for services.

Jim, a 25-year-old White male vocational rehabilitation counselor, was assigned Berice's case. Jim had worked at the state vocational rehabilitation office for several years, and he had had a few clients with head injuries. Jim finds Berice to be pleasant and motivated to become employed again. Berice expresses an interest in employment as an alarm system installer. He wants to receive training for this type of occupation and requests that the state vocational rehabilitation program fund the training. Jim does not know whether this is a viable goal given Berice's head injury and the residual effects. Berice gives permission for Jim to speak to his physician, family, and former employer as part of the initial information-gathering process.

A review of job tasks shows that the occupation of alarm system installer involves

- consulting with clients to assess risks and to determine security requirements;
- drilling holes for wiring in wall studs, joists, ceilings, and floors;
- feeding cables through access holes;
- inspecting installation sites; and
- studying work orders, building plans, and installation manuals (Occupational Information Network, n.d.).

Jim questions whether Berice has the ability and skills to perform such job tasks. He decides to obtain further formal assessment information and determines that a neuropsychological assessment would be helpful. His office typically uses a psychologist, Dr. Kinney, who is knowledgeable in neuropsychological assessment but who does not use any assessments that account for cultural differences. Counselors in the office know this is a limitation of Dr. Kinney. Jim decides to use Dr. Kinney despite these limitations because Jim has a large caseload and does not have the time to locate another neuropsychologist who might provide a more culturally sensitive assessment.

Berice completes the assessment with Dr. Kinney and then meets with Jim to discuss the results. Jim explains to Berice that the results indicate that Berice has limitations that prevent him from pursuing employment as an alarm system installer. Berice is upset with the results and states that he does not believe Dr. Kinney understood him. Jim decides to discuss the case of Berice with his supervisor, Shirley, to decide if he acted ethically and whether he should take additional steps to obtain another assessment.

The elements of the horizon that are possibly relevant to the case of Berice include the ethical dilemma; the counselor's values, race, gender, personal history, and so forth; the client's values, race, gender, personal history, and so forth; the supervisor's values, race, gender, personal history, and so forth; counseling agency policies; applicable local, state, and federal laws; professional knowledge; geographic region; professional codes of ethics; and ethical theories.

Ethical Dilemma

Jim and Shirley discuss whether Berice's referral to Dr. Kinney was ethical and appropriate or whether another assessment is warranted. Several questions are identified by Jim and Shirley as important to determine whether the assessment process was ethical. First, did the referral by Jim constitute an appropriate referral based on Dr. Kinney's known skills and the knowledge Dr. Kinney has demonstrated in past assessments? Jim and Shirley are aware of Dr. Kinney's limitations in the use of culturally sensitive assessments. For most of their referrals to Dr. Kinney, this is not an issue; they provide services to relatively homogeneous ethnic and racial groups. A second related question is whether the results are valid enough to use to make reasonable decisions and determine whether Berice is able to pursue the type of occupation he wants, that is, as an alarm system installer. The answer to the second question will determine whether they decide to order a second assessment, which will cost the organization more money.

Jim: The Counselor's Personal Values, Race, Gender, and Personal History

Jim has worked for the state vocational rehabilitation agency since his graduation from a master's program 2 years ago. He is married, and his spouse is also White. He grew up in a homogeneous ethnic and racial community that is a suburb of a large urban area that was a predominantly White community. His family did not travel far outside the community, so he had minimal exposure to other ethnic and racial groups.

He completed an internship during his master's program in a state vocational rehabilitation agency serving the same area where he grew up. His exposure to primarily homogeneous racial and ethnic groups continued with this internship. He took courses in cross-cultural counseling, and he did not feel he was prejudiced against minority groups. He had not grown up hearing any negative stereotypes expressed toward individual minority groups in his family or the schools he attended.

After completing his internship, he was hired to work in an urban state vocational rehabilitation office where he had his first significant exposure to minorities and different racial and ethnic groups. After a few years working as a vocational rehabilitation counselor, he believes he understands the issues facing those from minority groups. Approximately 10% of his caseload comprises members of minority groups, and of these clients he has a few who are Jamaican. Jim scored in the postconventional, social contract, stage of moral development on the Defining Issues Test. He is a member of his professional association, the American Rehabilitation Counseling Association, and he attends professional conferences. He frequently reviews Commission on Rehabilitation Counselor Certification professional codes of ethics in conducting his practice.

Berice: The Client's Personal Values, Race, Gender, and Personal History

Berice is married with two children, a boy and girl, ages 8 and 10. He grew up in rural Jamaica near Mandeville. He is the youngest of three sons. He was employed in odd jobs including taxi driving prior to coming to the United States. He also worked in maintenance positions and maintained apartment complexes. He speaks English and a patois that is a combination of English, Portuguese, Spanish, and African words. Jamaica was one of the first areas in the Western Hemisphere to receive slaves, and the island residents have been oppressed for centuries, both physically, through slavery, and later economically.

Berice has been married for 12 years, and his spouse is from the same rural community where he grew up. The two children attend public schools. His spouse, Olivia, works as a secretary at a local university. Berice sees his brother and his family on a regular basis, so there is a connection to extended family.

Shirley: The Supervisor's Personal Values, Race, Gender, and Personal History

Shirley is a 50-year-old African American woman who is married and has worked at the state vocational rehabilitation agency for more than 20 years. She has one child, and she grew up in the urban area where she works. During her years of experience, she has worked with members of numerous minority groups, including many Jamaicans. Prior to coming to the current office, Shirley worked for 5 years in a state vocational rehabilitation office in which more than half of the clients were members of minority groups. She grew up in a middle-class family and was the oldest of three children. She has been a supervisor for the past 8 years and supervises 10 counselors in her office.

She completed her master's degree in rehabilitation counseling more than 25 years ago, and she had courses in testing but no courses in multicultural counseling or ethics. However, she has attended several workshops and conferences addressing multicultural counseling and ethics. She believes she is knowledgeable about current issues in these areas. She encourages her counselors to attend various workshops that address competence in multiculturalism and ethics.

Source: Adapted from Houser, Wilczenski, and Ham (2006). Reprinted with permission.

Use Figure 16.1 to identify relevant elements of the horizon. Fill in the appropriate elements to help with your understanding and ethical decision.

Figure 16.1 Ethical Dilemma

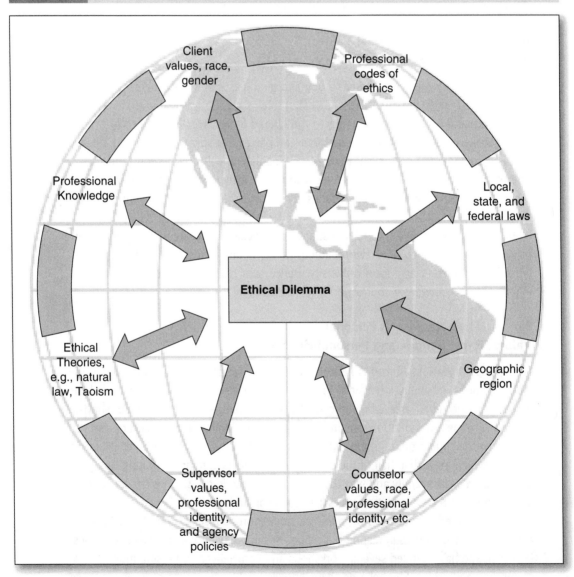

Additional Recommended Readings

Native American Ethics

Arvizu, D. R. (1995). The care voice and American Indian college students: An alternative perspective for student development professionals. *Journal of American Indian Education, 34*(3). Retrieved from http://jaie.asu.edu/v34/V34S3car.htm

Cohen, K. (2003). *Honoring the medicine: The essential guide to Native American healing.* New York, NY: Ballantine Books.

Cordova, V. F. (2003). Ethics: From an artist's point of view. In A. Waters (Ed.), *American Indian thought: Philosophical essays* (pp. 251–255). Malden, MA: Blackwell.

Cordova, V. F. (2003). Ethics: The we and the I. In A. Waters (Ed.), *American Indian thought: Philosophical essays* (pp. 173–181). Malden, MA: Blackwell.

Davis, M. B. (Ed.). (1994). *Native Americans in the twentieth century: An encyclopedia.* New York, NY: Garland.

Deloria, V. (2005). Indigenous peoples. In W. Schweiker (Ed.), *The Blackwell companion to religious ethics* (pp. 552–559). Malden, MA: Blackwell.

DuFour, J. (2003). Ethics and understanding. In A. Waters (Ed.), *American Indian thought: Philosophical essays* (pp. 34–42). Malden, MA: Blackwell.

The Good Red Roads—Code of Ethics. (n.d.). Retrieved from http://www.angelfire.com/biz2/turquoisebutterfly/roadintro.html

Kidwell, C. S., Noley, H., & Tinker, G. E. (2001). *A Native American theology.* Maryknoll, NY: Orbis.

Native American ethics: How do Native Americans address right and wrong? (n.d.). Retrieved from http://home.earthlink.net/~glbtrainbow/id9.html

Nerburn, K. (Ed.). (1999). *The wisdom of the Native American.* Novato, CA: New World Library.

Waters, A. (Ed.). (2003). *American Indian thought: Philosophical essays.* Malden, MA: Blackwell.

Hispanic/Latino Ethics

Arciniega, G., Anderson, T., Tovar-Blank, Z. G., & Tracey, T. (2008). Toward a fuller conception of machismo: Development of a traditional machismo and caballerismo scale. *Journal of Counseling Psychology, 55*(1), 19–33.

Baez, A., & Hernandez, D. (2001). Complementary spiritual beliefs in the Latino community: The interface with psychotherapy. *American Journal of Orthopsychiatry, 71,* 408–415.

Binderle, S., & Montoya, D. (2008). Hispanic/Latino identity labels: An examination of cultural values and personal experiences. *Howard Journal of Communications, 19,* 144–164.

Brackley, D., & Schubeck, T. L. (2002). Moral theology in Latin America. *Theological Studies, 63,* 123–160.

Deloria, V. (2005). Indigenous peoples. In W. Schweiker (Ed.), *The Blackwell companion to religious ethics* (pp. 552–559). Malden, MA: Blackwell.

Estrada, F., Rigali-Oiler, M., Arciniega, G., & Tracey, T. (2011). Machismo and Mexican American men: An empirical understanding using a gay sample. *Journal of Counseling Psychology, 58*(3), 358–367.

Garcia, I. (1997). *Dignidad: Ethics through Hispanic eyes.* Nashville, TN: Abingdon Press.

Gil, R., & Vasquez, C. (1996). *The Maria paradox: How Latinas can merge old world traditions with new world self-esteem.* New York, NY: G. P. Putnam.

Gracia, J. J. E. (2000). *Hispanic/Latino identity: A philosophical perspective.* Malden, MA: Blackwell.

Harrison, A. O., Wilson, M. N., Pine, C. J., Chan, S. Q., & Buriel, R. (1990). Family ecologies of ethnic minority children. *Child Development, 61,* 347–362.

African Ethics

African Ethics Initiative of the Unilever Ethics Centre for Comparative and Applied Ethics, University of Natal, Scottsville, South Africa. (n.d.). Retrieved from http://www .africanethics.org

Barboza, S. (Ed.). (1998). *The African American book of values.* New York, NY: Doubleday.

Bujo, B. (2001). *Foundations of an African ethic: Beyond the universal claims of Western morality* (B. McNeil, Trans.). New York, NY: Crossroad.

Bujo, B. (2005). Differentiation in African ethics. In W. Schweiker (Ed.), *The Blackwell companion to religious ethics* (pp. 423–437). Malden, MA: Blackwell.

Gyekye, K. (1996). *African cultural values.* Philadelphia, PA: Sankofa.

Hallen, B. (2002). *Short history of African philosophy.* Bloomington: Indiana University Press.

Hallen, B. (2005). African ethics? In W. Schweiker (Ed.), *The Blackwell companion to religious ethics* (pp. 406–412). Malden, MA: Blackwell.

Karenga, M. (2004). *MAAT, the moral ideal in ancient Egypt: A study in classical African ethics.* New York, NY: Routledge.

Walker, V., & Snarey, J. (Eds.). (2004). *Race-ing moral formation: African-American perspectives on care and justice.* New York, NY: Teachers College Press.

APPENDIX A

DUTY TO WARN/DUTY TO PROTECT STATE LAWS

State	Specific Law?	Website
Alabama	No specific law on duty to warn or protect	http://www.abec.alabama.gov/PDFs/Code.pdf
Alaska		http://www.dced.state.ak.us/occ/pub/CounselorStatutes.pdf
Arizona		http://www.magellanofaz.com/media/156838/7-7_duty_to_warn.pdf
Arkansas	No specific law on duty to warn or protect	
California		http://www.leginfo.ca.gov/cgi-bin/displaycode?section=civ&group=00001-01000&file=43-53
Colorado	Colorado state statute 13-21.117	
Connecticut		• http://www.ohpsych.org/resources/1/files/Ethics%20Committee/DutyToProtectHB71120303.pdf • http://www.cga.ct.gov/2009/pub/Chap899.htm#Sec52-146c.htm
Delaware		http://codes.lp.findlaw.com/decode/16/54/5402
Florida		http://www.flsenate.gov/Laws/Statutes/2010/491.0147
Georgia	No statutes, but a judicial decision	http://www.leagle.com/xmlResult.aspx?xmldoc=1982449250Ga199_1383.xml&docbase=CSLWAR1-1950-1985
Hawaii	No specific law on duty to warn or protect	
Idaho		http://www.legislature.idaho.gov/idstat/Title6/T6CH19SECT6-1903.htm

(Continued)

(Continued)

State	Specific Law?	Website
Illinois		http://www.wct-law.com/CM/Publications/publications13.asp
Indiana		http://www.in.gov/judiciary/cadp/docs/hb/legislation/related-statutes.pdf
Iowa	No specific law on duty to warn or protect	
Kansas	No specific law on duty to warn or protect	
Kentucky		http://www.lrc.state.ky.us/KRS/202A00/400.PDF
Louisiana		http://law.justia.com/codes/louisiana/2006/123/107255.html
Maine	No specific law on duty to warn or protect	http://www.nhdlaw.com/28C1B9/assets/files/News/43.NHD_News_Summer_2008.pdf
Maryland	HIV protection	http://gateway.nlm.nih.gov/MeetingAbstracts/ma?f=102181024.html
Massachusetts	Follows *Tarasoff* duty to protect	
Michigan	HIV threat link	http://michigan.gov/documents/mihivlaws_49845_7.pdf
Minnesota		https://www.revisor.mn.gov/statutes/?id=148.975
Nevada	No specific law on duty to warn or protect	
New Hampshire	Duty to protect laws (follows *Tarasoff*)	
New Jersey	Duty to protect laws (follows *Tarasoff*)	
New Mexico	No specific law on duty to warn or protect	
New York	No specific duty to protect laws	
North Carolina	No specific law on duty to warn or protect, but legal decision	http://www.capefearpsych.org/documents/TarasoffrulingforNC_001.pdf

State	Specific Law?	Website
North Dakota	No law on duty to warn/protect	
Ohio	Duty to protect law	http://www.ohpsych.org/resources/1/files/Ethics%20 Committee/DutyToProtectHB71120303.pdf
Oklahoma	Follows *Tarasoff* duty to protect	
Oregon	No specific duty to protect laws	
Pennsylvania		http://www.swlearning.com/blaw/cases/mental_health .html
Rhode Island	No specific duty to protect laws	
South Carolina	Follows *Tarasoff* duty to protect	
South Dakota		http://legis.state.sd.us/statutes/DisplayStatute.aspx?Type =Statute&Statute=36-33-32
Tennessee		• http://www.lexisnexis.com/hottopics/tncode/ • http://www.state.tn.us/mental/omd/omd_docs/ suicideliability.pdf
Texas	No duty to warn	http://www.law.uh.edu/healthlaw/law/StateMaterials/ Texas/TexasCases/thapar.PDF
Utah		http://law.justia.com/codes/utah/2006/title78/78_14003 .html
Virginia	No specific law on duty to warn or protect	
Washington	Follows *Tarasoff* duty to protect	
West Virginia	No specific law on duty to warn or protect	
Wisconsin	Follows *Taraoff* duty to protect	
Wyoming	No specific law on duty to warn or protect	

APPENDIX B

WEBSITES FOR STATE AND FEDERAL LAWS AFFECTING COUNSELING PRACTICE

Federal Laws

Child Protection—Native Americans: http://straylight.law.cornell.edu/uscode/html/uscode25/usc_sup_01_25_10_21.html

Family Education Rights and Privacy Act: http://www.ed.gov/policy/gen/guid/fpco/ferpa/index.html

Privacy in Substance Abuse Treatment: http://www.access.gpo.gov/nara/cfr/waisidx_00/42cfr2_00.html

Genetic Counseling: http://www.genome.gov/10002336
Health Insurance Portability and Accountability Act: http://www.hhs.gov/ocr/hipaa/

Laws Affecting Veterans: http://www.dol.gov/vets/regs/main.htm

Federal Special Education Laws: http://www.cec.sped.org/law_res/doc/law/index.php

Summaries of State Laws (All States)

State Laws Summary of Domestic Violence: http://www.ilj.org/dv/98legis.html

State Laws and Mental Health Coverage: http://www.ncsl.org/programs/health/Mentalben.htm

State Child Abuse Laws Summary: http://nccanch.acf.hhs.gov/general/legal/statutes/resources.pdf

State Laws Mandatory Child Abuse Reporters: http://nccanch.acf.hhs.gov/general/legal/statutes/manda.pdf

State Laws for Involuntary Commitment: http://www.psychlaws.org/LegalResources/statechart.htm

State Laws for Minors' Access to Health Services: http://www.guttmacher.org/statecenter/spibs/spib_MACS.pdf

Summary of State Laws Governing Confidentiality (Surgeon General's Report): http://www.mentalhealth.samhsa.gov/features/surgeongeneralreport/chapter7/sec3.asp

State Laws

Alabama

Child Abuse and Mandatory Reporting Laws: See "Summaries of State Laws," above

Confidentiality and Rights: http://www.legislature.state.al.us/CodeofAlabama/1975/coatoc.htm

Domestic Violence: http://www.legislature.state.al.us/CodeofAlabama/1975/coatoc.htm

Elder and Disabled Abuse Laws: http://www.legislature.state.al.us/CodeofAlabama/1975/coatoc.htm

Involuntary Commitment Law: http://mentalillnesspolicy.org/studies/state-standards-involuntary-treatment.html

Licensure Law: http://www.archives.state.al.us/officials/rdas/examcounseling.pdf

Mental Health Laws: http://www.legislature.state.al.us/CodeofAlabama/1975/coatoc.htm

Alaska

Child Abuse and Mandatory Reporting Laws: See "Summaries of State Laws," above

Licensure Law: http://www.dced.state.ak.us/occ/pub/pco4403.pdf

Involuntary Commitment Law: http://mentalillnesspolicy.org/studies/state-standards-involuntary-treatment.html

Arizona

Child Abuse and Mandatory Reporting Laws: See "Summaries of State Laws," above

Licensure Law: http://www.azca.org/government.html

Involuntary Commitment Law: http://mentalillnesspolicy.org/studies/state-standards-involuntary-treatment.html

Arkansas

Child Abuse and Mandatory Reporting Laws: See "Summaries of State Laws," above

Domestic Violence Laws: http://www.womenslaw.org/AR/AR_statutes.htm

Licensure Law: http://www.ark.org/abec/

Involuntary Commitment Law: http://mentalillnesspolicy.org/studies/state-standards-involuntary-treatment.html

California

Child Abuse and Mandatory Reporting Laws: See "Summaries of State Laws," above

Domestic Violence Laws: http://www.caadv.org/docs/2005leg.pdf

Involuntary Commitment Law: http://mentalillnesspolicy.org/studies/state-standards-involuntary-treatment.html

Licensure Law: http://www.bbs.ca.gov/lpcc_program/

Colorado

Child Abuse and Mandatory Reporting Laws: See "Summaries of State Laws," above

Domestic Violence Laws: http://www.womenslaw.org/CO/CO_statutes.htm#13-14

Licensure Law: http://www.counseling.org/Content/NavigationMenu/JOIN RENEW/STATELICENSURECERTIFICATIONDETAILEDCHART/ Colorado.htm

Involuntary Commitment Law: http://mentalillnesspolicy.org/studies/state-standards-involuntary-treatment.html

Connecticut

Child Abuse and Mandatory Reporting Laws: See "Summaries of State Laws," above

Domestic Violence Laws: http://www.womenslaw.org/CT/ct_statutes.htm

HIV Privacy Laws: http://www.glad.org/rights/connecticut_hiv.shtml# confidentiality

Involuntary Commitment Law: http://mentalillnesspolicy.org/studies/state-standards-involuntary-treatment.html

Licensure Law: http://www.counseling.org/Content/NavigationMenu/ JOINRENEW/STATELICENSURECERTIFICATIONDETAILEDCHART/ Connecticut.htm

Delaware

Child Abuse and Mandatory Reporting Laws: See "Summaries of State Laws," above

Domestic Violence Laws: http://courts.delaware.gov/How%20To/ Protection%20From%20Abuse/

Involuntary Commitment Law: http://mentalillnesspolicy.org/studies/state-standards-involuntary-treatment.html

Licensure Law: http://www.counseling.org/Content/NavigationMenu/JOIN RENEW/STATELICENSURECERTIFICATIONDETAILEDCHART/Delaware .htm

Florida

Child Abuse and Mandatory Reporting Laws: See "Summaries of State Laws," above

Domestic Violence Laws: http://www.dcf.state.fl.us/domesticviolence/

Involuntary Commitment Law: http://mentalillnesspolicy.org/studies/state-standards-involuntary-treatment.html

Licensure Law: http://www.doh.state.fl.us/mqa/491/soc_home.html

Georgia

Child Abuse and Mandatory Reporting Laws: See "Summaries of State Laws," above

Domestic Violence Laws: http://www.womenslaw.org/GA/GA_statutes.htm#1

Involuntary Commitment Law: http://mentalillnesspolicy.org/studies/state-standards-involuntary-treatment.html

Licensure Law: http://www.counseling.org/Content/NavigationMenu/JOIN RENEW/STATELICENSURECERTIFICATIONDETAILEDCHART/Georgia .htm

Hawaii

Child Abuse and Mandatory Reporting Laws: See "Summaries of State Laws," above

Domestic Violence Laws: http://www.hscadv.org/laws.asp#709-906

Involuntary Commitment Law: http://mentalillnesspolicy.org/studies/state-standards-involuntary-treatment.html

Licensure Law: http://www.counseling.org/Content/NavigationMenu/JOIN RENEW/STATELICENSURECERTIFICATIONDETAILEDCHART/Hawaii .htm

Idaho

Child Abuse and Mandatory Reporting Laws: See "Summaries of State Laws," above

Domestic Violence Laws: http://www3.state.id.us/cgi-bin/newidst?sctid=1800 90018.K

Involuntary Commitment Law: http://mentalillnesspolicy.org/studies/state-standards-involuntary-treatment.html

Licensure Law: http://www.counseling.org/Content/NavigationMenu/JOIN RENEW/STATELICENSURECERTIFICATIONDETAILEDCHART/Idaho.htm

Illinois

Child Abuse and Mandatory Reporting Laws: See "Summaries of State Laws," above

Domestic Violence Laws: http://www.ilcadv.org/legal/Booklet.pdf

Involuntary Commitment Law: http://mentalillnesspolicy.org/studies/state-standards-involuntary-treatment.html

Licensure Law: http://www.idfpr.com/dpr/WHO/prfcns.asp

Indiana

Child Abuse and Mandatory Reporting Laws: See "Summaries of State Laws," above

Domestic Violence Laws: http://www.womenslaw.org/IN/IN_statutes.htm

Involuntary Commitment Law: http://mentalillnesspolicy.org/studies/state-standards-involuntary-treatment.html

Licensure Law: http://www.counseling.org/Content/NavigationMenu/JOIN RENEW/STATELICENSURECERTIFICATIONDETAILEDCHART/Indiana .htm

Iowa

Child Abuse Laws: http://www.dhs.state.ia.us/dhs2005/dhs_homepage/ children_family/abuse_reporting/child_abuse.html

Domestic Violence Laws: http://www.judicial.state.ia.us/families/domviol/ dvlaws.asp

Involuntary Commitment Law: http://mentalillnesspolicy.org/studies/state-standards-involuntary-treatment.html

Licensure Law: http://www.counseling.org/Content/NavigationMenu/JOIN RENEW/STATELICENSURECERTIFICATIONDETAILEDCHART/Iowa .htm

Kansas

Child Abuse and Mandatory Reporting Laws: See "Summaries of State Laws," above

Domestic Violence Laws: http://www.womenslaw.org/KS/KS_statutes.htm

Involuntary Commitment Law: http://mentalillnesspolicy.org/studies/state-standards-involuntary-treatment.html

Licensure Law: http://www.ksbsrb.org/pro-counselors.html

Kentucky

Child Abuse and Mandatory Reporting Laws: See "Summaries of State Laws," above

Domestic Violence Laws: http://www.womenslaw.org/KY/KY_statutes.htm

Involuntary Commitment Law: http://mentalillnesspolicy.org/studies/state-standards-involuntary-treatment.html

Licensure Law: http://www.counseling.org/Content/NavigationMenu/JOIN RENEW/STATELICENSURECERTIFICATIONDETAILEDCHART/Kentucky .htm

Louisiana

Child Abuse and Mandatory Reporting Laws: See "Summaries of State Laws," above

Domestic Violence Laws: http://www.womenslaw.org/LA/LA_statutes.htm

Involuntary Commitment Law: http://mentalillnesspolicy.org/studies/state-standards-involuntary-treatment.html

Licensure Law: http://www.counseling.org/Content/NavigationMenu/ JOINRENEW/STATELICENSURECERTIFICATIONDETAILEDCHART/ Louisiana.htm

Maine

Child Abuse and Mandatory Reporting Laws: See "Summaries of State Laws," above

Domestic Violence Laws: http://janus.state.me.us/legis/statutes/19-A/title19-Ach101sec0.html

HIV Privacy and Counseling Laws: http://www.glad.org/rights/maine_hiv. shtml#Testing%20Issues

Involuntary Commitment Law: http://mentalillnesspolicy.org/studies/state-standards-involuntary-treatment.html

Licensure Law: http://www.state.me.us/pfr/olr/categories/cat13.htm

Maryland

Child Abuse and Mandatory Reporting Laws: See "Summaries of State Laws," above

Domestic Violence Laws: http://www.womenslaw.org/MD/MD_statutes.htm

Involuntary Commitment Law: http://mentalillnesspolicy.org/studies/state-standards-involuntary-treatment.html

Licensure Law: http://www.counseling.org/Content/NavigationMenu/JOINRENEW/STATELICENSURECERTIFICATIONDETAILEDCHART/Maryland.htm

Massachusetts

Child Abuse and Mandatory Reporting Laws: See "Summaries of State Laws," above

General Privacy Rights: http://www.bakernet.com/ecommerce/massachusetts-p.htm

HIV Privacy Rights: http://www.glad.org/rights/massachusetts_hiv.shtml#hivprivacy

Involuntary Commitment Law: http://mentalillnesspolicy.org/studies/state-standards-involuntary-treatment.html

Licensure Law: http://www.mass.gov/dpl/home.htm

Privileged Communication Laws: http://www.mass.gov/legis/laws/mgl/233-20b.htm

Special Education Laws: http://www.doe.mass.edu/lawsregs/

Michigan

Child Abuse and Mandatory Reporting Laws: See "Summaries of State Laws," above

Domestic Violence Laws: http://www.cityofmarysvillemi.com/police/Laws%20in%20Michigan.htm

Involuntary Commitment Law: http://mentalillnesspolicy.org/studies/state-standards-involuntary-treatment.html

Licensure Law: http://www.counseling.org/Content/NavigationMenu/JOINRENEW/STATELICENSURECERTIFICATIONDETAILEDCHART/Michigan.htm

Minnesota

Child Abuse and Mandatory Reporting Laws: See "Summaries of State Laws," above

Domestic Violence Laws: http://www.revisor.leg.state.mn.us/stats/518B/01 .html

Involuntary Commitment Law: http://mentalillnesspolicy.org/studies/state-standards-involuntary-treatment.html

Licensure Law: http://www.bbht.state.mn.us/

Mississippi

Child Abuse and Mandatory Reporting Laws: See "Summaries of State Laws," above

Domestic Violence Laws: http://www.womenslaw.org/MS/MS_statutes.htm

Involuntary Commitment Law: http://mentalillnesspolicy.org/studies/state-standards-involuntary-treatment.html

Licensure Law: http://www.lpc.state.ms.us/

Missouri

Child Abuse and Mandatory Reporting Laws: See "Summaries of State Laws," above

Domestic Violence Laws: http://www.moga.state.mo.us/STATUTES/C455 .HTM

Involuntary Commitment Law: http://mentalillnesspolicy.org/studies/state-standards-involuntary-treatment.html

Professional Licensure Laws: http://www.moga.state.mo.us/STATUTES/C337 .HTM

Montana

Child and Elder Protection Laws: http://data.opi.state.mt.us/bills/mca/52/1/52-1-103.htm

Domestic Violence Laws: http://data.opi.state.mt.us/bills/mca_toc/40_15.htm

Involuntary Commitment Law: http://mentalillnesspolicy.org/studies/state-standards-involuntary-treatment.html

Mental Health Laws: http://arm.sos.state.mt.us/37/37-14579.htm

Protection for Persons with Disabilities: http://data.opi.state.mt.us/bills/mca_toc/49_4_2.htm

Nebraska

Domestic Violence Laws: http://www.womenslaw.org/NE/NE_statutes.htm

Involuntary Commitment Law: http://mentalillnesspolicy.org/studies/state-standards-involuntary-treatment.html

Nevada

Child Abuse Laws: http://www.leg.state.nv.us/NRS/NRS-200.html#NRS200 Sec495

Child Confidentiality Laws: http://www.leg.state.nv.us/NRS/NRS-062H.html

Involuntary Commitment Law: http://www.whavins.com/nplh26.htm

Professional Licensure Laws: http://www.leg.state.nv.us/NRS/NRS-641A.html

Protection of elderly and those with disabilities: http://www.leg.state.nv.us/NRS/NRS-200.html#NRS200Sec495

Protection of Patients: http://www.leg.state.nv.us/NRS/NRS-200.html#NRS 200Sec495

New Hampshire

Child Abuse and Mandatory Reporting Laws: See "Summaries of State Laws," above

HIV Privacy Laws: http://www.glad.org/rights/newhampshire_hiv.shtml#testing

Involuntary Commitment Law: http://mentalillnesspolicy.org/studies/state-standards-involuntary-treatment.html

Licensure Law: http://www.state.nh.us/mhpb/index.html

New Jersey

Involuntary Commitment Law: http://mentalillnesspolicy.org/studies/state-standards-involuntary-treatment.html

Licensure Law: http://www.state.nj.us/lps/ca/medical/procounsel.htm

Special Education: http://www.state.nj.us/njded/specialed/reg/

New Mexico

Child Abuse and Mandatory Reporting Laws: See "Summaries of State Laws," above

Domestic Violence Laws: http://www.womenslaw.org/NM/NM_statutes.htm

Involuntary Commitment Law: http://mentalillnesspolicy.org/studies/state-standards-involuntary-treatment.html

New York

Child Abuse and Mandatory Reporting Laws: See "Summaries of State Laws," above

Involuntary Commitment Law: http://mentalillnesspolicy.org/studies/state-standards-involuntary-treatment.html

Mental Health Licensure Law: http://www.op.nysed.gov/mhpques-ans.htm

North Carolina

Child Abuse and Mandatory Reporting Laws: See "Summaries of State Laws," above

Domestic Violence Law: http://www.ncleg.net/enactedlegislation/statutes/html/bysection/chapter_50b/gs_50b-1.html

Involuntary Commitment Law: http://mentalillnesspolicy.org/studies/state-standards-involuntary-treatment.html

Licensure Law: http://www.ncblpc.org/

North Dakota

Child Abuse and Mandatory Reporting Laws: See "Summaries of State Laws," above

Involuntary Commitment Law: http://mentalillnesspolicy.org/studies/state-standards-involuntary-treatment.html

Domestic Violence Law: http://www.state.nd.us/lr/cencode/t14c071.pdf

Ohio

Child Abuse and Mandatory Reporting Laws: See "Summaries of State Laws," above

Involuntary Commitment Law: http://mentalillnesspolicy.org/studies/state-standards-involuntary-treatment.html

Licensure Law: http://cswmft.ohio.gov/

Oklahoma

Child Abuse and Mandatory Reporting Laws: See "Summaries of State Laws," above

Domestic Abuse Laws: http://www.oscn.net/applications/oscn/deliverdocument.asp?citeID=70255

Involuntary Commitment Law: http://mentalillnesspolicy.org/studies/state-standards-involuntary-treatment.html

Licensure Law: http://www.health.state.ok.us/program/lpc/

Oregon

Child Abuse and Mandatory Reporting Laws: See "Summaries of State Laws," above

Domestic Violence Laws: http://www.womenslaw.org/OR/OR_statutes.htm

Involuntary Commitment Law: http://mentalillnesspolicy.org/studies/state-standards-involuntary-treatment.html

Licensure Law: http://www.oblpct.state.or.us/

Mandatory Reporting: http://transcoder.usablenet.com/tt/http://www.oregon.gov/DHS/abuse/mandatory_report.shtml

Pennsylvania

Child Abuse and Mandatory Reporting Laws: See "Summaries of State Laws," above

Domestic Violence Laws: http://members.aol.com/StatutesP8/23.Cp.61.html

Involuntary Commitment Law: http://mentalillnesspolicy.org/studies/state-standards-involuntary-treatment.html

Licensure Law: http://www.pacode.com/secure/data/049/chapter49/chap49toc.html

Rhode Island

Child Abuse and Mandatory Reporting Laws: See "Summaries of State Laws," above

HIV Privacy Protection Laws: http://www.glad.org/rights/rhodeisland_hiv.shtml#confidentiality

Involuntary Commitment Law: http://mentalillnesspolicy.org/studies/state-standards-involuntary-treatment.html

Licensure Law: http://www.rules.state.ri.us/rules/released/pdf/DOH/DOH_277_.pdf

Mandatory Reporting: http://www.rilin.state.ri.us/statutes/title40/40%2D11/40%2D11%2D3.htm

South Carolina

Child Abuse Laws: http://www.scstatehouse.net/code/t20c007.htm

Domestic Violence Laws: http://www.scstatehouse.net/code/t20c004.htm

Involuntary Commitment Law: http://mentalillnesspolicy.org/studies/state-standards-involuntary-treatment.html

Licensure Law: http://www.llr.state.sc.us/POL/Counselors/

South Dakota

Child Abuse and Mandatory Reporting: http://legis.state.sd.us/statutes/DisplayStatute.aspx?Type=Statute&Statute=26-8A

Domestic Violence: http://legis.state.sd.us/statutes/DisplayStatute.aspx?Type=Statute&Statute=25-10

Involuntary Commitment Law: http://mentalillnesspolicy.org/studies/state-standards-involuntary-treatment.html

Licensure Law: http://www.state.sd.us/dhs/boards/counselor/

Tennessee

Adult Protective Services: http://www.state.tn.us/humanserv/adpro.htm

Child Abuse and Mandatory Reporting: http://www.tennessee.gov/sos/rules/0250/0250-04/0250-04-11.pdf

Domestic Violence Laws: http://www.womenslaw.org/TN/TN_statutes.htm

Involuntary Commitment Law: http://mentalillnesspolicy.org/studies/state-standards-involuntary-treatment.html

Licensure Law: http://state.tn.us/sos/rules/0450/0450.htm

Texas

Child Abuse Laws: http://www.capitol.state.tx.us/cgi-bin/statutes/pdfframe.cmd?filepath=/statutes/docs/FA/content/pdf/fa.005.00.000261.00.pdf&title=FAMILY%20CODE%20-%20CHAPTER%20261

Domestic Violence Laws: http://www.capitol.state.tx.us/cgi-bin/statutes/pdfframe.cmd?filepath=/statutes/docs/FA/content/pdf/fa.004.00.000071.00.pdf&title=FAMILY%20CODE%20-%20CHAPTER%2071

Involuntary Commitment Law: http://mentalillnesspolicy.org/studies/state-standards-involuntary-treatment.html

Licensure Law: http://www.dshs.state.tx.us/counselor/default.shtm

Minor Abortion Rights: http://www.capitol.state.tx.us/cgi-bin/statutes/pdfframe.cmd?filepath=/statutes/docs/FA/content/pdf/fa.002.00.000033.00.pdf&title=FAMILY%20CODE%20-%20CHAPTER%2033

Special Education: http://www.tea.state.tx.us/special.ed/rules/tec.html

Utah

Child Abuse and Mandatory Reporting Laws: See "Summaries of State Laws," above

Domestic Violence Laws: http://www.womenslaw.org/UT/UT_statutes.htm

Involuntary Commitment Law: http://mentalillnesspolicy.org/studies/state-standards-involuntary-treatment.html

Licensure Law: http://www.dopl.utah.gov/licensing/professional_counselor.html

Vermont

Child Abuse and Mandatory Reporting Laws: See "Summaries of State Laws," above

HIV Privacy Protection Laws: http://www.glad.org/rights/vermont_hiv.shtml#privacy

Involuntary Commitment Law: http://mentalillnesspolicy.org/studies/state-standards-involuntary-treatment.html

Mandatory Reporting: http://www.leg.state.vt.us/statutes/fullsection.cfm?Title=33&Chapter=049&Section=04913

Virginia

Child Abuse and Mandatory Reporting Laws: See "Summaries of State Laws," above

Domestic Violence Laws: http://www.womenslaw.org/VA/VA_statutes.htm

Involuntary Commitment Law: http://mentalillnesspolicy.org/studies/state-standards-involuntary-treatment.html

Licensure Law: http://www.dhp.state.va.us/counseling/

Washington

Child Abuse and Mandatory Reporting Laws: See "Summaries of State Laws," above

Confidentiality Laws: http://www.leg.wa.gov/RCW/index.cfm?fuseaction=section&section=18.225.105

Domestic Violence Laws: http://www.courts.wa.gov/dv/

Involuntary Commitment Law: http://mentalillnesspolicy.org/studies/state-standards-involuntary-treatment.html

Licensure Law: https://fortress.wa.gov/doh/hpqa1/hps7/Registered_Counselor/default.htm

Mental Health Laws: http://www1.dshs.wa.gov/mentalhealth/mentalaw.shtml

West Virginia

Child Abuse Laws: http://www.legis.state.wv.us/WVCODE/49/masterfrm2Frm.htm

Domestic Violence Laws: http://www.legis.state.wv.us/WVCODE/48/masterfrm2Frm.htm

Involuntary Commitment Law: http://mentalillnesspolicy.org/studies/state-standards-involuntary-treatment.html

Licensure Law: http://www.wvbec.org/

Wisconsin

Child Abuse Laws: http://www.legis.state.wi.us/statutes/Stat0813.pdf

Child Privacy Laws: http://www.legis.state.wi.us/statutes/Stat0048.pdf

Confidentiality Laws: http://www.dhfs.state.wi.us/clientrights/ConfidTrmtRecs.htm

Domestic Abuse Laws: http://www.legis.state.wi.us/statutes/Stat0813.pdf

Involuntary Commitment Law: http://mentalillnesspolicy.org/studies/state-standards-involuntary-treatment.html

Licensure Law: http://drl.wi.gov/prof/coun/def.htm

Wyoming

Child Abuse Laws: http://legisweb.state.wy.us/statutes/titles/title14/c03a02.htm

Involuntary Commitment Law: http://mentalillnesspolicy.org/studies/state-standards-involuntary-treatment.html

License Law: http://plboards.state.wy.us/mentalhealth/index.asp

REFERENCES

Adler, N., Ozer, E., & Tschann, J. (2003). Abortion among adolescents. *American Psychologist, 58,* 211–217.

Alhazo, R., Upton, T., & Cioe, N. (2011). Duty to warn versus duty to protect confidentiality: Ethical and legal considerations relative to individuals with AIDS/HIV. *Journal of Applied Rehabilitation Counseling, 42*(1), 43–49.

Ali, A., & Toner, B. (2001). Self-esteem as a predictor of attitudes toward wife abuse among Muslim women and men in Canada. *Journal of Social Psychology, 14,* 23–30.

Alkhatib, A., Regan, J., & Jackson, J. (2008). Informed assent and informed consent in the child and adolescent. *Psychiatric Annals, 38*(5), 337–339.

Alleman, J. (2002). Online counseling: The Internet and mental health treatment. *Psychotherapy: Theory/Research/Practice/Training, 39*(2), 199–209.

American Academy of Pediatrics. (1996). The adolescent's right to confidential care when considering abortion. *Pediatrics, 97,* 746–751.

American Association for Marriage and Family Therapy. (2001). *AAMFT code of ethics.* Alexandria, VA: Author.

American Association of Pastoral Counselors. (2010). *AAPC code of ethics.* Fairfax, VA: Author.

American Civil Liberties Union. (2001). *Laws restricting teenagers' access to abortion.* New York: Author.

American Counseling Association. (1996). *ACA code of ethics.* Alexandria, VA: Author.

American Counseling Association. (2005). *ACA code of ethics.* Alexandria, VA: Author.

American Mental Health Counseling Association. (2010). *Principles for AMHCA code of ethics.* Alexandria, VA: Author.

American Psychiatric Association. (2000). *Diagnostic and statistical manual of mental disorders* (4th ed., text rev.). Washington, DC: Author.

American Psychological Association. (1997). *Resolution on appropriate therapeutic responses to sexual orientation.* Washington, DC: Author.

American Psychological Association. (2007). *Guidelines for psychological practice with girls and women.* Washington, DC: Author.

American Psychological Association. (2010). *Ethical principles of psychologists and code of conduct.* Washington, DC: Author.

American School Counselor Association. (2010). *Ethical standards for school counselors.* Alexandria, VA: Author.

Americans United for Life. (2003). *State parental involvement laws for minors seeking abortion.* Chicago, IL: Author.

Ancis, J., & Marshall, D. (2010). Using a multicultural framework to assess supervisees' perceptions of culturally competent supervision. *Journal of Counseling & Development, 88,* 277–285.

Ang, R., & Goh, D. (2010). Cyberbulling among adolescents: The role of affective and cognitive empathy, and gender. *Child Psychiatry and Human Development, 41*(4), 387–397.

APA Presidential Task Force on Evidence-Based Practice. (2006). Evidence-based practice in psychology. *American Psychologist, 61,* 271–285.

Appelbaum, P. (2001). Law and psychiatry: Third party suits against therapist in recovered memories cases. *Psychiatric Services, 52,* 27–28.

Aquino, K., Freeman, D., Reed, A., Lim, V., & Felps, W. (2009). Testing a social-cognitive model of moral behavior: The interactive influence of situations and moral identity centrality. *Journal of Personality and Social Psychology, 97*(1), 123–141.

Aquino, K., & Reed, A. (2002). The self-importance of moral identity. *Journal of Personality and Social Psychology, 83*(6), 1423–1440.

Arciniega, G., Anderson, T., Tovar-Blank, Z. G., & Tracey, T. (2008). Toward a fuller conception of machismo: Development of a traditional machismo and caballerismo scale. *Journal of Counseling Psychology, 55*(1), 19–33.

Arizmendi, T., Beutler, L., Shandfield, S., Crago, M., & Hagaman, R. (1985). Client-therapist value similarity and psychotherapy outcome: A microscopic analysis. *Psychotherapy: Theory, Research, Practice, Training, 22*(1), 16–21.

Arredondo, P., Toporek, R., Brown, S., Jones, J., Locke, D., Sanchez, J., & Sadler, H. (1996). Operationalization of the multicultural counseling competencies. *Journal of Multicultural Counseling and Development, 24*(1), 42–78.

Association for Counselor Education and Supervision. (1993). *Ethical guidelines for counseling supervisors.* Washington, DC: Author.

Association for Specialists in Group Work. (2007). *Best practice guidelines 2007 revisions.* St Cloud, MN: Author.

Atkinson, D., & Lowe, S. (1995). Asian-American acculturation, gender, and willingness to seek counseling. *Journal of Multicultural Counseling and Development, 23,* 130–139.

Aubry, T., Flynn, R., Gerber, G., & Dostaler, T. (2005). Identifying the core competencies of community support providers working with people with psychiatric disabilities. *Psychiatric Rehabilitation Journal, 28,* 346–353.

Baban, A., & Craciun, C. (2007). Changing health-risk behaviors: A review of theory and evidence-based interventions in health psychology. *Journal of Cognitive and Behavioral Psychotherapies, 7*(1), 45–66.

Baca, C., Alverson, D., Manuel, J., & Blackwell, G. (2007). Telecounseling in rural areas for alcohol problems. *Alcoholism Treatment Quarterly, 25*(4), 31–44.

Balcazar, F., Suarez-Balcazar, Y., & Taylor-Ritzler, T. (2009). Cultural competence: Development of a conceptual framework. *Disability and Rehabilitation, 31*(14), 1153–1160.

Banja, J. (1990). Rehabilitation and empowerment. *Archives of Physical Medicine and Rehabilitation, 71,* 614–615.

Banks, J. (2009). *The Routledge international companion to multicultural education.* London, UK: Routledge.

Barbee, P., Combs, D., Ekleberry, F., & Villalobos, S. (2007). Duty to warn: Not in Texas. *Journal of Professional Counseling, 35*(1), 18–25.

Bargh, J., & Alvarez, J. (2001). The road to hell: Good intentions in the face of nonconscious tendencies to misuse power. In A. Lee-Chai (Ed.), *The use and abuse of power: Multiple perspectives on the causes of corruption* (pp. 41–56). Philadelphia, PA: Psychological Press.

Barnett, J., & Scheetz, K. (2003). Technological advances and telehealth: Ethics, law, and the practice of psychotherapy. *Psychotherapy: Theory, Research, Practice, Training, 40,* 86–93.

Barrett, M., & Berman, J. (2001). Is psychotherapy more effective when therapists disclose information about themselves? *Journal of Consulting and Clinical Psychology, 69*(4), 397–603.

Barstow, A. (1994). *Witchcraze: A new history of the European witch hunts.* London, UK: Pandora.

Batavia, A. (2001). The new paternalism. *Journal of Disability Policy Studies, 12,* 107–117.

Beauchamp, T., & Childress, J. (1989). *Principles of biomedical ethics* (3rd ed.). New York, NY: Oxford University Press.

Beauchamp, T., & Childress, J. (2001). *Principles of biomedical ethics* (5th ed.). New York, NY: Oxford University Press.

Beauchamp, T., & Childress, J. (2008). *Principles of biomedical ethics* (6th ed.). New York, NY: Oxford University Press.

Bebeau, M. (1994). Influencing the moral dimensions of dental practice. In J. Rest & D. Narvaez (Eds.), *Moral development in the professions: Psychology and applied ethics* (pp. 121–146). Hillsdale, NJ: Lawrence Erlbaum.

Bebeau, M. (2002). The Defining Issues Test and the four component model: Contributions to professional education. *Journal of Moral Education, 31*(3), 271–295.

Bebeau, M. (2008). Promoting ethical development and professionalism: Insights from educational research in the professions. *University of St. Thomas Law Journal, 5*(2), 367–403.

Bebeau, M. (2009). Enhancing professionalism using ethics education as part of a dental licensure board's disciplinary action: Pt. 1. An evidence-based process. *Journal of American College of Dentistry, 76*(2), 38–50.

Bebeau, M., Rest, J., & Yamoor, C. (1985). Measuring the ethical sensitivity of dental students. *Journal of Dental Education, 49*(4), 225–235.

Bebeau, M., & Thoma, S. (1999). "Intermediate" concepts and the connection to moral education. *Educational Psychology Review, 11,* 343–368.

Belar, C., Brown, R., Hersch, L., Hornyak, L., Rozensky, R., Sheridan, E., . . . Reed, G. (2001). Self-assessment in clinical health psychology: A model for ethical expansion of practice. *Professional Psychology: Research and Practice, 32*(2), 135–141.

Bellini, J. (2002). Correlates of multicultural counseling competencies of vocational rehabilitation counselors. *Rehabilitation Counseling Bulletin, 45,* 66–75.

Belt, D. (2002). The world of Islam. *National Geographic, 201,* 76–86.

Benjamin, L. (1994). SASB: The bridge between personality theory and clinical psychology. *Psychological Inquiry, 5*(4), 273–316.

Berberoglu, B. (1994). *Class structure and social transformation.* Westport, CT: Praeger.

Bergeron, R., & Gray, B. (2003). Ethical dilemmas of reporting suspected elder abuse. *Social Work, 48,* 96–105.

Berke, D., Rozell, C., Hogan, T., Norcross, C., & Karpiak, C. (2011). What clinical psychologists know about evidence-based practice: Familiarity with online resources and research methods. *Journal of Clinical Psychology, 67*(4), 329–339.

Berlin, I. (1983). Prevention of emotional problems among Native-American children: Overview of development. In S. Chess & A. Thomas (Eds.), *Annual progress in child psychiatry and child development* (pp. 320–333). New York, NY: Brunner/Mazel.

Bernard, I., & Goodyear, R. (1998). *Fundamentals of clinical supervision* (2nd ed.). Needham Heights, MA: Allyn & Bacon.

Bernard, J., Clingerman, T., & Gilbride, D. (2011). Personality type and clinical supervision. *Counselor Education and Supervision, 50,* 154–170.

Besel, L., & Yuille, J. (2010). Individual differences in empathy: The role of facial expression recognition. *Personality and Individual Differences, 49*(2), 107–112.

Betan, E. (1997). Toward a hermeneutic model of ethical decision making in clinical practice. *Ethics & Behavior, 7,* 347–365.

Beutler, L., & Harwood, T. (2004). Virtual reality in psychotherapy training. *Journal of Clinical Psychology, 60*(3), 317–330.

Bevan, E., & Higgins, D. (2002). Is domestic violence learned? The contribution of five forms of child maltreatment to men's violence and adjustment. *Journal of Family Violence, 17,* 223–245.

Bever, P. (2002). Witchcraft, female aggression, and power in the modern community. *Journal of Social History, 35,* 955–990.

Binderle, S., & Montoya, D. (2008). Hispanic/Latino identity labels: An examination of cultural values and personal experiences. *Howard Journal of Communications, 19,* 144–164.

Blair-Loy, M. (2001). Cultural constructions of family schemas: The case of women finance executives. *Gender & Society, 15,* 687–709.

Blasi, A. (1980). Bridging moral cognition and moral action. *Psychological Bulletin, 88,* 1–45.

Blasi, A. (1983). *The self as subject: Its dimensions and development.* Unpublished manuscript.

Bloom, J. (1998). The ethical practice of webcounseling. *British Journal of Guidance & Counseling, 26,* 53–60.

Blum, R., & Resnick, M. (1982). Adolescent sexual decision-making: Contraception, pregnancy, abortion, motherhood. *Pediatric Annals, 11,* 797–805.

Blummer, R. (2000, December 19). Whose constitutional rights at risk of being trampled? *Milwaukee Journal Sentinel,* p. 19a.

Bodenhorn, N. (2006). Exploratory study of common and challenging dilemmas experienced by professional school counselors. *Professional School Counseling, 10,* 195–202.

Bopp, J., Bopp, M., Brown, L., & Lane, P. (1985). *The sacred tree* (2nd ed.). Lethbridge, AB: Four Winds Development Press.

Bopp, J., Lane, P., Brown, L., & Bopp, M. (1989). *The sacred tree* (3rd ed.). Wilmont, WI: Lotus Light.

Borders, L., & Brown, L. (2005). *New handbook of counseling supervision* (2nd ed.). Mahwah, NJ: Lawrence Erlbaum.

Bordin, E. (1979). The generalizability of the psychoanalytic concept of the working alliance. *Psychotherapy: Theory, Research, Practice, Training, 16,* 252–260.

Bordin, E. (1983). A working alliance based model of supervision. *The Counseling Psychologist, 11,* 35–42.

Bowlby, J. (1969). *Attachment and loss* (Vol. 1). London, UK: Hogarth.

Bradley, L., & Hendricks, C. (2008). Ethical decision making: Basic issues. *Family Journal, 16*(3), 261–263.

Bragg, M. (2009). *HIPAA for the general public.* Chicago, IL: American Bar Association.

Brener, M. (2008). *Evolution and empathy.* Jefferson, NC: McFarland.

Brewer, M., & Gardner, W. (1996). Who is this "we"? Levels of collective identity and self representations. *Journal of Personality and Social Psychology, 71,* 83–93.

Brown, P., & O'Leary, K. (2000). Therapeutic alliance: Predicting continuance and success in group treatment for spouse abuse. *Journal of Consulting and Clinical Psychology, 68,* 340–345.

Bryan, K., & Lyons, H. (2003). Experiential activities and multicultural counseling competence training. *Journal of Counseling and Development, 81,* 400–409.

Bryceland, C., & Stam, H. (2005). Empirical validation and professional codes of ethics: Description or prescription. *Journal of Constructivist Psychology, 18*(2), 131–155.

Buckner, F., & Firestone, M. (2000). Where the public peril begins: 25 years after Tarasoff. *Journal of Legal Medicine, 21*(2), 187–222.

Bucky, S., Marques, S., Daly, J., Alley, J., & Karp, A. (2010). Supervision characteristics related to the supervisory working alliance as rated by doctoral-level supervisees. *Clinical Supervisor, 29,* 149–163.

Bujo, B. (2005). Differentiation in African ethics. In W. Schweiker (Ed.), *The Blackwell companion to religious ethics* (pp. 423–437). Malden, MA: Blackwell.

Burien, B. (2000). Social dual-role relationships during internships: A decision-making model. *Professional Psychology: Research and Practice, 31,* 332–378.

Burkard, A. W., Johnson, A. J., Madson, M., Pruitt, N., Contreras-Tadych, D., Kozlowski, J. M., . . . Knox, S. (2006). Supervisor responsiveness and unresponsiveness in cross-cultural supervision. *Journal of Counseling, 53,* 288–301.

Burkemper, E. (2002). Family therapists' ethical decision-making processes in two duty-to-warn situations. *Journal of Marital and Family Therapy, 28*(2), 203–211.

Burnouf, E. (2010). *Introduction to the history of Indian Buddhism.* Chicago, IL: University of Chicago Press.

Bussey, K., & Bandura, A. (1999). Social cognitive theory of gender development and differentiation. *Psychological Review, 106,* 676–713.

Butcher, J., Graham, J., Ben-Porath, Y., Tellegen, Y., Dahlsom, W., & Kraemmer, B. (2001). Minnesota Multiphasic Personality Inventory–2: Manual for administration and scoring (Rev. ed.). Minneapolis: University of Minnesota Press.

Butcher, J., Perry, J., & Hahn, J. (2004). Computers in clinical assessment: Historical developments, present status, and future challenges. *Journal of Clinical Psychology, 60*(3), 331–345.

Calderbank, R. (2000). Abuse and disabled people: Vulnerability or social indifference? *Disability and Society, 15,* 521–534.

Campbell, C., & Fox, G. (2003). Acknowledging the inevitable: Understanding multiple relationships in rural practice. *Professional Psychology: Research and Practice, 34,* 430–434.

Capozza, D., & Brown, R. (Eds.). (2000). *Social identity processes.* Thousand Oaks, CA: Sage.

Cappell, C., & Heiner, B. (1990). The intergenerational transmission of family aggression. *Journal of Family Violence, 5,* 135–152.

Carey, B. (2005). *Straight, gay or lying? Bisexuality revisited.* New York: New York Times.

Carey, J., & Dimmitt, C. (2008). A model for evidence-based elementary school counseling: Using school data, research, and evaluation to enhance practice. *Elementary School Journal, 108*(5), 422–430.

Carleton, R. (2006). Does the mandate make a difference? Reporting decisions in emotional abuse. *Child Abuse Review, 15*(1), 19–37.

Carp, R., & Stidham, R. (1998). *Judicial process in America.* Washington, DC: CQ Press.

Carr, D., & Steutel, J. (1999). *Virtue ethics and moral education.* Florence, KY: Psychology Press.

Carroll, L., & Gilroy, P. (2001). Teaching "outside the box": Incorporating queer theory in counselor education. *Journal of Humanistic Counseling, Education & Development, 40*(1), 49–58.

Carter, D., & Rashidi, A. (2003). Theoretical model of psychotherapy: Eastern Asian-Islamic women with mental illness. *Health Care for Women International, 24*(5), 399–413.

Cashwell, C., Shcherbakova, J., & Cashwell, T. (2003). Effect of client and counselor ethnicity on preference for counselor self disclosure. *Journal of Counseling & Development, 81,* 196–201.

Casile, W., Gruber, E., & Rosenblatt, S. (2007). Implementation of a collaborative supervision model. In J. Gregoire & C. Jungers (Eds.), *The counselor's companion: What every beginning counselor needs to know* (pp. 86–110). Mahwah, NJ: Lawrence Erlbaum.

Casper, F. (2004). Technological developments and applications in clinical psychology and psychotherapy: Introduction. *Journal of Clinical Psychology, 60*(3), 221–238.

Castillo, L., & Cano, M. (2007). Mexican American psychology: Theory and clinical application. In C. Negy (Ed.), *Cross-cultural psychotherapy: Toward a critical understanding of diverse client populations* (2nd ed., pp. 85–102). Reno, NV: Bent Tree Press.

Castillo, L., Perez, F., Castillo, R., & Ghosheh, M. (2010). Construction and initial validation of the Marianismo Beliefs Scale. *Counselling Psychology Quarterly, 23*(2), 163–175.

Catholic Medical Association. (2000). *Homosexuality and hope.* Retrieved from http://narth.com/docs/hope.html

Cattaneo, L., & Chapman, A. (2010). The process of empowerment. *American Psychologist, 65*(7), 646–659.

Chadrow, N. (1978). *The reproduction of mothering.* Berkeley: University of California Press.

Chan, F., Tarvydas, V., Blalock, K., Strauser, D., & Atkins, B. (2009). Unifying and elevating rehabilitation counseling through model-driven, diversity-sensitive evidence-based practice. *Rehabilitation Counseling Bulletin, 52*(2), 114–119.

Chang, F. (1994). School teachers' moral reasoning. In J. Rest & D. Narvaez (Eds.), *Moral development in the professions: Psychology and applied ethics* (pp. 51–70). Hillsdale, NJ: Lawrence Erlbaum.

Chang, T., & Yeh, C. (2003). Using online groups to support Asian American men: Racial, cultural, gender and treatment issues. *Professional Psychology: Research and Practice, 34,* 634–643.

Chao, R., Chu-Lien, W., Good, G., & Flores, L. (2011). Race/ethnicity, color-blind racial attitudes, and multicultural counseling competence: The moderating effects of multicultural counseling training. *Journal of Counseling Psychology, 58*(1), 72–82.

Chessick, R. (1990). Hermeneutics for psychotherapists. *American Journal of Psychotherapy, 44,* 245–274.

Chi-Ying Chung, R., & Bemak, F. (2002). The relationship of culture and empathy in cross-cultural counseling. *Journal of Counseling and Development, 80,* 154–160.

Clark, A. (2010). Young children as protagonists and the role of participatory, visual methods in engaging multiple perspectives. *American Journal of Community Psychology, 46*(1/2), 115–123.

Clark, C., & Krupa, T. (2002). Reflections on empowerment in community mental health: Giving shape to an elusive idea. *Psychiatric Rehabilitation Journal, 25,* 341–349.

Cockburn, T. (2005). Children and the feminine ethic of care. *Childhood: A Global Journal of Child Research, 12*(1), 71–89.

Cohen, K. (2003). *Honoring the medicine: The essential guide to Native American healing.* New York, NY: Random House.

Colangelo, J. (2007). Recovered memory debate revised: Practice implications for mental health counselors. *Journal of Mental Health Counseling, 29*(2), 93–120.

Colby, A. (2002). Moral understanding, motivation and identity. *Human Development, 45*(2), 130–135.

Commission on Rehabilitation Counselor Certification. (2009). *Code of professional ethics for rehabilitation counselors.* Schaumburg, IL: Author.

Commission on Rehabilitation Counselor Certification. (2010). *Code of professional ethics for rehabilitation counselors.* Schaumburg, IL: Author.

Connor, P., & Becker, B. (2003). Personal value systems and decision-making styles of public managers. *Public Personnel Management, 32,* 155–181.

Constantine, M. (1997). Facilitating multicultural competency in counseling supervision: Operationalizing a practical framework. In D. Pope-Davis & H. Coleman (Eds.), *Multicultural counseling competencies: Assessment, education and training, and supervision* (pp. 310–324). Thousand Oaks, CA: Sage.

Constantine, M. (2001). Multicultural training, theoretical orientation, empathy, and multicultural case conceptualization ability in counselors. *Journal of Mental Health Counseling, 23*(4), 357–372.

Constantine, M. (2002). Predictors of satisfaction with counseling: Racial and ethnic minority clients' attitudes towards counseling and ratings of their counselors' general and multicultural competence. *Journal of Counseling Psychology, 49,* 255–263.

Cook, J., Mulkern, V., Grey, D., Burke-Miller, J., Blyer, C., Razzano, L., . . . Steigman, P. (2006). Effects of local unemployment rate on vocational outcomes in a randomized trial of supported employment for individuals with psychiatric disabilities. *Journal of Vocational Rehabilitation, 25,* 71–84.

Cooper, C., & Gottlieb, M. (2000). Ethical issues with managed care: Challenges facing counseling psychology. *Counseling Psychologist, 28,* 179–236.

Cooper, S., Benton, S., Benton, S., & Phillips, J. (2008). Evidence-based practice in psychology among college counseling center clinicians. *Journal of College Student Psychotherapy, 22*(4), 28–50.

Cooper, T. (1998). *A time before deception: Truth in communication, culture, and ethics.* Santa Fe, NM: Clear Light.

Corey, G., Corey, M., & Callanan, P. (2007). *Issues and ethics in the helping professions* (7th ed.). Pacific Grove, CA: Brooks/Cole.

Corey, G., Corey, M., & Callanan, P. (2010). *Issues and ethics in the helping professions* (8th ed.). Belmont, CA: Brooks/Cole.

Cornish, J., Gorgens, K., Olkin, R., Palombi, B., & Abels, A. (2008). Perspectives on ethical practice with people who have disabilities. *Professional Psychology: Research and Practice, 39*(5), 488–497.

Cottone, R. (2001). A social constructivism model of ethical decision making in counseling. *Journal of Counseling & Development, 79*(1), 39–45.

Cottone, R., & Claus, R. (2000). Ethical decision-making models: A review of the literature. *Journal of Counseling and Development, 78,* 275–283.

Cottone, R., & Tarvydas, V. (2006). *Counseling ethics and decision-making* (3rd ed.). Upper Saddle River, NJ: Prentice Hall.

Council for Accreditation of Counseling and Related Educational Programs. (2009). *2009 standards.* Alexandria, VA: Author.

Creel, A. (1977). *Dharma in Hindu ethics.* Columbia, MO: South Asia Books.

Crowell, C., Narvaez, D., & Gomberg, A. (2004). Information ethics from a developmental perspective. In L. A. Freeman & A. G. Peace (Eds.), *Information ethics: Privacy and intellectual property* (pp. 19–37). Hershey, PA: Information Science.

Cruess, S., Johnston, S., & Cruess, R. (2004). Profession: A working definition for medical educators. *Teaching and Learning in Medicine, 16*(1), 74–76.

Cummings, A. (2000). Teaching feminist counselor responses to novice female counselors. *Counselor Education and Supervision, 40,* 47–58.

Curtis, J. (1982). Principles and techniques of non-disclosure by the therapist during psychotherapy. *Psychological Reports, 51,* 907–914.

Cush, D., Robinson, C., & Robinson, M. (2008). *Encyclopedia of Hinduism.* London, UK: Routledge.

Dalla-Vorgia, P., Lascaratos, P., Skiadas, P., & Garanis-Papadatos, T. (2001). Is consent in medicine a concept only of modern times? *Journal of Medical Ethics, 27,* 59–61.

Danish, S., D'Augelli, A., & Hauer, A. (1980). *Helping skills: A basic training program.* New York, NY: Human Sciences Press.

Davis, L., Hoffman, N., Morse, R., & Luehr, J. (1992). Substance use disorder diagnostic schedule (SUDDS): The equivalence and validity of a computer-administered and interviewer-administered format. *Alcoholism: Clinical & Experimental Research, 16*(2), 250–254.

Day, A., Casey, S., & Gerace, A. (2010). Interventions to improve empathy awareness in sexual and violent offenders: Conceptual, empirical, and clinical issues. *Aggression and Violent Behavior, 15*(3), 201–208.

De Lauretis, T. (1991). Queer theory: Lesbian and gay sexualities: An introduction. *Differences: A Journal of Feminist Cultural Studies 3*(2), iiix–viii.

Decety, J., Michalska, K., & Akitsuki, Y. (2008). Who caused the pain? An fMRI investigation of empathy and intentionality in children. *Neuropsychologia, 46,* 2607–2614.

DeLettre, J., & Sobell, L. (2010). Keeping psychotherapy notes separate from the patient record. *Clinical Psychology & Psychotherapy, 17*(2), 160–163.

Dell Orto, A., & Power, P. (2007). *The psychological and social impact of illness and disability* (5th ed.). New York, NY: Springer.

Denney, R., Aten, J., & Gingrich, F. (2008). Using spiritual self-disclosure in psychotherapy. *Journal of Psychology and Theology, 36*(4), 294–302.

Detert, J., Trevino, L., & Sweitzer, V. (2008). Moral disengagement in ethical decision making: A study of antecedents and outcomes. *Journal of Applied Psychology, 93*(2), 374–391.

Dilthey, W. (1978). *The critique of historical reason* (M. Emarth, Trans.). Chicago, IL: University of Chicago Press.

DiMarco, M., & Zoline, S. (2004). Duty to warn and HIV-related psychotherapy: Decision-making and biases among psychologists. *Counseling and Clinical Psychology Journal, 1*(2), 68–85.

Doniger-O'Flaherty, W. (1990). *Textual sources for the study of Hinduism.* Chicago, IL: University of Chicago Press.

Dorff, E. (2000). Ethics of Judaism. In N. Neusner & A. Avery-Peck (Eds.), *The Blackwell companion to Judaism* (pp. 373–388). Malden, MA: Blackwell.

Dorff, E. N. (2003). *Love your neighbor and yourself: A Jewish approach to modern personal ethics.* Philadelphia, PA: Jewish Publication Society.

Draycott, S., & Dabbs, A. (1998). Cognitive dissonance 2: A theoretical grounding of motivational interviewing. *British Journal of Clinical Psychology, 37*(3), 355–364.

Drotar, D. (2008). Ethical issues in treatment and intervention research with children and adolescents with behavioral and mental disorders. *Ethics & Behavior, 18*(2/3), 119–126.

Duncan, L. (2003). Understanding leaders of repressive social movements. *Analysis of Social Issues and Public Policy, 3,* 181–184.

Dye, A., & Borders, D. (1990). Counseling supervisors: Standards for preparation and practice. *Journal of Counseling and Development, 69,* 27–29.

Eagley, A. (1987). *Sex differences in social behavior: A social-role interpretation.* Hillsdale, NJ: Lawrence Erlbaum.

Eagly, A. (2009). The his and hers of prosocial behavior: An examination of the social psychology of gender. *American Psychologist, 64*(8), 644–658.

Egan, G. (2009). *The skilled helper.* Florence, KY: Brooks/Cole.

Eisenberg, N., Cumberland, A., Guthri, I., Murphy, B., & Shepard, S. (2005). Age changes in prosocial responding and moral reasoning in adolescence and early adulthood. *Journal of Research on Adolescence, 15*(3), 235–260.

Eisenberg, N., & Miller, P. (1987). The relation of empathy to prosocial and related behaviors. *Psychological Bulletin, 101*(1), 91–119.

Elleven, R., & Allen, J. (2004). Applying technology to online counseling: Suggestions for the beginning E-therapist. *Journal of Instructional Psychology, 31,* 223–228.

Elliot, A., & Devine, P. (1994). On the motivational nature of cognitive dissonance: Dissonance as psychological discomfort. *Journal of Personality and Social Psychology, 67*(3), 382–394.

Enright, R., Lapsley, D., Harris, D., & Shauver, D. (1983). Moral development interventions in early adolescence. *Theory into Practice, 22,* 134–144.

Epstein, J., & Klinkenberg, W. (2001). From Eliza to Internet: A brief history of computerized assessment. *Computers in Human Behavior, 17,* 295–314.

Epstein, R., & Hundert, E. (2002). Defining and assessing professional competence. *Journal of the American Medical Association, 287*(2), 226–235.

Erdynast, A., & Rapgay, L. (2009). Developmental levels of conceptions of compassion in the ethical decision-making of Western Buddhist practitioners. *Journal of Adult Development, 16*(1), 1–12.

Erickson, E. (1968). *Identity: Youth and crisis.* New York: New York Times.

Erickson-Schroth, L., & Mitchell, J. (2009). Queering queer theory, or why bisexuality matters. *Journal of Bisexuality, 9,* 297–315.

Eriksen, K., Marston, G., & Korte, T. (2002). Working with God: Managing conservative Christian beliefs that may interfere with counseling. *Counseling and Values, 47,* 48–68.

Esposito, J. (1999). *The Islamic threat: Myth of reality?* (3rd ed.). New York, NY: Oxford University Press.

Estrada, F., Rigali-Oiler, M., Arciniega, G., & Tracey, T. (2011). Machismo and Mexican American men: An empirical understanding using a gay sample. *Journal of Counseling Psychology, 58*(3), 358–367.

Evans, M., Boothroyd, R., Armstrong, M., Greenbaum, P., Brown, E., & Kuppinger, A. (2003). An experimental study of the effectiveness of intensive and in-home crisis services for children and their families: Program outcomes. *Journal of Emotional and Behavioral Disorders, 11,* 92–102.

Faden, R., Beauchamp, T., & King, N. (1986). *History and theory of informed consent.* Oxford, UK: Oxford University Press.

Falcov, C. (1988). Learning to think culturally. In H. Liddle, D. Breunlin, & R. Schwartz (Eds.), *Handbook of family therapy training and supervision* (pp. 335–357). New York, NY: Guilford.

Fawcett, S., White, G., Balcazar, F., Suarez-Balcazar, Y., Mathews, E., Paine-Andrews, P., . . . Smith, J. F. (1994). A contextual-behavioral model of empowerment: Case studies involving people with physical disabilities. *American Journal of Community Psychology, 22,* 471–496.

Festinger, L. (1957). *A theory of cognitive dissonance.* Stanford, CA: Stanford University Press.

Fisher, C. (2004). Ethical issues in therapy: Therapist self-disclosure of sexual feelings. *Ethics & Behavior, 14*(2), 105–121.

Fisher, C., & Fried, A. (2003). Internet-mediated psychological services and the American Psychological Association ethics code. *Psychotherapy: Theory, Research, Practice, Training, 40,* 103–111.

Fisher, C., & Oransky, M. (2008). Informed consent to psychotherapy: Protecting the dignity and respecting the autonomy of client. *Journal of Clinical Psychology, 64*(5), 576–588.

Fiske, S., & Taylor, S. (1991). *Social cognition* (2nd ed.). New York, NY: McGraw-Hill.

Follesdal, D. (2001). Hermeneutics. *International Journal of Psychoanalysis, 82,* 375–379.

Ford, J., & Beveridge, A. (2004). "Bad" neighbors, fast food, "sleaky" businesses and drug dealers: Relations between the location of licit and illicit businesses and environment. *Journal of Drug Issues, 34,* 51–81.

Forehand, M., Deshpande, R., & Reed, A. (2002). Identity salience and the influence of differential activation of the social self-schema on advertising response. *Journal of Applied Psychology, 87,* 1086–1099.

Fowler, M. (2009). Preface to thematic section: Religions, spirituality, ethics and nursing. *Nursing Ethics, 16,* 391–392.

Frame, W., Flanagan, C., Gold, R., & Harris, S. (1997). You're in the hot seat: An ethical decision-making simulation for counseling students. *Simulation & Gaming, 28*(1), 107–115.

Franklin, K. (2000). Antigay behaviors among young adults: Prevalence, patterns and motivators in a non-criminal population. *Journal of Interpersonal Violence, 15*(4), 339–362.

Freeman, S. J. (2000). *Ethics: An introduction to philosophy and practice.* Belmont, CA: Wadsworth/Thomson Learning.

Freuchen, D. (Ed.). (1957). *Book of the Eskimos.* Cleveland, OH: World.

Fuertes, J. (2001). Future research directions in the study of counselor multicultural competency. *Journal of Multicultural Counseling and Development, 29,* 3–13.

Fuertes, J., & Brobst, K. (2002). Client's ratings of counselor multicultural competency. *Cultural Diversity and Ethnic Minority Psychology, 8,* 214–223.

Gabriel, L. (2005). *Speaking the unspeakable: The ethics of dual relationships in counselling and psychotherapy.* New York, NY: Routledge.

Gadamer, H. (1975). *Truth and method* (G. Barden & J. Cummings, Trans.). New York, NY: Crossroad.

Gadamer, H. (1984). *Reason in the age of science.* Cambridge, MA: MIT Press.

Gale Group. (2002, May). Key moments of Islamic civilization. *New Internationalist Magazine, 345,* 10–26.

Gallup, G., & Lindsay, D. (1999). *Surveying the religious landscape: Trends in U.S. beliefs.* Harrisburg, PA: Morehouse.

Ganote, S. (1990). A look at counseling in long term-care settings. *Generations, 14,* 31–34.

Garcia, I. (1997). *Dignidad: Ethics through Hispanic eyes.* Nashville, TN: Abington Press.

Gardner, W., Scherer, D., & Tester, M. (1989). Asserting scientific authority: Cognitive development and adolescent legal rights. *American Psychologist, 44,* 895–902.

Garner, B. (2004). *Black's law dictionary* (8th ed.). Eagan, MN: Thomson West.

Garrett, T. (2010). The prevalence of boundaries violations between mental health professionals and their clients. In F. Subotsky, S. Bewley, & M. Crow (Eds.), *Abuse of the doctor-patient relationship* (pp. 51–63). London, UK: RCPsych.

Gbadegesin, S. (2007). Origins of African ethics. In W. Schweiker (Ed.), *The Blackwell companion to religious ethics* (pp. 413–422). Indianapolis, IN: John Wiley.

Geldhart, W., & Yardley, D. (1995). *Introduction to English law.* New York, NY: Oxford University Press.

Geraerts, E., Schooler, J., Merckelbach, H., Marko, J., Hauer, B., & Ambadar, A. (2007). The reality of recovered memories: Corroborating continuous and discontinuous memories in childhood abuse. *Psychological Science, 18*(7), 564–568.

Gil, R., & Vasquez, C. (1996). *The Maria paradox: How Latinas can merge Old World traditions with New World self-esteem.* New York, NY: G. P. Putnam.

Gilligan, C. (1982). *In a different voice: Psychological theory and women's development.* Cambridge, MA: Harvard University Press.

Gladding, S. (2007). *Groups: A counseling specialty* (5th ed.). Englewood Cliffs, NJ: Prentice-Hall.

Glantz, K., Durlach, N., Barnett, R., & Aviles, W. (1996). Virtual reality (VR) for psychotherapy: From the physical to the social environment. *Psychotherapy, 33*(3), 464–473.

Gloria, A., Hird, J., & Tao, K. (2008). Self-reported multicultural supervision competence of White predoctoral intern supervisors. *Training in Education in Professional Psychology, 2*(3), 129–136.

Glosoff, H., Herlihy, B., & Spence, E. (2000). Privileged communication in the counselor-client relationship. *Journal of Counseling & Development, 78*(4), 454–462.

Glosoff, H., Herlihy, S., Herlihy, B., & Spence, E. (1997). Privileged communication in the psychologist-client relationship. *Professional Psychology: Research and Practice, 28*(6), 573–581.

Goetz, J., Keltner, D., & Simon-Thomas, E. (2010). Compassion: An evolutionary analysis and empirical review. *Psychological Bulletin, 136*(3), 351–374.

Goldstein, J., & Kornfield, J. (1987). *Seeking the heart of wisdom.* Boston, MA: Shambhala.

Gomez, M. (1994). Muslims in early America. *Journal of Southern History, 60*(4), 671–710.

Gone, J. (2004). Mental health services for Native Americans in the 21st century United States. *Professional Psychology: Research and Practice, 35,* 10–18.

Gone, J. (2010). Psychotherapy and traditional healing for American Indians: Exploring the prospects for therapeutic integration. *The Counseling Psychologist, 38,* 166–235.

Gostin, L., Lazzarini, Z., & Flaherty, K. (1995). *Legislative survey of state confidentiality laws, with specific emphasis on HIV and immunization.* Atlanta, GA: Centers for Disease Control and Prevention.

Gowers, S. (2006). Evidence-based research in CBT with adolescent eating disorders. *Child and Adolescent Mental Health, 11*(1), 9–12.

Granello, D. (2002). Assessing the cognitive development of counseling students: Changes in epistemological assumptions. *Counselor Education & Supervision, 41,* 279–292.

Green, R. M. (2005). Foundations of Jewish ethics. In W. Schweiker (Ed.), *The Blackwell companion to religious ethics* (pp. 166–175). Malden, MA: Blackwell.

Greene, J., & Baron, J. (2001). Intuitions about declining marginal utility. *Journal of Behavioral Decision Making, 14,* 243–255.

Greist, J., Gustafson, D., Strauss, F., Rowse, G., Laughren, T., & Chiles, J. (1973). A computer interview for suicide risk prediction. *American Journal of Psychiatry, 130,* 1327–1332.

Griffin-Carlson, M., & Schwanenflugel, P. (1998). Adolescent abortion and parental notification: Evidence for the importance of family functioning on the perceived quality of parental involvement in U.S. families. *Journal of Child Psychology and Psychiatry, 39,* 543–553.

Grimshaw, J. (1993). The idea of a female ethic. In P. Singer (Ed.), *A companion to ethics* (pp. 491–499). Malden, MA: Blackwell.

Grove, J. (2009). How competent are trainee and newly qualified counselors to work with lesbian, gay and bisexual clients and what do they perceive as their most effective learning experience. *Counselling & Psychotherapy Research, 9*(2), 78–85.

Gruber, E., & Anderson, M. (1990). Legislating parental involvement in adolescent abortion: Reexamining the arguments of Worthington and his colleagues. *American Psychologist, 45,* 1174–1176.

Guest, C., & Dooley, K. (1999). Supervisor malpractice: Liability to the supervisee in clinical supervision. *Counselor Education and Supervision, 39,* 269–279.

Guilamo-Ramos, V., Dittus, P., Jaccard, J., Johansson, M., Bouris, A., & Acosta, N. (2007). Parenting practices among Dominican and Puerto Rican mothers. *Social Work, 52*(1), 17–30.

Gurtman, M., & Lee, D. (2009). Sex differences in interpersonal problems: A circumplex analysis. *Psychological Assessment, 21*(4), 515–527.

Gushue, G. (2004). Race, color-blind racial attitudes, and judgments about mental health: A shifting standards perspective. *Journal of Counseling Psychology, 51,* 398–407.

Haberstroh, S., Duff, T., Evans, M., Gee, R., & Trepal, H. (2007). The experience of online counseling. *Journal of Mental Health Counseling, 29,* 269–282.

Haddad, Y. (1991). *The Muslims in America.* New York, NY: Oxford University Press.

Haddad, Y. (1999). The globalization of Islam: The return of Muslims to the West. In J. Esposito (Ed.), *The Oxford history of Islam* (pp. 549–600). Oxford, UK: Oxford University Press.

Hadjistavropoulos, T., Malloy, D., Sharpe, D., Green, S., & Fuchs-Lacelle, S. (2002). The relative importance of the ethical principles adopted by the American Psychological Association. *Canadian Psychology, 43,* 254–259.

Haidt, J. (2001). The emotional dog and its rational tail: A social intuitionist approach to moral judgment. *Psychological Review, 108*(4), 814–834.

Haidt, J. (2010). Moral psychology must not be based on faith and hope: Commentary on Narvaez. *Perspectives on Psychological Science, 5*(2), 182–184.

Haidt, J., & Bjorkland, F. (2007). Social intuitionists answer six questions about moral psychology. In W. Sinnott-Armstrong (Ed.), *Moral psychology: Vol. 2. The cognitive science of morality: Intuition and diversity* (pp. 182–217). Boston, MA: MIT Press.

Hall, A., & Lin, M. (1994). An integrative consultation framework: A practical tool for elementary school counselors. *Elementary School Guidance & Counseling, 29*(1), 16–27.

Halperin, D. (2003). The normalization of queer theory. *Journal of Homosexuality, 45*(2/4), 339–343.

Hamilton, P. (2008). The educational psychologist and primary prevention or a "shotgun wedding." *Educational and Child Psychology, 25*(4), 26–33.

Hansen, C. (1992). *A Daoist theory of Chinese thought: A philosophical interpretation.* New York, NY: Oxford University Press.

Hansen, J. (2010). Consequences of the postmodernist vision: Diversity as the guiding value for the counseling profession. *Journal of Counseling & Development, 88*(1), 101–107.

Hardy, S., & Carlo, G. (2005). Identity as a source of moral motivation. *Human Development, 48*(4), 232–256.

Hare, R. (1991). The philosophical basis of psychiatric ethics. In S. Block & P. Chodoff (Eds.), *Psychiatric ethics* (2nd ed., pp. 14–42). Oxford, UK: Oxford University Press.

Harlow, H. (1958). The nature of love. *American Psychologist, 13*(12), 673–685.

Harris, C. (1997). *Applying moral theories* (3rd ed.). Belmont, CA: Wadsworth.

Harris, C. E. (2002). *Applying moral theories* (4th ed.). Belmont, CA: Wadsworth.

Harris, C. E. (2007). *Applying moral theories* (5th ed.). Belmont, CA: Wadsworth.

Harris, M., & Mertlich, D. (2003). Piloting home-based behavioral family systems therapy for adolescents with poorly controlled diabetes. *Children's Health Care, 32,* 65–79.

Harris, S., Kemmerling, R., & North, M. (2002). Brief virtual reality therapy for public speaking anxiety. *Cyberpsychology & Behavior, 5*(6), 543–550.

Harrison, L. (1956). The Oslo study of untreated syphilis: Review and commentary. *British Journal of Venereal Diseases, 32,* 70–79.

Hart, D. (2005). Adding identity to the moral domain. *Human Development, 48*(4), 257–261.

Hartung, C., & Widiger, T. (1998). Gender differences in the diagnosis of mental disorders: Conclusions and controversies of the DSM-IV. *Psychological Bulletin, 123,* 260–278.

Hassouneh-Phillips, D. (2001). Polygamy and wife abuse: A qualitative study of Muslim women in America. *Healthcare for Women International, 22,* 735–748.

Hathaway, W. (2002). Integration as interpretation: A hermeneutical-realist view. *Journal of Psychology and Christianity, 21,* 205–218.

Hathaway, W., Scott, S., & Garvey, S. (2004). Assessing religious/spiritual functioning: A neglected domain in clinical practice? *Professional Psychology: Research and Practice, 35,* 97–104.

Hauser, M. (2006). *Moral minds: The nature of right and wrong.* New York, NY: Harper Perennial.

Heaven, P., & Oxman, L. (1999). Human values, conservatism and stereotypes of homosexuals. *Personality and Individual Differences, 27,* 109–118.

Hein, L., & Matthews, A. (2010). Reparative therapy: The adolescent, the psych nurse, and the issues. *Journal of Child and Adolescent Psychiatric Nursing, 23*(1), 29–35.

Held, V. (1987). Feminism and moral theory. In E. Kittay & D. Meyers (Eds.), *Women and moral theory* (pp. 111–128). Totowa, NJ: Rowman & Littlefield.

Hendey, N., & Pascall, G. (1998). Independent living: Gender, violence, and the threat of violence. *Disability and Society, 13,* 415–427.

Hendrick, S. (1990). A client perspective on counselor disclosure. *Journal of Counseling & Development, 69*(2), 184–185.

Hendricks, C. (2008). Introduction: Who are we? The role of ethics in shaping counselor Identity. *Family Journal: Counseling and Therapy for Couples and Families, 16*(3), 258–260.

Henkelman, J., & Everall, R. (2001). Informed consent with children: Ethical and practical implications. *Canadian Journal of Counseling, 35*(2), 109–121.

Henry, C. (1996). Taking an ethical position on standards. *British Journal of Guidance and Counselling, 24,* 35–45.

Herlihy, B., Gray, N., & McCollum, V. (2002). Legal and ethical issues in school counselor supervision. *Professional School Counseling, 6,* 55–61.

Herlihy, B., & Sheeley, V. (1987). Privileged communication in selected helping professions: A comparison among statutes. *Journal of Counseling & Development, 65*(9), 479–483.

Herrera, C. (2006). Restraint use and autonomy in psychiatric care. *Journal of Ethics in Mental Health, 1*(1), 1–4.

Hilton, N., Harris, G., & Rice, M. (2001). Predicting violence by serious wife assaulters. *Journal of Interpersonal Violence, 16,* 408–423.

Hite, R., & Fraser, C. (1988). Meta-analyses of attitudes toward advertising by professionals. *Journal of Marketing, 52,* 95–105.

Hoffman, M. (1975). Developmental synthesis of affect and cognition and its implications for altruistic motivation. *Developmental Psychology, 11,* 607–622.

Hoffman, M. (1981). Is altruism part of human nature? *Journal of Personality and Social Psychology, 40*(1), 121–137.

Hoffman, M. (2000). *Empathy and moral development.* Cambridge, UK: Cambridge University Press.

Horowitz, L., Wilson, K., Turan, B., Zolotsev, P., & Constantino, M. (2006). How interpersonal motives clarify the meaning of interpersonal behavior: A revised circumplex model. *Personality and Social Psychology Review, 10*(1), 67–86.

Hourani, G. (1971). *Islamic rationalism: The ethics of Abd al-Jabbar.* Oxford, UK: Clarendon Press.

Houser, R. (2009). *Counseling and educational research: Evaluation and application.* Thousand Oaks, CA: Sage.

Houser, R., & Domokos-Cheng Ham, M. (2004). *Gaining power and control through diversity and group affiliation.* Westport, CT: Praeger.

Houser, R., Hampton, N., & Carriker, C. (2000). Implementing the empowerment concept in rehabilitation: Contributions of social role theory. *Journal of Applied Rehabilitation Counseling, 31*(2), 18–23.

Houser, R., Wilczenski, F. L., & Ham, M. (2006). *Culturally relevant ethical decision-making in counseling.* Thousand Oaks, CA: Sage.

Huebner, B., Lee, J., & Hauser, M. (2010). The moral-conventional distinction in mature moral competence. *Journal of Cognition and Culture, 10*(1/2), 1–26.

Hunsberger, B., Owusu, V., & Duck, R. (1999). Religion and prejudice in Ghana and Canada: Religious fundamentalism, right-wing authoritarianism, and attitudes toward homosexuals and women. *International Journal for the Psychology of Religion, 9,* 181–194.

Hunsley, J. (2007). Addressing the key challenges in evidence-based practice in psychology. *Professional Psychology: Research and Practice, 38*(2), 113–121.

Huprich, S., Fuller, K., & Schneider, R. (2003). Divergent ethical perspectives on the duty-to-warn principle with HIV patients. In D. Bersoff (Ed.), *Ethical conflicts in psychology* (4th ed., pp. 207–213). Washington, DC: American Psychological Association.

Ibrahim, F. (1996). A multicultural perspective on principle and virtue ethics. *The Counseling Psychologist, 24,* 78–85.

Ingersoll, R. (2000). Teaching a psychopharmacology course to counselors: Justification structure, and methods. *Counselor Education and Supervision, 40,* 58–69.

Isaacs, M., & Stone, C. (2001). Confidentiality with minors: Mental health counselors' attitudes toward breaching or preserving confidentiality. *Journal of Mental Health Counseling, 23,* 342–357.

Jaffee, S. (2002). Pathways to adversity in young adulthood among early childbearers. *Journal of Family Psychology, 16,* 38–49.

Jagose, A. (2009). Feminism's queer theory. *Feminism & Psychology, 19*(2), 157–174.

Johansson, I., & Lundman, B. (2002). Patients' experience of involuntary psychiatric care. *Journal of Psychiatric and Mental Health Nursing, 9,* 639–647.

Johnson, S., Podratz, K., Dipboye, R., & Gibbons, E. (2010). Physical attractiveness biases in ratings of employment suitability: Tracking down the "beauty is beastly" effect. *Journal of Social Psychology, 15*(3), 301–318.

Jones, G., & Stokes, A. (2009). *Online counseling: A handbook for practitioners.* New York, NY: Macmillan.

Jones, W., & Markos, P. (1997). Client rating of counselor effectiveness: A call for caution. *Journal of Applied Rehabilitation Counseling, 29,* 23–28.

Jordon, A., & Meara, N. (1990). Ethics and professional practice of psychologists: The role of virtues and principles. *Professional Psychology: Research and Practice, 21,* 107–114.

Kagan, J. (2005). Human morality and temperament. In C. Gustavo (Ed.), *Moral motivation through the life span* (pp. 1–32). Lincoln: University of Nebraska Press.

Kahneman, D., & Klein, G. (2009). Conditions for intuitive expertise. *American Psychologist, 64*(6), 515–526.

Kaiser, A. (2007). Addressing challenging behavior: Systematic problems, systematic solutions. *Journal of Early Intervention, 29,* 114–118.

Kaiser, A., & McIntyre, L. (2010). Editorial: Introduction to special section on evidence-based practices for persons with intellectual and developmental disabilities. *American Journal on Intellectual and Developmental Disabilities, 115*(5), 357–363.

Kanel, K. (2003). *Manual to accompany a guide to crisis intervention* (2nd ed.). Pacific Grove, CA: Brooks/Cole.

Kant, I. (1953). *The moral law; or groundwork of the metaphysic of morals* (Rev. ed., H. Patton, Trans.). London, UK: Hutchinson. (Original work published 1785)

Keel, P., & Haedt, A. (2008). Evidence-based psychosocial treatments for eating problems and eating disorders. *Journal of Clinical Child & Adolescent Psychology, 37*(1), 39–61.

Keller, P., & Block, L. (1999). The effect of affect-based dissonance versus cognition-based dissonance on motivated reasoning and health-related persuasion. *Journal of Experimental Psychology, Applied, 5*(3), 302–313.

Kelly, M. (1984). *Islam: The religious and political life of a world community.* Westport, CT: Praeger.

Keltner, D., & Haidt, J. (2003). Approaching awe, a moral, spiritual and aesthetic emotion. *Cognition & Emotion, 17*(2), 297–315.

Keown, D. (2005). *Buddhist ethics: A short introduction.* New York, NY: Oxford University Press.

Kermani, E., & Drob, S. (1987). Tarasoff decision: A decade later dilemma still faces psychotherapists. *American Journal of Psychotherapy, 41,* 271–285.

Kettlewell, P. (2004). Development, dissemination, and implementation of evidence-based treatments: Commentary. *Clinical Psychology: Science and Practice, 11*(2), 190–194.

Kiesler, D. (1983). The 1982 interpersonal circle: A taxonomy for complementarity in human transactions. *Psychological Review, 90*(3), 185–212.

Killen, M., & Smetana, J. (Eds.). (2006). *Handbook of moral psychology* (pp. 67–91). Mahwah, NJ: Lawrence Erlbaum.

Kim, B., Hill, C., Gelso, C., Goates, M., Asay, P., & Harbin, J. (2003). Counselor self-disclosure, East Asian American client adherence to Asian cultural values and counseling process. *Journal of Counseling Psychology, 50*(3), 324–332.

Kim, B., & Lyons, H. (2003). Experiential activities and multicultural competence training. *Journal of Counseling and Development, 81,* 400–409.

Kinzbrunner, B. (2004). Jewish medical ethics and end-of-life care. *Journal of Palliative Medicine, 7*(4), 558–573.

Kirk-Greene, A. (2001). The concept of the good man in Hausa. In E. Eze (Ed.), *African philosophy: An anthology* (pp. 121–129). Chicago, IL: Encyclopedia Britannica.

Knapp, S. (1999). Utilitarianism and the ethics of professional psychologists. *Ethics and Behavior, 9,* 383–393.

Knapp, S., Gottlieb, M., Berman, J., & Handelsman, M. (2007). When laws and ethics collide: What should psychologists do? *Professional Psychology: Research and Practice, 38*(1), 54–59.

Kocarek, C., Talbot, D., Batka, J., & Anderson, M. (2001). Reliability and validity of three measures of multicultural competency. *Journal of Counseling and Development, 79,* 486–498.

Kohlberg, L. (1969). Stage and sequence: The cognitive-development approach to socialization. In D. A. Goslin (Ed.), *Handbook of socialization theory and research* (pp. 347–480). Chicago, IL: Rand McNally.

Kohlberg, L. (1984a). *Essays on moral development: Vol. 2. The psychology of moral development: Moral stages, their nature and validity.* San Francisco, CA: Harper & Row.

Kohlberg, L. (1984b). *The psychology of moral development: The nature and validity of moral stages.* San Francisco, CA: Harper & Row.

Kohlberg, L., & Hersh, R. (1977). Moral development: A review of the theory. *Theory Into Practice, 16*(2), 53–59.

Kohn, L. (2001). *Daoism and Chinese culture.* Cambridge. MA: Three Pines Press.

Kollar, I., Fischer, F., & Hesse, F. (2006). Collaboration scripts: A conceptual analysis. *Educational Psychology Review, 18,* 159–185.

Kottler, J. (1986). *On being a therapist.* San Francisco, CA: Jossey-Bass.

Krishnamurthy, R., VandeCreek, L., Kaslow, N., Tazeau, Y., Miville, M., Kerns, R., . . . Benton, S. (2004). Achieving competency in psychological assessment: Directions for education and training. *Journal of Clinical Psychology, 60*(7), 725–739.

Kropp, P., Hart, S., Webster, C., & Eaves, D. (1999). *Manual for the spousal assault risk assessment guide.* Toronto, Canada: Multi-Health Systems.

Kuntze, M., Stoermer, R., Mueller-Spahn, F., & Bullinger, A. (2002). Ethical codes and values in a virtual world. *Cyber Psychology and Behavior, 5,* 203–206.

Kurtines, W., & Gewritz, J. (1987). *Moral development through social interaction.* New York, NY: John Wiley.

Kuykendall, R., & Day, A. (1967). *Hawaii: A history, from Polynesian kingdom to American state.* Englewood Cliffs, NJ: Prentice Hall.

Ladany, N., & Bradley, L. (2010). *Counselor supervision* (4th ed.). New York, NY: Routledge.

Ladany, N., Lehman-Waterman, D., Molinaro, M., & Wolgast, B. (1999). Psychotherapy supervisor ethical practices: Adherence to guidelines, the supervisory working alliance, and supervisee satisfaction. *The Counseling Psychologist, 27,* 443–475.

Lafferty, P., Beutler, L., & Crago, M. (1989). Differences between more and less effective psychotherapists: A study of select therapist variables. *Journal of Consulting and Clinical Psychology, 57*(1), 76–80.

Lakin, M. (1988). *Ethical issues in psychotherapy.* New York, NY: Oxford University Press.

Lamb, D., & Catanzaro, S. (1998). *Ethical issues in psychotherapy.* New York, NY: Oxford University Press.

Lamb, D., Catanzaro, S., & Moorman, A. (2003). Psychologists reflect on their sexual relationships with clients, supervisees, and students: Occurrence, impact, rationales and collegial intervention. *Professional Psychology, Research and Practice, 34*(1), 102–107.

Lange, A., & Rietdijk, D. (2003). Interapy: A controlled randomized trial of the standardization treatment of posttraumautic stress through the Internet. *Journal of Consulting and Clinical Psychology, 71,* 901–909.

Lanza, M. (2001). Setting fees: The conscious and unconscious meaning of money. *Perspectives in Psychiatric Care, 37,* 69–72.

Lawrence, G., & Robinson Kurpius, S. (2000). Legal and ethical issues involved when counseling minors in non school settings. *Journal of Counseling and Development, 78,* 130–137.

Leeder, E. (1996). Speaking rich people's words: Implications of a feminist class analysis and psychotherapy. In M. Hill & E. Rothblum (Eds.), *Classism and feminist therapy: Counting costs* (pp. 45–58). New York, NY: Haworth.

Leibert, T., Archer, A., Munson, M., & York, Y. (2006). An exploratory study of client perceptions of Internet counseling and the therapeutic alliance. *Journal of Mental Health Counseling, 28,* 69–83.

Levin, B. (2002). From slavery to hate crime laws: The emergence of race and status-based protection in American criminal law. *Journal of Social Issues, 58,* 227–245.

Lewis, M. (2008). Familias in the heartland: Exploration of the social, economic, and cultural realities of Latino immigrants. *Families in Society, 89*(2), 193–201.

Liebman, C., & Fishman, S. (2000). Jewish communal policy toward outmarried families. *Journal of Jewish Communal Service, 77,* 117–127.

Liebowitz, A., Eisen, M., & Chow, W. (1984). *An economic model of teenage pregnancy decision making* (Research Report No. 5.009). Austin: University of Texas Population Research Center.

Lilienfeld, S. (2007). Psychological treatments that cause harm. *Perspectives on Psychological Science, 2,* 53–68.

Limb, G., & Hodge, D. (2009). Utilizing spiritual ecograms with Native American families and children to promote cultural competence in family therapy. *Journal of Marital and Family Therapy, 37*(1), 81–94.

Linzer, N. (1992). The role of values in determining agency policy. *Journal of Contemporary Human Services, 73*(9), 553–558.

Littrell, J., & Littrell, M. (1982). American Indian and Caucasian students' preferences for counselors: Effects of counselor dress and sex. *Journal of Counseling Psychology, 29,* 48–57.

Lombardi, F., & Lombardi, G. (1982). *Circle without end.* Happy Camp, CA: Naturegraph.

Lorant, V., Deliege, D., Eaton, W., Robert, A., Philipott, P., & Ansseau, M. (2003). Socioeconomic inequalities in depression: A meta-analysis. *American Journal of Epidemiology, 157,* 98–112.

Lunt, I. (1999). The professionalization of psychology in Europe. *European Psychologist, 4,* 240–247.

Lyons, C., & Hazler, R. (2002). The influence of student development level on improving counselor student empathy. *Counselor Education & Supervision, 42,* 119–130.

Magnuson, S., Norem, K., & Wilcoxon, A. (2000). Clinical supervision of prelicensed counselors: Recommendations for consideration and practice. *Journal of Mental Health Counseling, 22,* 176–190.

Mahalik, J., Van Ormer, A., & Simi, N. (2000). Ethical issues in using self-disclosure in feminist therapy. In M. Brabeck (Ed.), *Practicing feminist ethics in psychology* (pp. 189–201). Washington, DC: American Psychological Association.

Maheu, M. (2003). The online clinical practice management model. *Psychotherapy: Theory, Research, Practice, Training, 40,* 20–32.

Mallen, M., & Vogel, D. (2005). Introduction to the major contribution: Counseling psychology and online counseling. *The Counseling Psychologist, 33,* 761–774.

Manese, J., Wu, J., & Nepomuceno, C. (2001). The effect of training on multicultural counseling competencies: An exploratory study over a ten-year period. *Journal of Multicultural Counseling and Development, 29*(1), 31–40.

Mantovani, F., Castelnuovo, G., Gaggiioli, A., & Riva, G. (2003). Virtual reality training for health-care professionals. *Cyberpsychology & Behavior, 6*(4), 389–395.

Margolin, G., Gordis, E., Medina, A., & Oliver, P. (2003). The co-occurrence of husband-to-wife aggression, family-of-origin aggression, and child abuse potential in a community sample. *Journal of Interpersonal Violence, 18,* 413–440.

Markey, P., & Markey, C. (2010). Vulnerability to violent video games: A review and integration of personality research. *Review of General Psychology, 14*(2), 82–91.

Marshall, J. (2001). *The Lakota way: Stories and lessons for living.* New York, NY: Viking Compass.

Martin, J., & Thompson, J. (2003). Psychotherapy as in interpretation of being: Hermeneutic perspectives on psychotherapy. *Journal of Constructivist Psychology, 16,* 1–16.

Maslach, C., & Jackson, S. (1981). The measurement of experienced burnout. *Journal of Occupational Behavior, 2,* 99–113.

Maslach, C., Schaufeli, W., & Leiter, M. (2001). Job burnout. *Annual Review of Psychology, 52,* 397–422.

Massachusetts Department of Children and Families. (2009). *Child abuse & neglect reporting: A guide for mandated reporters.* Boston: Massachusetts Department of Children and Families.

Mayer, D. (2004). *Essential evidence-based medicine.* New York, NY: Cambridge University Press.

Mbiti, J. (1969). *African religions and philosophy.* London, UK: Henemann.

McCabe, D. (1993). Faculty responses to academic dishonesty: The influence of student honor codes. *Research in Higher Education, 34,* 647–658.

McCarthy, P. (1982). Differential effects of counselor self-referent responses and counselor status. *Journal of Counseling Psychology, 29*(2), 125–131.

McCullough, L. (1983). The development of a microcomputer based information system for psychotherapy research. *Problem Oriented Systems & Treatment Post, 6*(1), 3–4.

McDaniel, M. (2006). In the eye of the beholder: The role of reporters in bringing families to the attention of child protective services. *Children and Youth Services Review, 28*(3), 306–324.

McLeod, J. (1992). What do we know about how best to assess counselor competence? *Counseling Psychology Quarterly, 5,* 359–373.

Melton, G. (1990). Knowing what we do know: APA and adolescent abortion. *American Psychologist, 45,* 1171–1173.

Merriam, S., Courtenay, B., & Baumgartner, L. (2003). On becoming a witch: Learning in a marginalized community of practice. *Adult Education Quarterly, 53,* 170–188.

Merriam-Webster's Collegiate Dictionary (11th ed.). (2005). Springfield, MA: Merriam-Webster.

Merskey, H. (1996). Ethical issues in the search for repressed memories. *American Journal of Psychotherapy, 50,* 323–336.

Meyer, H., Taiminen, T., Vuori, T., Aijala, A., & Helenius, H. (1999). Posttraumatic stress disorder symptoms related to psychosis and acute involuntary hospitalization in schizophrenic and delusional patients. *Journal of Nervous and Mental Disease, 187*(6), 343–351.

Meyerbroker, K., & Emmelkamp, P. (2010). Virtual reality exposure therapy in anxiety disorders: A systematic review of process-and-outcome studies. *Depression and Anxiety, 27,* 933–944.

Meyersburg, C., Bogdan, R., Gallo, D., & McNally, R. (2009). False memory propensity in people reporting recovered memories of past lives. *Journal of Abnormal Psychology, 118*(2), 399–404.

Milan, S., Ickovics, J., Kershaw, T., Lewis, J., Meade, C., & Eithier, K. (2004). Prevalence, course, and predictors of emotional distress in pregnant and parenting adolescents. *Journal of Consulting and Clinical Psychology, 72,* 328–340.

Mill, J. (1863). *Utilitarianism.* London, UK: Parker, Son and Bourn.

Mitchell, D. (2002). *Buddhism: Introducing the Buddhist experience.* New York, NY: Oxford University Press.

Moldoveanu, M., & Stevenson, H. (1998). Ethical universals in practice: An analysis of five principles. *Journal of Socio-Economics, 27,* 721–753.

Momaday, N. (1987). *The names: A memoir.* Tucson: University of Arizona Press.

Moore-Thomas, C., & Day-Vines, N. (2010). Culturally competent collaboration: School counselor collaboration with African-American families and communities. *Professional School Counseling, 14*(1), 53–62.

Morgan, D. (2001). *The best guide to Eastern philosophy and religion.* New York, NY: St. Martin's Griffin.

Morland, I., & Willox, A. (2005). *Queer theory.* New York: NY: Palgrave Macmillan.

Morrison, J., Clutter, S., Pritchett, E., & Demmitt, A. (2009). Perceptions of clients and counseling professionals regarding spirituality in counseling. *Counseling and Values, 53,* 183–194.

Morton, K., Worthley, J., Testerman, J., & Mahoney, M. (2006). Defining features of moral sensitivity and moral motivation: Pathways to moral reasoning in medical students. *Journal of Moral Education, 35*(3), 387–406.

Muratori, M. (2001). Examining supervisor impairment from the counselor trainee's perspective. *Counselor Education and Supervision, 41,* 41–56.

Murphy, L., & Mitchell, D. (1998). When writing helps to heal: E-mail as therapy. *British Journal of Guidance and Counseling, 26*(1), 21–32.

Myers, D., & Hayes, J. (2006). Effects of therapist general self-disclosure and countertransference disclosure on ratings of the therapist and session. *Psychotherapy: Theory, Research, Practice, Training, 45*(2), 173–185.

Narvaez, D., & Vaydich, J. (2008). Moral development and behavior under the spotlight in the neurobiological sciences. *Journal of Moral Education, 37*(3), 289–313.

National Career Development Association. (2007). *Code of ethics.* Broken Arrow, OK: Author.

Neimeyer, G., Taylor, J., & Wear, D. (2010). Continuing education in psychology: Patterns of participation and aspects of selection. *Professional Psychology: Research and Practice, 41*(4), 281–287.

Neukrug, E., & Lowell, C. (1996). Employing ethical codes and ethical decision-making models: A developmental process. *Counseling and Values, 40,* 98–104.

Neukrug, E., Milliken, T., & Walden, S. (2001). Ethical complaints made against credentialed counselors: An updated survey of state licensing boards. *Counselor Education and Supervision, 41,* 57–71.

Neville, H., Spanierman, L., & Doan, B. (2006). Exploring the association between color-blind racial ideology and multicultural counseling competencies. *Cultural Diversity and Ethnic Minority Psychology, 12*(2), 275–290.

New York Office of Children & Family Services. (2002). *Summary guide for mandated reporters in New York State* (Publication No. 1159). Albany: Author.

Nicolosi, J., Byrd, D., & Potts, R. (2000). Retrospective self-reports of changes in sexual orientation: A consumer survey of conversion therapy clients. *Psychological Reports, 86,* 1071–1088.

Nodding, N. (2003). *Caring: A feminine approach to ethics and moral education* (2nd ed.). Berkeley: University of California Press.

Norcross, J., Hedges, M., & Prochaska, J. (2002). The face of 2010: A Delphi poll on the future of psychotherapy. *Professional Psychology: Research and Practice, 33*(3), 316–322.

Novicevic, M., Harvey, M., Budkley, R., & Fung, H. (2008). Self-evaluation bias of social comparisons in ethical decision making: The impact of accountability. *Journal of Applied Social Psychology, 38*(4), 1061–1091.

Nyman, S., & Daugherty, T. (2001). Congruence of counselor self-disclosure and perceived effectiveness. *Journal of Psychology, 135*(3), 269–276.

Nystul, M. (1999). *Integrative approach to teaching counseling psychology.* Boston, MA: Allyn & Bacon.

Occupational Information Network. (n.d.). Retrieved from http://www.onetonline.org/

O'Dell, J., & Dickson, J. (1984). ELIZA as a "therapeutic" tool. *Journal of Clinical Psychology, 40*(4), 942–945.

Office of Civil Rights. (2003). *OCR privacy brief: Summary of the HIPAA privacy rule.* Washington, DC: Author.

Okamoto, S. (2003). The function of professional boundaries in the therapeutic relationship between male practitioners and female youth clients. *Child and Adolescent Social Work Journal, 20,* 303–313.

Oldstone-Moore, J. (2002). *Confucianism.* New York, NY: Oxford University Press.

Omonzejele, P. (2005). *African ethics and voluntary euthanasia.* Retrieved from http://216.239.51.104/search?q=cache:F9WgOjC3aGIJ:www.ruhr-uni-bochum.de/zme/healthliteracy/africanethics.pdf+african+ethics+and+vountary+euthanasia&hl=en

Osborn, C. (2004). Seven salutary suggestions for counselor stamina. *Journal of Counseling & Development, 82,* 319–328.

Ottens, A., Shank, G., & Long, R. (1995). The role of adjective logic in understanding and using advanced empathy. *Counselor Education and Supervision, 34*(3), 199–211.

Oveis, C., Horberg, E., & Keltner, D. (2010). Compassion, pride, and social intuitions of self-other similarity. *Journal of Personality and Social Psychology, 98*(4), 618–630.

Owen, J., Wong, Y., & Rodolfa, E. (2009). Empirical search for psychotherapists' gender competence in psychotherapy. *Psychotherapy: Theory, Research, Practice, Training, 46*(4), 448–458.

Ozer, E., & Bandura, A. (1990). Mechanisms governing empowerment effects: A self-efficacy analysis. *Journal of Personality and Social Psychology, 58,* 472–486.

Pandey, S., Zhan, M., & Collier-Tenison, S. (2004). Families' experience with welfare reform on reservations in Arizona. *Social Work Research, 28,* 93–103.

Park, Y., Kim, B., Chiang, J., & Ju, C. (2010). Acculturation, enculturation, parental adherence to Asian cultural values, parenting styles, and family conflicts among Asian American college students. *Asian American Journal of Psychology, 1*(1), 67–79.

Parsons, T. (1961). *Theories of society: Foundations of modern sociological theory.* New York, NY: Free Press.

Pearson, B., & Piazza, N. (1997). Classification of dual relationships in the helping professions. *Counselor Education and Supervision, 37*(2), 89–99.

Pederson, P. (1998). *Multiculturalism as a fourth force.* Levittown, PA: Brunner/Mazel.

Pedersen, P. (2007). Ethics, competence, and professional issues in cross-cultural counseling. In P. Pedersen, W. Lonner, J. Draguns, & J. Trimble (Eds.), *Counseling across cultures* (pp. 5–20). Thousand Oaks, CA: Sage.

Perkins, D., Hudson, B., Gray, D., & Stewart, M. (1998). Decisions and justifications by community mental health providers about hypothetical ethical dilemmas. *Psychiatric Services, 49*(10), 1317–1322.

Peterson, C., & Seligman, M. (2004). *Character strengths and virtues: A handbook and classification.* Washington, DC: American Psychological Association and Oxford University Press.

Piaget, J. (1932). *The moral judgment of the child* (M. Gabain, Trans). New York, NY: Free Press.

Pinsoneault, T. (1996). Rationally developed fake-good and fake-bad scales for the Jesness Inventory. *Journal of Psychopathology and Behavioral Assessment, 18*(3), 255–273.

Pipes, R., Holstein, J., & Aguirre, M. (2005). Examining the personal-professional distinction: Ethics codes and the difficulty of drawing a boundary. *American Psychologist, 60*(4), 325–334.

Plato. (1956). *Euthyphro, Apology, Crito* (F. Church, Trans.). New York, NY: Liberal Arts Press.

Ponton, R., & Duba, J. (2009). The ACA code of ethics: Articulating counseling's professional covenant. *Journal of Counseling & Development, 87,* 117–121.

Pope, J., & Arthur, N. (2009). Socioeconomic status and class: A challenge for the practice of psychology in Canada. *Counseling Psychology, 50*(2), 55–65.

Pope, K., Tabachmick, B., & Keith-Spiegel, P. (1987). Ethics of practice: The beliefs and behaviors of psychologists as therapists. *American Psychologist, 42,* 993–1006.

Prochaska, J., & Norcross, J. (2010). *Systems of psychotherapy: A transtheoretical analysis.* Belmont, CA: Brooks/Cole.

Rachels, J. (1998). *The elements of moral philosophy.* New York, NY: McGraw-Hill.

Radhakrishnan, S. (1922). The Hindu dharma. *International Journal of Ethics, 33*(1), 1–22.

Ragusea, A., & VandeCreek, L. (2003). Suggestions for the ethical practice of online psychotherapy. *Psychotherapy: Theory, Research, Practice, Training, 40,* 94-102.

Rassau, A., & Arco, L. (2003). Effects of chat-based online cognitive behavior therapy on study related behavior and anxiety. *Behavioural and Cognitive Psychotherapy, 31,* 377–381.

Reese, L. (2001). Morality and identity in Mexican immigrant parents' visions of the future. *Journal of Ethnic and Migration Studies, 27,* 455–472.

Remley, T., & Herlihy, B. (2005). *Ethical, legal, and professional issues in counseling* (2nd ed.). Upper Saddle River, NJ: Merrill Prentice Hall.

Rennison, C., & Welchans, S. (2002). *Intimate partner violence.* Washington, DC: U.S. Department of Justice.

Rest, J. (1983). Morality. In P. Mussen (Ed.), *Handbook of child psychology* (4th ed., pp. 560–629). New York, NY: John Wiley.

Rest, J. (1984). Research on moral development: Implications for training counseling psychologists. *Counseling Psychologist, 12,* 19–29.

Rest, J. (1986). *Moral development.* New York, NY: Praeger.

Rest, J., & Narvaez, D. (1994). Summary—What's possible? In J. R. Rest & D. Narvaez (Eds.), *Moral development in the professions: Psychology and applied ethics* (pp. 213–224). Hillsdale, NJ: Lawrence Erlbaum.

Rest, J., Narvaez, D., Bebeau, M., & Thoma, S. (1999a). A neo-Kohlbergian approach to moral judgment: An overview of Defining Issues Test research. *Educational Psychology Review, 11*(4), 291–324.

Rest, J., Narvaez, D., Bebeau, M., & Thoma, S. (1999b). *Postconventional moral thinking: A neo-Kohlbergian approach.* Mahwah, NJ: Lawrence Erlbaum.

Reynolds, S., & Ceranic, T. (2007). The effects of moral judgment and moral identity on moral behavior: An empirical examination of the moral individual. *Journal of Applied Psychology, 92*(6), 1610–1624.

Richards, M. (2009). Electronic medical records: Confidentiality issues in the time of HIPAA. *Professional Psychology: Research and Practice, 40*(6), 550–556.

Riva, G. (2009). Virtual reality: An experiential tool for clinical psychology. *British Journal of Guidance & Counselling, 37*(3), 337–345.

Riva, G., & Vincelli, F. (2001). Virtual reality as an advanced imaginal system: A new experiential approach for counseling and therapy. *International Journal of Action Methods: Psychodrama, Skill Training, and Role Playing, 54*(2), 51–64.

Roberts, A., Monferrari, I., & Yeager, K. (2008). Avoiding malpractice lawsuits by following risk assessment and suicide prevention guidelines. *Brief Treatment and Crisis Intervention, 8*(1), 5–14.

Roberts, M., Borden, K., Christiansen, M., & Lopez, S. (2005). Fostering a culture shift: Assessment of competence in the education and careers of professional psychologists. *Professional Psychology: Research and Practice, 36*(4), 355–361.

Robiner, W., Fuhrman, M., & Bobbitt, B. (1990). Supervision in the practice of psychology: Toward the development of a supervisory instrument. *Psychotherapy in Private Practice, 8*(1), 87–98.

Robinet, I. (1997). *Taoism: Growth of a religion.* Palo Alto, CA: Stanford University Press.

Rochlen, A., Land, L., & Wong, Y. (2004). Male restrictive emotionality and evaluations of online versus face-to-face counseling. *Psychology of Men and Masculinity, 5,* 190–200.

Rochlen, A., Zack, J., & Speyer, C. (2004). Online therapy: Review of relevant definitions, debates, and current empirical support. *Journal of Clinical Psychology, 60,* 269–283.

Rodolfa, E., Bent, R., Eisman, E., Nelson, P., Rehm, L., & Ritchie, P. (2005). A cube model for competency development: Implications for psychology educators and regulators. *Professional Psychology: Research and Practice, 36*(4), 347–354.

Ronnestad, M., & Skovholt, T. (1993). Supervision of beginning and advanced graduate students of counseling and psychotherapy. *Journal of Counseling & Development, 71*(4), 396–405.

Ronnestad, M., & Skovholt, T. (2003). The journey of the counselor and therapist: Research findings and perspectives on professional development. *Journal of Career Development, 30*(1), 5–42.

Rosenbaum, A., & Leisring, P. (2003). Beyond power and control: Towards an understanding of partner abusive men. *Journal of Comparative Family Studies, 34,* 7–22.

Ross, M. (1989). Feminism and the problem of moral character. *Journal of Feminist Studies in Religion, 5,* 57.

Rousseau, D., & McCarthy, S. (2007). Educating managers from an evidence-based perspective. *Academy of Management Learning & Education, 6*(1), 84–101.

Rozin, P., Haidt, J., & McCauley, C. (1993). Disgust. In M. Lewis & J. Haviland (Eds.), *Handbook of emotions* (pp. 575–594). New York, NY: Guilford.

Rubel, D., & Ratts, M. (2011). Diversity and social justice issues in counseling and psychotherapy. In D. Capuzzi & D. Gross (Eds.), *Counseling and psychotherapy* (5th ed.). Alexandria, VA: American Counseling Association.

Rubin, S., & Roessler, R. (2008). *Foundations of the vocational rehabilitation process* (6th ed.). Austin, TX: Pro-Ed.

Ruggiero, V. (2004). *Thinking critically about ethical issues* (6th ed.). Boston, MA: McGraw-Hill.

Rule, J., & Bebeau, M. (2005). *Dentists who care: Inspiring stories of professional commitment.* Hanover Park, IL: Quintessence.

Russell, G. (1996). Internalized classim: The role of class in the development of self. In M. Hill & E. Rothblum (Eds.), *Classism and feminist therapy: Counting costs* (pp. 59–72). New York, NY: Haworth.

Rutter, P., Estrada, D., Ferguson, L., & Diggs, G. (2008). Sexual orientation and counselor competency: The impact of training on enhancing awareness, knowledge and skills. *Journal of LGBT Issues in Counseling, 2*(2), 109–125.

Saccuzzo, D. (2002). *Liability for failure to supervise adequately: Let the master beware.* San Diego: California School of Law.

Saccuzzo, D. (2005). *Liability for failure to supervise adequately: Let the master beware.* Retrieved from e-psychologist.nationalregister.org/module14.pdf

Sackett, D., Rosenberg, W., Gray, W., Haynes, R., & Richardson S. (1996). Evidence based medicine: What it is and what it isn't. *British Medical Journal, 312,* 71–72.

Saltzstein, H., & Kasachkoff, T. (2004). Haidt's moral intuitionist theory: A psychological and philosophical critique. *Review of General Psychology, 8*(4), 273–282.

Sampson, R. (2002). Transcending tradition: New directions in community research, Chicago style. *Criminology, 40,* 213–241.

Sanchez-Page, D. (2005). The online-counseling debate: A view toward the underserved. *The Counseling Psychologist, 33,* 891–899.

Satcher, D. (1999). *Mental health: A report of the surgeon general.* Rockville, MD: Office of the Surgeon General.

Satcher, D. (2001). *Mental health: Culture, race, and ethnicity.* Rockville, MD: Department of Health and Human Services.

Savani, K., Markus, H., Naidu, N., Kumar, S., & Berlia, N. (2010). What counts as a choice? U.S. Americans are more likely than Indians to construe actions as choice. *Psychological Science, 21*(3), 391–398.

Schlachter, R. H. (1975). Home counseling of adolescents and parents. *Social Work, 20*(6), 427–481.

Schlenker, B. (2008). Integrity and character: Implications of principled expedient ethical ideologies. *Journal of Social and Clinical Psychology, 27*(10), 1078–1125.

Schnall, S., Haidt, J., Clore, G. L., & Jordon, A. (2008). Disgust as embodied moral judgment. *Personality and Social Psychology Bulletin, 34,* 1096–1109.

Schank, J., & Skovholt, T. (1997). Dual-relationship dilemmas of rural and small-community psychologists. *Professional Psychology: Research and Practice, 28,* 44–49.

Scheffler, R., Garrett, H., Zarin, D., & Pincus, H. (2000). Managed care and fee discounts in psychiatry: New evidence. *Journal of Behavioral Health Services and Research, 27,* 1094–3412.

Schlaefli, A., Rest, J., & Thoma, S. (1985). Does moral education improve moral judgment: A meta-analysis of intervention studies using the DIT. *Review of Educational Research, 55,* 319–352.

Schneewind, J. (1992). Autonomy, obligation, and virtue: An overview of Kant's moral philosophy. In P. Guyer (Ed.), *The Cambridge companion to Kant* (pp. 309–341). New York, NY: Cambridge University Press.

Scott, C. (2000). Ethical issues in addiction counseling. *Rehabilitation Counseling Bulletin, 43,* 209–219.

Sears, S., Evans, G., & Perry, N. (1998). Innovations in training: The University of Florida rural psychology program. *Professional Psychology: Research and Practice, 29,* 504–507.

Seidman, S. (1996). *Queer theory/sociology.* Cambridge, MA: Blackwell.

Shanahan, T., & Wang, R. (2003). *Reason and insight: Western and Eastern perspectives on the pursuit of moral wisdom* (2nd ed.). Belmont, CA: Wadsworth.

Shanahan, T., & Wang, R. (2006). *Reason and insight: Western and Eastern perspectives on the pursuit of moral wisdom.* Florence, KY: Wadsworth.

Shapiro, E., & Ginsberg, R. (2003). To accept or not to accept: Referrals and the maintenance of boundaries. *Professional Psychology: Research and Practice, 34,* 258–263.

Shattuck, C. (1999). *Hinduism.* London, UK: Routledge.

Shepard, M. (1992). Predicting batterer recidivism five years after community intervention. *Journal of Family Violence, 7,* 167–178.

Sheppard, S., Macatangay, K., Colby, A., & Sullivan, W. (2008). *Educating engineers: Designing for the future of the field.* Hoboken, NJ: John Wiley.

Shidlo, A., & Schroeder, M. (2002). Changing sexual orientation: A consumer's report. *Professional Psychology: Research and Practice, 33,* 249–259.

Silk, J., Sessa, F., Morris, A., Steinberg, L., & Avenevoli, S. (2004). Neighborhood cohesion as a buffer against hostile maternal parenting. *Journal of Family Psychology, 18,* 135–146.

Silverman, S. (2010). What is diversity? An inquiry into preservice teacher beliefs. *American Educational Research Journal, 47*(2), 292–329.

Silverman, W., Pina, A., & Viswesvaran, C. (2008). Evidence-based psychosocial treatments for phobic and anxiety disorders in children and adolescents. *Journal of Clinical Child & Adolescent Psychology, 37*(1), 105–130.

Singer, P. (1993). Ethics. In *The new encyclopedia Britannica* (Vol. 18, pp. 492–521). Chicago, IL: Encyclopedia Britannica.

Singh, A. K. (2008, October 19). *Dharma—The universal law of morality.* Retrieved from http://ezinearticles.com/?Dharma---The-Universal-Law-of-Morality&id=1597760

Sinnott, J. (2009). Introduction to this special issue: Complex thought and construction of identity. *Journal of Adult Development, 16*(3), 129–130.

Sioui, G. (1995). *For an Amerindian autohistory: An essay on the foundations of a social ethic* (S. Fischman, Trans.). Montreal, Canada: McGill-Queen's University Press.

Skarderud, F. (2003). Shame in cyperspace. Relationships without faces: The e-media and eating disorders. *European Eating Disorders Review, 11,* 155–169.

Smedley, A. (1999). "Race" and the construction of human identity. *American Anthropologist, 100*(3), 690–701.

Smith, H. (1991). *The world's religions: Our great wisdom traditions.* New York, NY: HarperCollins.

Smith, H., & Novak, P. (2003). *Buddhism.* New York, NY: HarperCollins.

Smith, L. (2008). Positioning classism within counseling psychology's social justice agenda. *The Counseling Psychologist, 36,* 895–924.

Smith, S., Gleaves, D., Pierce, B., Williams, T., Gilliland, T., & Gerkens, D. (2003). Eliciting and comparing false and recovered memories: An experimental approach. *Applied Cognitive Psychology, 17,* 251–279.

Somer, E. (1999). Therapist-client sex: Retrospective reports. *Professional Psychology: Research and Practice, 30,* 504–509.

Spruill, J., Rozensky, R., Stigall, T., Vasquez, M., Bingham, R., & Olvey, C. (2004). Becoming a competent clinician: Basic competencies in intervention. *Journal of Clinical Psychology, 60*(7), 741–754.

Standard, R., Sandhu, D., & Painter, L. (2000). Assessment of spirituality in counseling. *Journal of Counseling & Development, 78,* 204–210.

Staub, E. (2005). The roots of goodness: The fulfillment of basic human needs and the development of caring, helping and nonaggression, inclusive caring, moral courage, active bystandership, and altruism born of suffering. In R. Dienstbier (Series Ed.), G. Carlo, & C. Edwards (Vol. Eds.), *Nebraska symposium on motivation: Vol. 51. Moral motivation through the life span: Theory, research, applications* (pp. 22–72). Lincoln: University of Nebraska Press.

Stebnicki, M. (2008). *Empathy fatigue: Healing the mind, body, and spirit of professional counselors.* New York, NY: Springer.

Stenhoff, D., & Lignugaris-Kraft, B. (2007). A review of the effects of peer tutoring on students with mild disabilities in secondary settings. *Exceptional Children, 74,* 8–30.

Stephens, N., Markus, H., & Townsend, S. (2007). Choice as an act of meaning: The case of social class. *Journal of Personality and Social Psychology, 93*(5), 814–830.

Steward, D., & Sprinthall, N. (1994). Moral development in public administration. In T. Cooper (Ed.). *Handbook of administrative ethics* (pp. 2325–2349). New York, NY: Marcel Dekker.

Stone, R. (1990). *Adolescents and abortion: Choice in crisis.* Washington, DC: Center for Population Options.

Storch, J., & Kenny, N. (2007). Shared moral work of nurses and physicians. *Nursing Ethics, 14*(4), 478–491.

Strike, D., Skovholt, T., & Hummel, T. (2004). Mental health professionals' disability competence: Measuring self-awareness, perceived knowledge, and perceived skills. *Rehabilitation Psychology, 49*(4), 321–327.

Stuart, E., & Campbell, J. (1989). Assessment of patterns of dangerousness with battered women. *Issues in Mental Health Nursing, 10,* 245–260.

Sue, D., Arredondo, P., & McDavis, R. (1992). Multicultural counseling competencies and standards: A call to the profession. *Journal of Counseling and Development, 70,* 477–486.

Sue, D., & Sue, D. (2008). *Counseling the culturally different: Theory and practice* (2nd ed.). New York, NY: John Wiley.

Sullivan, G. (1999). Political opportunism and the harassment of homosexuals in Florida. *Journal of Homosexuality, 37*(4), 57–81.

Taijfel, H. (1982). Social psychology of intergroup relations. *Annual Review of Psychology, 33,* 1–39.

Taijfel, H. (2010). *Social identity and intergroup relations* (European studies in social psychology). Cambridge, UK: Cambridge University Press.

Tannenbaum, R., & Berman, M. (1990). Ethical and legal issues in psychotherapy supervision. *Psychotherapy in Private Practice, 8,* 65–77.

Tarasoff v. Regents of the University of California, 17 Cal. 3rd 425 (Cal. Supreme Court, 1976).

Taylor, C. (1997). *North American Indians.* Bristol, UK: Sienna.

Taylor, L., McMinn, M. R., Bufford, R., & Chang, K. (2010). Psychologists' attitudes and ethical concerns regarding the use of social networking web sites. *Professional Psychology: Research & Practice, 41*(20), 153–159.

Thapar v. Zezulka, Texas Supreme Court, No. 97-1208 (1998–1999).

Thomas, B., Veach, P. M., & LeRoy, B. (2006). Is self-disclosure part of the genetic counselor's clinical role? *Journal of Genetic Counseling, 15*(3), 163–177.

Thomason, T. (2010). The trend toward evidence-based practice and the future of psychotherapy. *American Journal of Psychotherapy, 64*(1), 29–38.

Thompson-Brenner, H., Glass, S., & Western, D. (2003). A multidimensional meta-analysis of psychotherapy for bulimia nervosa. *Clinical Psychology: Science and Practice, 10*(3), 269–287.

Tjeltveit, A. (2006). To what ends: Psychotherapy goals and outcomes, the good life and the principle of beneficence. *Psychotherapy: Theory, Research, Practice, Training, 43,* 186–200.

Tong, R. (1998). The ethics of care: A feminist virtue ethics of care for healthcare practitioners. *Journal of Medicine and Philosophy, 23,* 131–152.

Tromski-Klingshirm, D. (2007). Should the clinical supervisor be the administrative supervisor? The ethics versus the reality. *Clinical Supervisor, 25*(1/2), 53–67.

Tromski-Klingshirm, D., & Davis, T. (2007). Supervisees' perceptions of their clinical experience: A study of the dual role of clinical and administrative supervision. *Counselor Education & Supervision, 46,* 294–304.

Tucci, G., Nakamura, H., & Reynolds, F. (1993). The Buddha and Buddhism. In *The new encyclopedia Britannica* (Vol. 15, pp. 269–270). Chicago, IL: Encyclopedia Britannica.

Turiel, E., & Killen, M. (2010). Taking emotion seriously: The role of emotions in moral development. In W. Arsenio & E. Lemerise (Eds.), *Emotions, aggression, and morality in children: Bridging development and psychopathology* (pp. 33–52). Washington, DC: American Psychological Association.

Turner, R. (1990). Role change. *Annual Review of Sociology, 16,* 87–110.

Tweed, R., & Lehman, D. (2002). Learning considered within a cultural context: Confucian and Socratic approaches. *American Psychologist, 57*(2), 89–99.

University of Pennsylvania. (2003). *National study of U.S. high school seniors finds religion good for their health.* Philadelphia: Author.

U.S. Census Bureau. (2000). *U.S. Census Bureau state and county quickfacts: Data derived from population estimates, 2000 census of population and housing.* Washington, DC: Author.

U.S. Census Bureau. (2001). *U.S. census 2000, summary files 1 and 2.* Retrieved from http://www.census.gov/Press-Release/www/2001/sumfile1.html and http://www.census.gov/Press-Release/www/2001/sumfile2.html

U.S. Census Bureau. (2004). *U.S. interim projections by age, sex, race, and Hispanic origin.* Retrieved from http://www.census.gov/ipc/www/usinterimproj

U.S. Census Bureau. (2010). *Overview of race and Hispanic origin: 2010.* Retrieved from http://www.census.gov/prod/cen2010/briefs/c2010br-02.pdf

U.S. Department of Health & Human Services. (2003). *Summary of the HIPAA privacy rule.* Retrieved from www.hhs.gov/ocr/privacysummary.pdf

U.S. Department of State. (n.d.). *Fact sheet: Islam in the United States.* Retrieved from http://www.islamfortoday.com/historyusa4htm

U.S. Surgeon General. (2001). *Report on mental health: Culture, race and ethnicity—A supplement to mental health: A report of the surgeon general.* Rockville, MD: Substance Abuse and Mental Health Services Administration.

Vashon, D., & Agresti, A. (1992). A training proposal to help mental health professionals clarify and manage implicit values in the counseling process. *Professional Psychology: Research and Practice, 23,* 509–514.

Vinski, E., & Tryon, G. (2009). Study of cognitive dissonance intervention to address high school students' cheating attitudes and behaviors. *Ethics & Behavior, 19*(3), 218–226.

Vitiello, B. (2008). Effectively obtaining informed consent for child and adolescent participation in mental health research. *Ethics & Behavior, 18*(2/3), 182–198.

Volker, J. (1984). Counseling experience, moral judgment, awareness of consequences and moral sensitivity in counseling practice. *Dissertation Abstracts International, 45*(3A), 793–794.

Walden, S., Herlihy, B., & Ashton, L. (2003). The evolution of ethics: Personal perspectives of ACA ethics committee chairs. *Journal of Counseling and Development, 81,* 106–111.

Waller, A. (1995). Health care issues in health care reform. *Whittier Law Review, 16,* 15–49.

Wampold, B., Goodheart, C., & Levant, R. (2007). Clarification and elaboration on evidence-based practice in psychology. *American Psychologist, 62,* 616–618.

Wang, R., Wang, H., & Hsu, M. (2003). Factors associated with adolescent pregnancy: A sample of Taiwanese female adolescents. *Public Health Nursing, 20,* 33–41.

Wang, S., & Kim, B. (2010). Therapist multicultural competence, Asian American participants' cultural values, and counseling process. *Journal of Counseling Psychology, 10,* 1–8.

Watkins, S. (1989). Confidentiality: An ethical and legal conundrum for family therapists. *American Journal of Family Therapy, 17,* 291–302.

Weaver, K. (2007). Ethical sensitivity: State of knowledge and needs for further research. *Nursing Ethics, 14*(2), 141–155.

Weaver, K., Morse, J., & Mitcham, C. (2008). Ethical sensitivity in professional practice: Concept analysis. *Journal of Advanced Nursing, 62*(5), 607–618.

Webb, L. (2008). Above these badlands: Delusions, autonomy, and individual beliefs in right to refuse psychotropic medication. *Journal of Ethics in Mental Health, 3*(1), 1–4.

Webber, D. (2004). Self-incrimination, partner notification, and the criminal law: Negatives for the CDS's "prevention for positives" initiative. *AIDS & Public Policy Journal, 19*(1/2), 54–65.

Weikel, W., & Palmo, A. (1996). *Foundations of mental health counseling* (2nd ed.). Springfield, IL: Charles C Thomas.

Weinrach, S., & Thomas, K. (2002). A critical analysis of the multicultural counseling competencies: Implications for the practice of mental health counseling. *Journal of Mental Health Counseling, 24*(1), 20–35.

Welfel, E. (1998). *Ethics in counseling and psychotherapy: Standards, research and emerging issues.* Pacific Grove, CA: Brooks/Cole.

Welfel, E. (2006). *Ethics in counseling and psychotherapy: Standards, research and emerging issues.* Pacific Grove, CA: Brooks/Cole.

Welfel, E. (2009). *Ethics in counseling & psychotherapy.* Florence, KY: Brooks/Cole.

Welfel, E., & Kitchner, K. (1992). Introduction to the special section: Ethics education—An agenda for the 90s. *Professional Psychology, Research and Practice, 23*(3), 179–181.

Wells, M., Mitchell, K., Finkelhor, D., & Becker-Blease, K. (2007). Online mental health treatment: Concerns and considerations. *Cyberpsychology & Behavior, 10*(3), 453–459.

Wells, T. (1994). Therapist self-disclosure: Its effects on clients and the treatment relationship. *Smith College Studies in Social Work, 65*(1), 23–41.

Wester, S., Vogel, D., & Archer, J. (2004). Males, supervisors, and counseling supervision. *Journal of Counseling & Development, 82,* 91–99.

Whaley, A., & David, K. (2007). Cultural competence and evidence-based practice in mental health services: A complementary perspective. *American Psychologist, 62*(6), 563–574.

Wheeler, S. (2007). What shall we do with the wounded healer? The supervisor's dilemma. *Psychodynamic Practice: Individuals, Groups and Organisations, 13*(3), 245–256.

Wheeler, S., & King, D. (2000). Do counseling supervisors want or need to have their supervision supervised? An exploratory study. *British Journal of Guidance and Counseling, 28,* 279–291.

White, V., & Queener, J. (2003). Supervisor and supervisee attachments and social provisions related to the supervisory working alliance. *Counselor Education and Supervision, 42,* 203–219.

Whitley, B. (2001). Gender-role variables and attitudes toward homosexuality. *Sex Roles: A Journal of Research, 45,* 691–700.

Wilcoxon, A., & Hawk, R. (1990). Continuing education services: A survey of state associations of AACD. *Journal of Counseling & Development, 69,* 93–94.

Williams, C., & Abeles, N. (2004). Issues and implications of deaf culture in therapy. *Professional Psychology: Research and Practice, 35*(6), 643–648.

Wise, R., King, A., Miller, J., & Pearce, M. (2011). When HIPAA and FERPA apply to university training clinics. *Training and Education in Professional Psychology, 5*(1), 48–56.

Wolfson, E. (1999). The fee in social work: Ethical dilemmas for practitioners. *Social Work, 44,* 269–274.

Woody, R. (1998). Bartering for psychological services. *Professional Psychology: Research and Practice, 29*(2), 174–178.

Worchel, S., Iussini, J., Coutant, D., & Ivaldi, M. (2000). A multimodal model of identity: Relating individual and group identities to intergroup behavior. In D. Capozza & R. Brown (Eds.), *Social identity processes* (pp. 15–32). Thousand Oaks, CA: Sage.

Worthington, E., Larson, D., Brubaker, M., Colecchi, C., Berry, J., & Morrow, D. (1989). The benefits of legislation requiring parental involvement prior to adolescent abortion. *American Psychologist, 44,* 1542–1545.

Yalom, I., & Leszcz, M. (2005). *Theory and practice of group counseling* (5th ed.). New York, NY: Basic Books.

Yao, X. (2000). *An introduction to Confucianism.* Cambridge, UK: Cambridge University Press.

Young, J., Wiggins-Frame, M., & Cashwell, C. (2007). Spirituality and counselor competence: A national survey of American Counseling Association members. *Journal of Counseling & Development, 85,* 47–52.

Young, K. (2005). An empirical examination of client attitudes towards online counseling. *Cyberpsychology & Behavior, 8,* 172–177.

Yum, J. (1988). The impact of Confucianism on interpersonal relationships and communication patterns in East Asia. *Communication Monographs, 55,* 374–388.

Yurkovich, E., Clairmont, J., & Grandbois, D. (2002). Mental health care providers' perception of giving culturally responsive care to American Indians. *Perspectives in Psychiatric Care, 38,* 147–156.

Zabin, L., Hirsch, M., & Emerson, J. (1989). When urban adolescents choose abortion: Effects on education, psychological status and subsequent pregnancy. *Family Planning Perspectives, 21,* 248–255.

Zea, M., Mason, M., & Murguia, A. (2000). Psychotherapy with members of Latino/Latina religions and spiritual traditions. In P. Richards & A. Bergin (Eds.), *Handbook of psychotherapy and religious diversity* (pp. 397–419). Washington, DC: American Psychological Association.

Zeddies, T. (2002). More than just words: A hermeneutic view of language in psychoanalysis. *Psychoanalytic Psychology, 19,* 3–23.

Zellman, G. (1990). Child abuse reporting and failure to report among mandated reporters: Prevalence, incidence, and reasons. *Journal of Interpersonal Violence, 5*(1), 3–22.

Zur, O. (2007). *Boundaries in psychotherapy: Ethical and clinical explorations.* Washington, DC: American Psychological Association.

Index

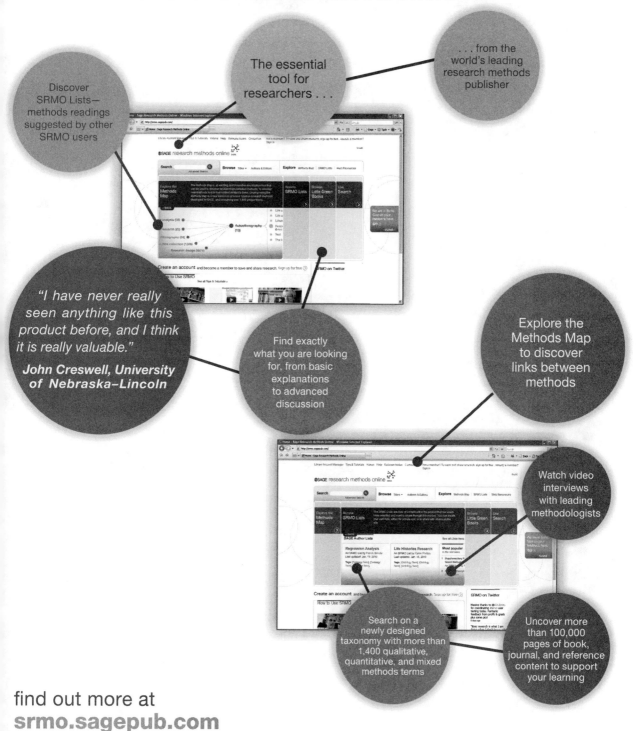